T0092050

Critical Care

Editor

LILY PARKINSON

VETERINARY CLINICS
OF NORTH AMERICA:
EXOTIC ANIMAL PRACTICE

www.vetexotic.theclinics.com

Consulting Editor
JÖRG MAYER

September 2023 • Volume 26 • Number 3

ELSEVIER

1600 John F. Kennedy Boulevard • Suite 1800 • Philadelphia, Pennsylvania, 19103-2899
http://www.vetexotic.theclinics.com

VETERINARY CLINICS OF NORTH AMERICA: EXOTIC ANIMAL PRACTICE Volume 26, Number 3 September 2023 ISSN 1094-9194, ISBN-13: 978-0-323-93995-9

Editor: Stacy Eastman
Developmental Editor: Axell Ivan Jade M. Purificacion

Veterinary Clinics of North America: Exotic Animal Practice (ISSN 1094-9194) is published in January, May, and September by Elsevier, Inc., 360 Park Avenue South, New York, NY 10010-1710. Subscription prices are $305.00 per year for US individuals, $614.00 per year for US institutions, $100.00 per year for US students and residents, $355.00 per year for Canadian individuals, $739.00 per year for Canadian institutions, $370.00 per year for international individuals, $739.00 per year for international institutions, $100.00 per year Canadian students/residents, and $165.00 per year for international students/residents. To receive student/resident rate, orders must be accompanied by name of affiliated institution, date of term, and the *signature* of program/residency coordinator on institution letterhead. Orders will be billed at individual rate until proof of status is received. Foreign air speed delivery is included in all *Clinics* subscription prices. All prices are subject to change without notice. **POSTMASTER:** Send address changes to *Veterinary Clinics of North America: Exotic Animal Practice*, Elsevier Health Sciences Division, Subscription Customer Service, 3251 Riverport Lane, Maryland Heights, MO 63043. **Customer Service: Telephone: 1-800-654-2452** (U.S. and Canada); **1-314-447-8871** (outside U.S. and Canada). **Fax: 1-314-447-8029. E-mail: journalscustomerservice-usa@elsevier.com (for print support); journalsonlinesupport-usa@elsevier.com (for online support).**

Reprints. For copies of 100 or more of articles in this publication, please contact the Commercial Reprints Department, Elsevier Inc., 360 Park Avenue South, New York, New York 10010-1710. Tel.: 212-633-3874; Fax: 212-633-3820; E-mail: reprints@elsevier.com.

Veterinary Clinics of North America: Exotic Animal Practice is covered in *MEDLINE/PubMed (Index Medicus).*

Contributors

CONSULTING EDITOR

JÖRG MAYER, Dr med vet, Msc
Diplomate, American Board of Veterinary Practitioners (Exotic Companion Mammals); Diplomate, European College of Zoological Medicine (Small Mammals); Diplomate, American College of Zoological Medicine; Associate Professor of Zoological Medicine, Department of Small Animal Medicine and Surgery, University of Georgia College of Veterinary Medicine, Athens, Georgia, USA

EDITOR

LILY PARKINSON, DVM, DACZM, Cert Aq V, DACVECC
Diplomate, American College of Zoological Medicine; Diplomate, American College of Veterinary Emergency and Critical Care; Clinical Veterinarian, Brookfield Zoo, Chicago Zoological Society, Brookfield, Illinois

AUTHORS

JULIET F. ARMSTRONG, DVM
Diplomate, American College of Veterinary Internal Medicine (Neurology); Veterinary Neurologist, Small Animal Specialty Medicine, NorthStar VETS, Robbinsville, New Jersey

NICOLA DI GIROLAMO, DMV, MSc (EBHC), PhD
Diplomate, European College of Zoological Medicine (Herpetology); Diplomate, American College of Zoological Medicine; Diplomate, American College of Veterinary Preventive Medicine; Department of Clinical Sciences, College of Veterinary Medicine, Cornell University, Ithaca, New York

SARA GARDHOUSE, DVM
Diplomate, American Board of Veterinary Practitioners (Exotic Companion Mammals); Diplomate, American College of Zoological Medicine; Evolution Veterinary Specialists, Lakewood, Colorado

NATALIE H. HALL, DVM
Diplomate, American College of Zoological Medicine; Clinical Veterinarian, Disney's Animals, Science, and Environment

LA'TOYA V. LATNEY, DVM, CertAqV
Diplomate, European College of Zoological Medicine; Diplomate, American Board of Veterinary Practitioners (Reptile/Amphibian); Avian and Exotic Medicine and Surgery, The Animal Medical Center, New York, New York

MARINA LILES, DVM
Department of Clinical Sciences, Cummings School of Veterinary Medicine at Tufts University, North Grafton, Massachusetts

LILY PARKINSON, DVM, DACZM, Cert Aq V, DACVECC
Diplomate, American College of Zoological Medicine; Diplomate, American College of Veterinary Emergency and Critical Care; Clinical Veterinarian, Brookfield Zoo, Chicago Zoological Society, Brookfield, Illinois

KATHRYN L. PERRIN, BVetMeD, PhD
Diplomate, American College of Zoological Medicine; Diplomate, European College of Zoological Medicine (Zoo Health Management); San Diego Zoo Wildlife Alliance, Veterinary Services, Escondido, California

H. NICOLE TRENHOLME, DVM, MS
Diplomate, American College of Veterinary Emergency and Critical Care (Small Animal); Diplomate, American College of Veterinary Anesthesia and Analgesia; Department of Veterinary Clinical Medicine, University of Illinois College of Veterinary Medicine, Urbana, Illinois

STACEY LEONATTI WILKINSON, DVM
Diplomate, American Board of Veterinary Practitioners in Reptile and Amphibian Practice, Avian and Exotic Animal Hospital of Georgia, Pooler, Georgia

Contents

Preface: Providing the Best Emergency and Critical Care for Exotic Patients ix

Lily Parkinson

Temperature Monitoring and Thermal Support in Exotic Animal Critical Care 525

Marina Liles and Nicola Di Girolamo

Body temperature measurement is one of the most important parameters to assess the health of a patient. In small exotic mammals, rectal temperature is obtained via a similar process as in dogs or cats, with a few specific differences. In reptiles and birds, measurement of body temperature can provide important information, albeit its accuracy may be limited. In most animals, temperature should be taken at the beginning of the examination to not artificially elevate the temperature during the physical exam. Heat support is typically indicated any time a patient's temperature is below the accepted core temperature range and cooling may be indicated whenever a patient's temperature exceeds a critical point.

Neurologic Assessment and Critical Care of Exotic Animals: Approach to the Neurologic Exam, Species Differences, Prognostic Scales, Commonly Encountered Conditions, Ancillary Diagnostic Tests, and Caring for Neurologically Impaired Patients 545

Juliet F. Armstrong

Many disorders of other body systems have been well characterized in exotic species; however, data regarding neurologic conditions is limited. Across some of these species, correlates between feline and canine neurology can be made, but variations in the nervous system anatomy make evaluation more challenging. With accurate neurolocalization a focused list of differential diagnoses can be created. Performing the neurologic examination should be methodical for all patients, and the order and extent of examination may depend upon the patient's clinical condition and cooperation. Applications of objective scale measures (such as coma scales), and ancillary diagnostics (electrodiagnostics, advanced imaging, biopsy techniques, and BAER testing) complement physical assessment and clinicopathologic assessment in these neurologic patients. Once a neurolocalization, likely diagnosis, and prognosis have been established, specific considerations for hospitalization and care of neurologic patients can be implemented while treatment is instituted.

Point of Care Ultrasound in Exotic Animal Emergency and Critical Care 567

Sara Gardhouse

Exotic pets are presented to veterinary clinics with increasing frequency for routine, urgent, and emergency needs. With these increased visits, owners' expectations for high-quality veterinary care are also increasing. Many presenting complaints of reptiles, birds, and small mammals can benefit from the use of point of care ultrasound (POCUS) to establish a minimum database, aid in triage, and help guide further diagnostics, treatment, and prognostic discussions with the owner. Hospitalized exotic patients can also have their progress tracked and better assessed with the aid of POCUS.

Sedation and Anesthesia in Exotic Animal Critical Care **591**

H. Nicole Trenholme

Sedation and anesthesia of exotic animals in inherently challenging, but often facilitates the best care for patients. Critical illness or injury adds on another layer of complexity to their management for obtaining diagnostics and providing treatments. This article serves to review some of the more recent literature of sedation and anesthesia within exotics practice, bringing to light some nuances and considerations for when those patients are critically ill or injured.

Fluid Therapy in Exotic Animal Emergency and Critical Care **623**

Lily Parkinson

Many new concepts are emerging in the understanding of fluid therapy in human and mammalian medicine, including the role of the glycocalyx, increased understanding of fluid, sodium, and chloride overload, and the advantages of colloid administration in the form of albumin. None of these concepts, however, appear to be directly applicable to non-mammalian exotic patients, and careful consideration of their alternate physiology is required when formulating fluid plans for these patients.

Urine Output Monitoring and Acute Kidney Injury in Mammalian Exotic Animal Critical Care **647**

Stacey Leonatti Wilkinson

Acute kidney injury (AKI) is a sudden, severe decrease in kidney function which can occur in any species. There are various causes of AKI, some of which are seen in domestic species and some that are unique to exotics. Exotic animals present unique challenges with AKI management such as differences in anatomy and physiology, intravenous and urinary catheterization, repeated blood sampling, and their tendency to present in advanced states of illness. This article will discuss AKI, diagnosis, treatment, and prognosis for exotic companion mammals. The following article will discuss the same in non-mammalian patients.

Urine Output Monitoring and Acute Kidney Injury in Non-mammalian Exotic Animal Critical Care **673**

Stacey Leonatti Wilkinson

Acute kidney injury (AKI) is a sudden, severe decrease in kidney function which can occur in any species. There are various causes of AKI, some of which are seen in domestic species and some that are unique to birds, reptiles, and amphibians. These species present unique challenges with AKI management, such as differences in anatomy and physiology, intravenous and urinary catheterization, repeated blood sampling, and their tendency to present in advanced states of illness. This article will discuss AKI, diagnosis, treatment, and prognosis for non-mammalian exotic species.

Nutritive Support for Critical Exotic Patients 711

La'Toya V. Latney

Malnutrition and need for nutritive support are both very common in exotic animals requiring critical care. Assessment and monitoring of body condition, weight, protein absorption, and catabolic loss is recommended to help guide restorative therapy. Several critical care diets are available based on digestive strategy. Fluid requirements and evaporative water loss can vary based on taxa; ectoderms suffer evaporative losses at a greater magnitude than endotherms. Enteral and parenteral nutrition strategies can be appropriate for patients, with natural history and anatomic and physiologic differences considered as much as possible.

Cerebro-Cardiopulmonary Resuscitation and Postarrest Care in Exotic Animal Critical Care 737

Natalie H. Hall

Evidence-based recommendations for performing cardiopulmonary resuscitation (CPR) in domestic species provide a foundation for application to nondomestic species. The exotic and zoo practitioner must consider human safety, species anatomy, physiology, and special techniques for performing CPR. Having the hospital and team prepared and trained for a CPR response can improve outcomes. Basic life support includes various techniques for chest compressions and ventilation support. Advanced life support includes means of intravascular and intraosseous access, rescue drug administration, and consideration of the patient presenting circumstances. Team debriefs and support for mental wellness are useful to optimize performance and maintain team resiliency through CPR events.

Coagulation Disorders, Testing, and Treatment in Exotic Animal Critical Care 751

Kathryn L. Perrin

Despite poor recognition in the literature, exotic companion animals are affected by many diseases that can result in disordered coagulation and fibrinolysis. This article outlines current knowledge of hemostasis, common diagnostic tests and reviews reported diseases associated with coagulopathy in small mammals, bird and reptiles. A range of conditions affect platelets and thrombocytes, endothelium and blood vessels, and plasma clotting factors. Improved recognition and monitoring of hemostatic disorders will enable targeted therapy and improved case outcomes.

VETERINARY CLINICS OF NORTH AMERICA: EXOTIC ANIMAL PRACTICE

FORTHCOMING ISSUES

January 2024
Exotic Animal Nutrition
Amanda Ardente, *Editor*

May 2024
Pediatrics
João Lemos Brandão and Peter M. DiGeronimo, *Editors*

September 2024
Exotic Animal Practice Around the World
Shangzhe Xie and Brian Speer, *Editors*

RECENT ISSUES

May 2023
Dermatology
Dario d'Ovidio and Domenico Santoro, *Editors*

January 2023
Pain Management
David Sanchez-Migallon Guzman, *Editor*

September 2022
Exotic Animal Clinical Pathology
J. Jill Heatley and Karen E. Russell, *Editors*

SERIES OF RELATED INTEREST

Veterinary Clinics: Small Animal Practice
https://www.vetsmall.theclinics.com/
Advances in Small Animal Care
https://www.advancesinsmallanimalcare.com

Preface

Providing the Best Emergency and Critical Care for Exotic Patients

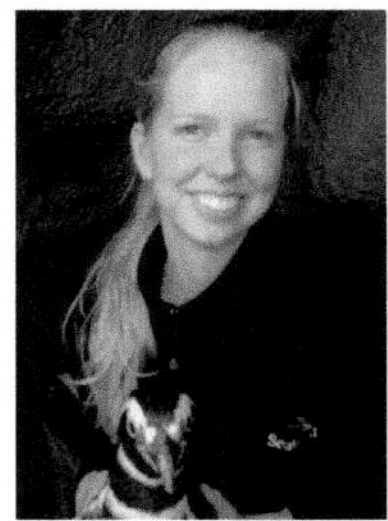

Lily Parkinson, DVM, DACZM, Cert Aq V, DACVECC
Editor

Thank you for your interest in this Emergency and critical care (ECC) focused *Veterinary Clinics of North America: Exotic Animal Practice.* I hope you and your sickest patients benefit from the excellent information compiled here. Our unique patients are extremely prone to hiding any signs of illness until they truly are a dire emergency; at that point, they require the most advanced diagnostics and intensive care. Exotic animal veterinarians have little to no margin for error when confronted with a critical patient, and, often, even with the most aggressive supportive care, exotic patients may fail to survive. In those situations, we often wonder if there was something else we could have done to better help our patient.My hope is that this issue helps you to feel current and as well-prepared as possible for many different ECC situations .

This issue focuses on newer emergency and critical care information emerging in human and domestic animal medicine and discusses possible applications in the exotic animal world. World experts contributed knowledge and articles on many situations you will encounter. From assessing non-traditional species neurologically or with point-of-care ultrasound to supporting them with nutrition and temperature management, this issue will help you navigate these challenging cases. When further diagnostics or treatments are needed, reviews of acute kidney injury, fluid therapy, coagulation, and sedation and anesthesia can help you accomplish top-notch care. Finally, when the worst happens, and cerebrocardiopulmonary resuscitation must be initiated, another excellent review will help you navigate that challenging time and procedure.

I would like to thank all of the outstanding authors in this issue and gratefully acknowledge the help of Elsevier. Their generous time and energy helped to provide

Vet Clin Exot Anim 26 (2023) ix–x
https://doi.org/10.1016/j.cvex.2023.05.011

a valuable resource for all clinicians confronted with a critical, exotic patient. We hope this helps you and your patients!

Lily Parkinson, DVM, DACZM, Cert Aq V, DACVECC
Brookfield Zoo
Chicago Zoological Society
3300 Golf Road
Brookfield, IL 60513, USA

E-mail address:
lily.parkinson@czs.org

Temperature Monitoring and Thermal Support in Exotic Animal Critical Care

Marina Liles, DVM[a],
Nicola Di Girolamo, DMV, MSc (EBHC), PhD, Dipl.ECZM (Herp), Dipl.ACZM, Dipl.ACVPM[b,*]

KEYWORDS

• Avian • Hyperthermia • Hypothermia • Guinea Pig • Monitoring • Rabbit • Reptile • Temperature

KEY POINTS

- In multiple species, it has been proven that upon examination, a high or low temperature can help stratify a patient's status and correlate with prognosis.
- In addition to obtaining a temperature on presentation, if an abnormal reading is identified, it should be reassessed routinely while appropriate interventions are made.
- Cloacal temperature acquisition in hospitalized reptiles can provide useful clinical information, when considered in light of specific hospitalization settings.
- The ideal way to assess temperature in birds is via a temperature probe in the crop/proventriculus, but this can only be performed in sedated or anesthetized animals.
- Temperature measurement is crucial in the perioperative period to ensure a safe anesthetic event and a smooth recovery for the patient.

INTRODUCTION

Body temperature measurement is one of the most important parameters to assess the health of a patient. In multiple species, it has been proven that upon examination, a high or low temperature can help stratify illness severity, including patient's prognosis.[1–3] In human medicine, body temperature has emerged as a critical vital sign to assess in cases of sepsis,[4–6] major trauma,[7–11] and in newborns[12–17] to determine mortality rates and severity of disease progression. Recent studies in rabbits[1] and guinea pigs[2] have shown that on presentation to veterinary hospitals, a low rectal temperature is associated with a higher likelihood of death compared to a normal rectal temperature.

[a] Department of Clinical Sciences, Cummings School of Veterinary Medicine at Tufts University, North Grafton, MA 01536, USA; [b] Department of Clinical Sciences, College of Veterinary Medicine, Cornell University, Ithaca, NY 14853, USA
* Corresponding author.
E-mail address: nicoladiggi@gmail.com

Vet Clin Exot Anim 26 (2023) 525–543
https://doi.org/10.1016/j.cvex.2023.05.001 vetexotic.theclinics.com
1094-9194/23/

Temperature measurement is also crucial in the perioperative period to ensure a safe anesthetic event and a smooth recovery for the patient.[18–24]

Temperature Measurement in Exotic Pets

Currently, most animals that are presented for veterinary care should have a temperature evaluated as part of an initial triage and examination. Methods to monitor temperature are similar across species, but their interpretation varies across species.

Small exotic mammals

In small exotic mammals, such as rabbits, rodents, and ferrets, rectal temperature is obtained similarly to a dog or a cat, with just a few specific differences (**Fig. 1**). Normal temperatures for various species are reported in **Table 1**. Studies have compared different techniques to achieve the most optimal, accurate temperature. In dogs, rectal thermometer readings were most consistent with core body temperature, compared to auricular readings,[25,26] and in cats, both auricular and rectal thermometer readings were in agreement with core body temperature.[27] Infrared transponders in microchips are commonly used in laboratory animal settings for temperature measurement. In both guinea pigs and rabbits, studies assessing the transponder's accuracy have found that they are more agreeable to rectal temperature compared to other infrared methods.[28,29] A study in client-owned guinea pigs assessed digital thermometer readings in both the inguinal and axillary regions compared to rectal temperatures. A wide difference between the techniques was found, indicating that rectal temperature should remain the reference standard measurement method.[30]

Among the small exotic patients, ferrets appear to react more vigorously to rectal temperature measurement. For this reason, in many practices, rectal temperature is not routinely obtained in ferrets, and this measurement is reserved for dull or comatose patients. Similar to cats, ferrets had good agreement between digital rectal thermometer readings and readings using a human infrared auricular thermometer, so this

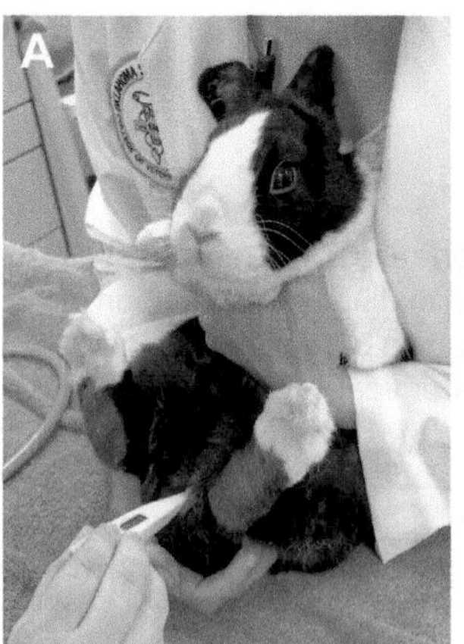

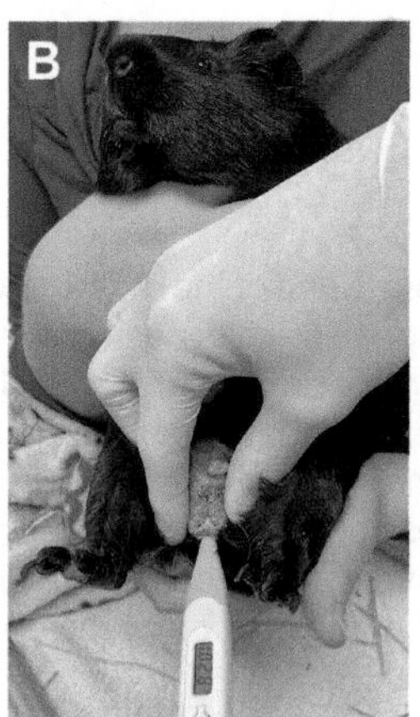

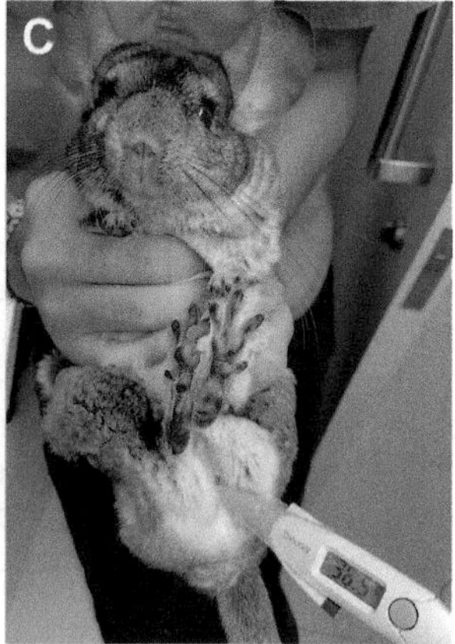

Fig. 1. Rectal temperature measurement in a rabbit (*A*), guinea pig (*B*) and chinchilla (*C*). In rabbits, temperature can be measured in the position shown, often referred as "C-position," or in abdominal recumbency. For measurement of temperature in C-position, while one operator holds the rabbit on the table, the other operator gently extroverts the anus with the nondominant hand and inserts the lubricated thermometer with the dominant hand. In guinea pigs, identification of the anus may be challenging due to the presence of a blind recess. The anus is the opening closer to the tail. Chincillas have a rectal temperature lower than other small mammals.

Table 1
Normal temperature range in commonly presented exotic animals from representative original research

Species	Rabbits	Ferrets	Guinea Pigs	Chinchillas	Bearded Dragon	Ball Python	Birds
Normal temperature range	38–40°C[84]	37.8–40°C[85]	37.2–39.5°C[86]	34.9–37.9°C[87]	29–33°C[39] (POTZ)	26–34°C[88] (POTZ)	35.0–47.7°C[46]
Ozawa[32] 2017				34.9–37.9°C			
Brattstrom[88] 1965						26–34°C	
Prinzinger[46] 1991							*Resting:* 37.58–39.96°C *Active:* 38.73–41.31°C *High activity:* 42.91–44.79°C

method can be used when a patient is not amenable to rectal temperature measurements.[31]

Chinchillas have a relatively low rectal temperature compared to other small exotic mammals (see **Table 1**). In chinchillas, a study showed that the insertion depth of a thermometer when measuring rectal temperature can result in significant variation.[32] At an insertion depth of 1 cm, the mean temperature was 35.3 ± 0.94°C (95.5 ± 1.69°F), and at 2 cm the mean temperature was 36.4 ± 0.77°C (97.5 ± 1.39°F), resulting in a mean difference of 1.14 ± 0.77°C (2.05 ± 1.39°F).[32] This study suggests using an insertion depth of 2 cm as a reference standard for rectal measurement. In addition, the study found that tympanic temperature readings were not reliable in chinchillas.[32] Other studies do not frequently report the depth of temperature probe placement when investigating rectal temperatures, but it is reasonable to assume that in small mammals, differences in thermometer depth could significantly affect the results that are obtained.

In addition to taking the temperature during triage of a patient, if an animal is found to have an abnormal temperature reading, it should be reassessed routinely after the appropriate interventions are made (ie, heating support or cooling). In human medicine, the recommendation is to obtain temperature measurements every 15 minutes until normothermia is reached.[33] If a small exotic patient is debilitated, obtunded, or easily handleable, where temperatures can be taken in a non-stressful manner, or a temperature probe can be left inserted, readings every 15 minutes is likely a good monitoring guideline. With many exotic patients however, the stress of being handled for frequent temperature readings, or having a probe left inserted, would counteract any positive effects of treatments, so recheck temperatures every hour in patients that react negatively to handling might be a more appropriate approach until normothermia is reached.

Reptiles

Reptiles are poikilothermic ectotherms, meaning their temperature is widely variable and fluctuates based on external environmental factors. This is in contrast to most[34,35] mammals or birds which are homeothermic endotherms, that is, animals who maintain their temperature constant in a narrow range and maintaining of the temperature is regulated by internal factors.[36,37] Because of this, reptiles have a preferred optimal temperature zone (POTZ) that allows maintaining of a preferred body temperature (PBT). When a reptile body temperature is in the PBT for that species, optimal biologic functions, immune response, and reproduction are possible. Conversely, a body temperature below this range does not allow normal physiological processes to be carried out, metabolism decreases, and the animal can become ill.[38,39] **Table 1** presents the POTZ of a few species of reptiles commonly kept as pets. A POTZ that results in a body temperature higher than normal is also detrimental and may result in acute cases of heat stroke.[40–43]

Because of the variation in temperature, which can also vary with season and time of day, it is difficult to provide “reference intervals” for body temperature in reptiles. Assessing core temperature can also be challenging because reptiles have a cloaca, unlike mammals. A study in leopard tortoises showed that cloacal temperature was significantly lower than all other parts of the body that were measured, including the core, rear skin, front skin, and carapace.[44]

Cloacal temperature is routinely obtained in many veterinary centers (**Fig. 2**). Measurement of cloacal temperature on admission can provide important information, including ruling in or out temperature-related behavior changes brought on by transport to the hospital. Similarly, acquiring a cloacal temperature in hospitalized reptiles can provide useful clinical information when considered in light of the specific hospitalization settings. A reptile must have a thermogradient to carry out normal functions

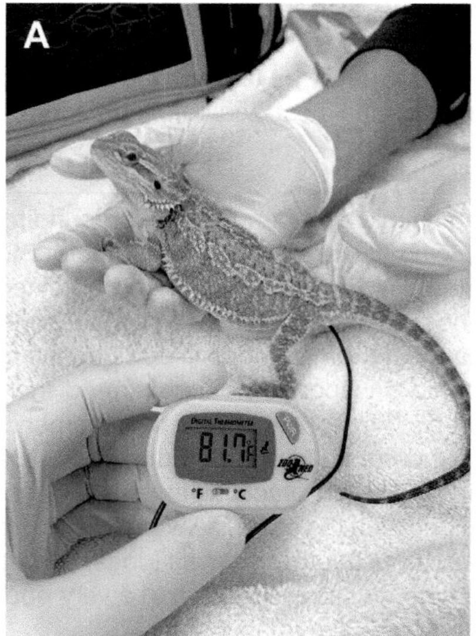

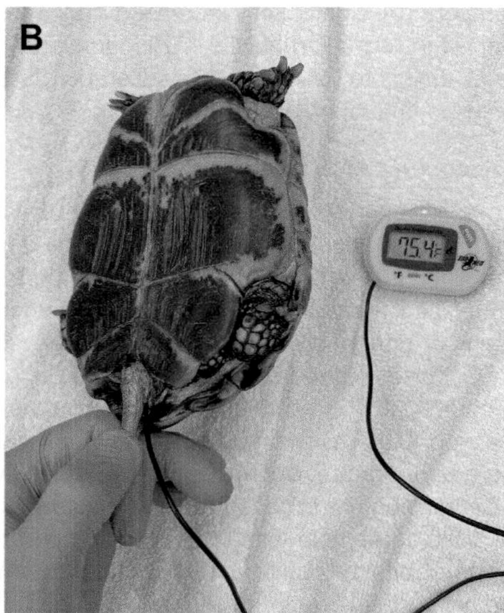

Fig. 2. Cloacal temperature measurement in a bearded dragon (*Pogona vitticeps*) (*A*) and in a Russian tortoise (*Testudo horsfieldii*) (*B*) with an environmental temperature probe. Standard thermometers for temperature measurement in mammals may not work in reptiles due to their narrow temperature reading ranges.

and recover from its illness. To help achieve this, multiple thermometers should be set up in the enclosure to make sure the proper gradient is available, according to their POTZ. Checking these temperatures throughout the day and adjusting them as needed are also recommended to assure the gradient is maintained. Hospitalization is best performed in a heat and humidity-controlled environment, such as specific terraria or incubators. In addition to daily cloacal temperature measurements, thermometers should always be present in a reptile enclosure to ensure that the temperature remains appropriate.[39]

Birds

Like mammals, avian species are homeothermic endotherms, but like reptiles, their temperature and biological functions vary depending on the time of day and season. Birds have a higher average body temperature compared to other animals (38–45°C; 100.4 - 113°F). Temperature is not routinely taken during physical examination because of its high variability, and because of the unclear clinical significance.[45,46] When environmental temperatures and food availability are not adequate, and a bird needs to conserve energy, some species can go into a state of torpor where their metabolism, heart rate, and respiratory rate drop significantly; therefore, their temperature decreases.[47] Although this is primarily seen in wild birds and species held in zoological collections rather than pet birds, this process can also make it difficult to determine if an animal is sick based on temperature. As in any other organism, temperatures obtained via a mucosal surface (eg, the cloaca), are likely to underestimate core body temperature.[44] This may not be an issue, as soon as specific reference intervals are developed for each reading site and the variation between core body temperature and cloacal temperature are not random.

If temperature is measured, care must be taken to not artificially elevate the temperature during the physical exam. In a study performed in barred owls, cloacal temperature significantly increased during manual restraint.[48] A similar finding was reported in red-tailed hawks,[49] Hispaniolan Amazon parrots,[50] Amazon parrots,[51] and cockatiels[52] to varying degrees. Temperature should ideally be taken at the beginning of the examination based on these findings to provide the most-accurate temperature.

Factors that Affect Temperature

To accurately assess temperature, the clinician should be aware of any confounding factors that can affect a temperature reading. One of the most important factors to consider is the temperature measurement method. Rectal temperatures obtained with digital thermometers have been the reference standard for temperature measurement, and there are several studies that evaluate different methods in comparison to this. These methods include implanted microchip transponder,[25,28,29] infrared thermometers,[28,29,31] and tympanic thermometers.[25,26,29,31,32] Although the microchip transponder was most consistent with rectal temperature in many studies to assess core temperature, during regular clinical activity, this is not practical. In ferrets, auricular thermometers measured on the dorsal skin between the scapulae was found to be in close agreement with core body temperature,[31] but in other animals (dogs, guinea pigs, rabbits, chinchillas), the auricular thermometers used in the ear had a very poor agreement and were not recommended.[25,28,29,32]

In addition to the type of thermometry that is used, temperature reading location also has an effect. As mentioned before, auricular readings are not recommended due to the variability and underestimation they give compared to core body temperature, and this is most likely due to the different conformation of animal ears compared to human ears.[25,28,29,32] However, even when assessing with the same thermometer for temperature readings in different areas in guinea pigs,[30] dogs, and cats,[53] axillary and inguinal varied widely from rectal temperature, were sometimes not repeatable, or underestimated rectal temperature by as much as 2°C.

Although not validated in other species, it has been shown that in chinchillas, the depth of the thermometer plays a major role in obtaining an accurate measurement. When using a digital rectal thermometer, changing the insertion depth from 1 to 2 cm increased the reading by 1.14 $\pm$ 0.77°C. (97.5 $\pm$ 1.39°F).[32] This finding is consistent with other studies in dairy cattle[54] and humans,[55] indicating that the depth of the thermometer is key in taking an accurate temperature. In our hospital, we mark rectal thermometers with a permanent marker at 2 cm from the tip to assure that temperature readings are always obtained at the same depth in every animal (**Fig. 3**).

Another factor to consider when assessing the presentation of an animal is if they are in shock. No matter which type of shock (cardiogenic, obstructive, distributive, and so forth), mechanisms are occurring in the body to compensate for that shock. There are two general phenotypes in shock: vasoconstrictive and vasodilatory, which both progress through stages of compensatory and decompensatory shock as an animal's disease process progresses. Both shock phenotypes at both stages will affect temperature readings in various areas of the body. Vasoconstrictive shock seeks to maintain tissue perfusion to the most essential tissues via peripheral vasoconstriction utilizing norepinephrine, epinephrine and, phenylephrine acting on different receptors during different shock states.[56,57] For a variety of reasons and through a variety of mechanisms, vasodilatory shock leads to an animal's peripheral vasculature becoming dilated.

In vasoconstrictive shock, during both decompensated and compensated shock, rectal temperature is decreased due to the peripheral vasoconstriction and shunting blood away from the gastrointestinal tract, although in the decompensation phase, temperature is lower than during the compensated state.[56] In vasodilatory shock, an

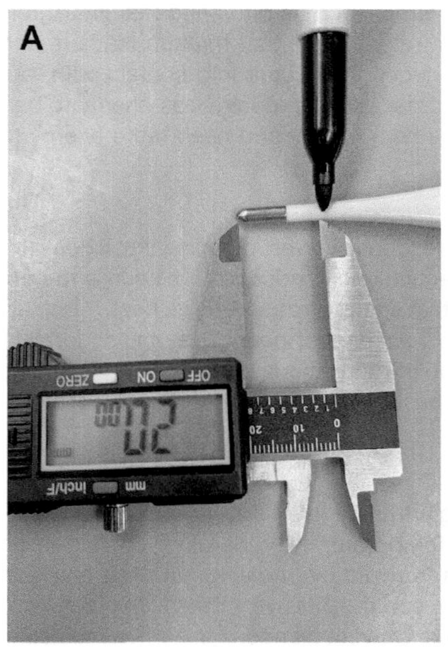

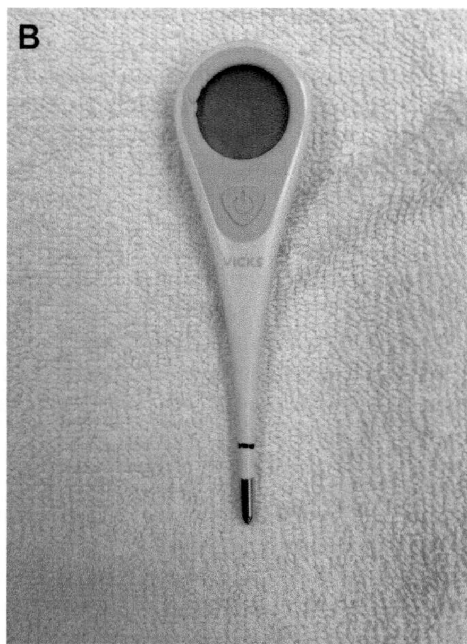

Fig. 3. Rectal temperature varies depending on the depth of insertion of thermometers. In our hospital, we mark rectal thermometers with a permanent marker at 2 cm from the tip, in order to have temperature always obtained at the same depth.

animal's peripheral temperature will be elevated during the compensatory phase, but will be markedly decreased in the decompensatory phase. Because of blood shunting, core body temperature may differ notably from peripheral temperatures, and this can either be assessed subjectively (eg, feeling that the limbs are cooler compared to the body) or with infrared thermography. Studies in children with shock have shown that different body sites have a decreased temperature, especially distal sites such as the feet and hands.[58] Although limited studies have been performed in animals, much less exotic animals, similar conclusions can be made and should be taken into account when caring for critical patients, especially those that are hypothermic.

Mechanisms of Heat Transfer

Heat is loss or gained via four mechanisms: convection, conduction, radiation, and evaporation, and these methods are important to understand when assessing the best method of heating or cooling your patient.

Convection

Convection is the process by which heat transfers from a fluid to either fluid or air or a different temperature through contact. When cooler air moves over the surface of a warmer animal, the animal is cooled. This also occurs within the body – warm blood is transferred from the core to the extremities, or cooled blood closer to the surface is moved to cool overheated areas of the body.[59]

Conduction

Conduction is the mechanism where heat is transferred between two solid objects. Heat travels down the thermal gradient to move from the warmer object to the cooler one. Ectotherms, such as reptiles, can regulate heat in this way by moving onto a warmed rock in a cool environment. Endotherms, such as birds and mammals, rely less on external sources of heat due to their retention of heat through feathers and fur.[59] Animals can lose heat via external surfaces they come into contact with, but also through internal mechanisms as well. Larger animals require less energy to balance heat loss whereas smaller animals lose heat rapidly and need more energy to maintain heat in comparison.[59]

Radiation

Radiation is energy that is emitted via electromagnetic waves, meaning that it does not need a medium to transfer heat unlike convection and conduction. The sun is the primary source of Earth's radiative energy and that energy is absorbed as heat,[59] but this can also be utilized via heat emitting devices (heat lamps, incubators, and so forth) to provide heat to an animal in a similar fashion to the sun. This is important in ectotherms who need a thermoregulatory gradient and a basking area to achieve a certain temperature for optimal metabolism.

Evaporation

Evaporation converts water to gas, allowing a transfer of energy even if the environmental heat is greater than the animal's temperature. Evaporative cooling is an important mechanism used by endotherms to avoid overheating, and this relies on environmental or body water. This process can be passive through the skin, and also through panting in animals that do not have sweat glands.[59] In human medicine, a major cause of hypothermia in newborns is through evaporative heat loss due to insensible water loss and an immature skin barrier. A study in premature infants showed that by placing infants in plastic bags reduce both evaporative and convective heat loss, insensible water loss, and the need for metabolic heat production. This was also done without producing hyperthermia or other complications.[60,61] This may be an important an inexpensive method to incorporate into exotic animal practice for the prevention of heat loss in our small patients.

HYPOTHERMIA

Hypothermia is defined as a subnormal body temperature in a homeothermic organism,[62] and it induces physiologic changes in different organ systems throughout the body. Hypothermia causes marked vasoconstriction, tachycardia, and an increase in cardiac output due to the need of perfusing the subject's core. When hypothermia is untreated and progresses, heart rate decreases, myocardial contractility decreases, and subsequently cardiac output decreases and cardiac arrest risk increases.[63–65] Coagulation is also altered and disseminated intravascular coagulation can ensue. Hemoglobin also has a decreased affinity for oxygen, but this is counterbalanced by the decreased tissue-oxygen demand and increased oxygen solubility of plasma.[63–65] In addition to cardiovascular effects, a progressive decrease in respiratory rate occurs. Level of consciousness becomes depressed due to a decrease in cerebral blood flow and acid-base abnormalities occur, which usually progress to metabolic acidosis, which can then further depress the neurologic system. Another important effect of hypothermia to consider also is gastrointestinal ileus,[66] which is especially important in hind-gut fermenter patients, such as rabbits, guinea pigs, and chinchillas.[63] In reptiles, hypothermia can also affect the absorption and metabolism of medications and fluids, reducing their effectiveness.[67]

For clinical purposes, hypothermia is characterized into two main categories: primary and secondary hypothermia. Primary hypothermia occurs due to environmental exposure, while secondary hypothermia occurs due to an illness, anesthesia, medications, or trauma. In animals under 5 kg, this loss is more significant due to the higher surface-area-to-volume ratio compared to larger animals.[22] Temperature loss can also be increased in emaciated animals, due to lack of subcutaneous fat for insulation.[22,33] In newborns, studies have shown that in the delivery room, hypothermia is a major concern as it increases oxygen consumption[12] and hypothermic newborns had a higher mortality rate compared to normothermic newborns.[14,17] A study evaluating oxygen consumption in newborn rabbits and kittens had similar findings.[15] There is an increase in oxygen consumption in the first day of life, compared to the tenth day, and this is due to poor thermoregulatory mechanisms in newborn animals.[15] In human patients, it has also shown that hypothermia in cases of major trauma[7–11] or sepsis[4–6] is a negative prognostic factor.

INDICATIONS FOR HEAT SUPPORT

Because of the risks associated with hypothermia, heat support is typically indicated any time a patient's temperature is below the accepted core temperature range, or if the temperature is decreasing and trending toward hypothermia. During anesthesia of exotic animals, heat support should be always provided to prevent perioperative hypothermia (**Fig. 4**). A study in small breed dogs evaluated the effect of pre-warming on perioperative hypothermia and recovery. The results showed that there was no difference in the incidence of perioperative hypothermia, and all dogs developed hypothermia regardless of pre-warming.[68] This study indicates that providing heat too early, such as just after induction, does not provide any benefit and emphasizes the need instead for heat support during anesthesia.

Heat support is, however, not indicated in every case. Most notably in human medicine, therapeutic hypothermia, or targeted temperature management, following cardiac arrest, traumatic brain injury, or a global ischemic event, has been shown to improve the neurologic status and chance of complete recovery.[69–73] There are limited studies of this in veterinary medicine describing its application,[74–76] but further research in the area of therapeutic hypothermia is definitely desirable.

METHODS OF THERMAL SUPPORT

In cases of primary hypothermia, rewarming is the mainstay of treatment. Based on current epidemiological research, it appears that the majority of the small exotic mammals with hypothermia are suffering from secondary rather than primary hypothermia.[2] In cases of secondary hypothermia, rewarming is still a significant component of

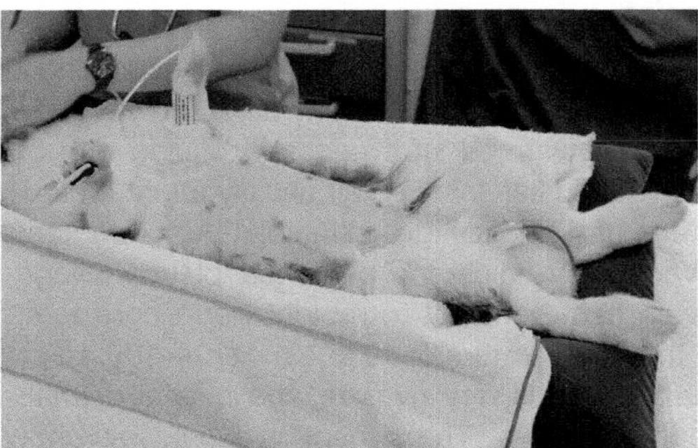

Fig. 4. Continuous rectal temperature measurement and active surface rewarming with a forced warm air device in a rabbit under anesthesia.

treatment, but identifying and treating underlying causes of hypothermia is key. There are three methods of rewarming: passive surface, active surface, and active core.

Passive Surface Rewarming

Passive surface rewarming allows the animal's own heat production to increase core temperature. This type of warming is done through shivering. In addition, tasks can be performed to prevent further heat loss, including drying any wet fur and covering the animal with blankets, towels, or bubble wrap to provide an insulating layer. If shivering is not present, the animal is not increasing its body temperature, and passive surface rewarming will not be effective as the sole mechanism of rewarming.[62] With this method in place, temperatures can increase by 0.5 to 4°C/h (approximately, 0.9 to 7.2°F/h) depending upon the animal's metabolic and thermoregulatory function.[33,77] If there is active movement occurring, this increase changes to 1 to 5°C/h (approximately, 1.8 to 9°F/h).[33]

Active Surface Rewarming

Active surface rewarming includes methods that apply heat to the surface of the animal to increase core body temperatures. This category comprises incubators, warm water blankets placed under or on top of the animal, forced warm air (such as the Bair Hugger, 3M, Maplewood, MN, USA) under blankets or bubble wrap, radiant heat sources such as heat lamps, warmed fluid bags/bottles, rice socks, and warmed towels (**Fig. 5**). Care must be taken not to place the warming device in direct contact with the patient if he or she is unable to move, such as under anesthesia or in a critical state, as this can lead to severe burns.[62] In small mammals, birds, and reptiles, incubators, and terraria can be used as they heat up quickly, and the heat is contained in a small area to provide a warm enclosed environment. These methods increase core body temperature by 0.5 to 4°C/h (approximately, 0.9 to 7.2°F/h) as well, but also prevents heat loss, unlike passive surface rewarming.[33,77] In anesthetized ringed turtle doves (*Streptopelia risorii*), three different methods of heat support were evaluated on their ability to maintain core body temperature: a warmed-water blanket, radiant heat (heat lamp), and an inspired warmed air humidified. The study found that core body temperature was easily maintained with the radiant heat source while there was a minimal to no effect from the water blanket and air humidifier, respectively.[78] Based on this, radiant heat sources can be recommended, or a combination of methods can be used to provide optimal warming to an anesthetized or hypothermic bird.

Active Core Rewarming

Active core rewarming is a more effective method of rewarming and involves directly supplying heat to the core of the animal. Many different types of interventions belong in this category including warmed intravenous (IV) fluids with or without a fluid line warmer, warmed and humidified inspired air usually for intubated or anesthetized patients, warm water enemas, and lavages in the bladder or peritoneal/pleural/coelomic cavity (**Fig. 6**).[62] Warmed IV fluids and peritoneal/pleural lavage are recommended because they provide heat centrally to rapidly warm core temperatures, and they should be warmed to a temperature of 40 to 43°C (104–109.4°F).[18] It should be noted that peritoneal/pleural lavage is very invasive, and in small animals may be contraindicated in the majority of cases. The exception would be under anesthesia when abdominal, thoracic, or coelomic surgery is being performed and there is direct access to those cavities already.

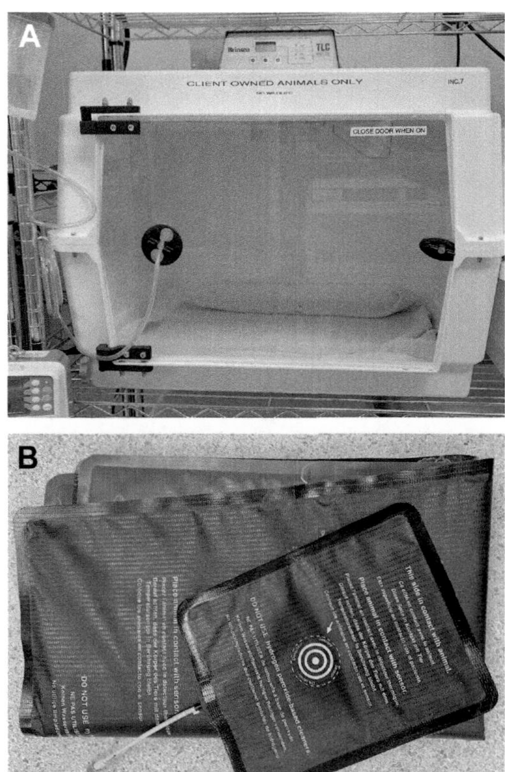

Fig. 5. Devices commonly used for active surface rewarming of exotic animals include incubators (*A*) and heating pads (*B*).

When using a fluid line warmer, it is important that it be placed as close the animal as possible to prevent further loss of heat through the line as it connects to the animal's IV catheter.[79] Heated-inspired air devices have been constructed for small companion animal use to address hypothermia (Darvall ZDS Heated Qubes, DarvallVet, Prescott, AZ, USA). Compared to devices meant for dogs, cats, and humans, these have zero dead space. They can attach directly to an anesthesia circuit and eliminate high scavenge system air flow around the animal as with a Bain circuit to reduce the risk of hypothermia.

CESSATION OF HEAT SUPPORT

In dogs and cats, it is recommended to continue active rewarming until the patient is at 37°C (98.6°F) to restore coagulation and cardiovascular function to normal without overwhelming the circulatory system.[64] Restoring to this temperature may also prevent the "afterdrop" phenomenon in which the core body temperature of an animal may continue to drop after the onset of rewarming due to the return of cooler peripheral blood to the body core and the movement of warmer core blood to the periphery. Other complications can occur associated with rewarming including acute respiratory distress syndrome, cerebral edema and ischemia, pneumonia, pulmonary edema, reperfusion injury, and shock.[64] These conditions should be closely monitored for

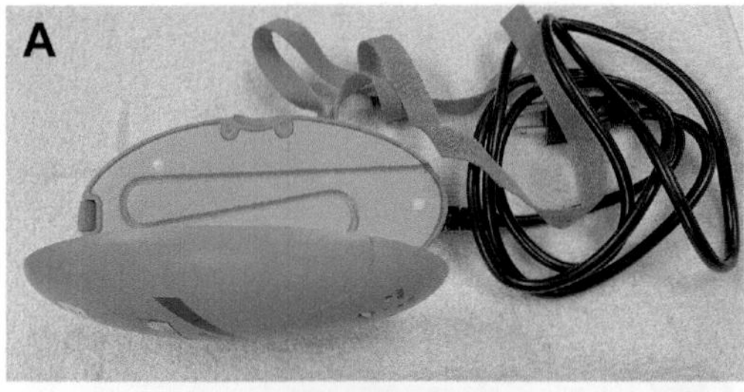

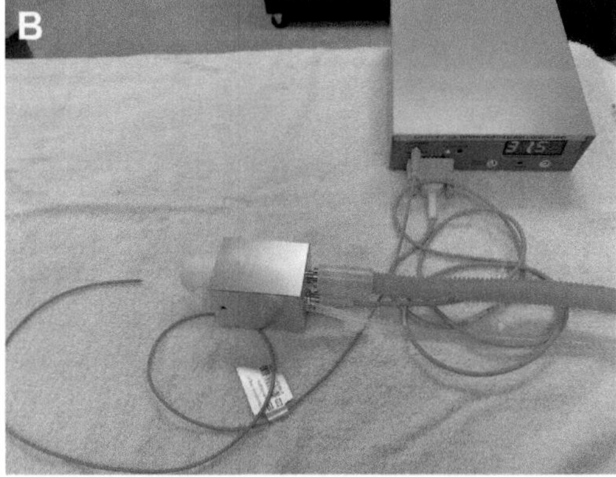

Fig. 6. Line warmers (*A*) can used for active core rewarming of exotic animals. If emergent anesthesia of a hypothermic animal is needed, air warmers can be used as active core rewarming increasing the temperature of inspired air (*B*).

both during and after the cessation of heat support. If kept in an incubator, the animal does not necessarily need to be removed, but the temperature should be reduced to prevent hyperthermia. In reptiles, temperature can be monitored continuously during active rewarming with a cloacal probe, if tolerated (**Fig. 7**).

HYPERTHERMIA

Hyperthermia is reported less commonly compared to hypothermia in exotic animal practice. Hyperthermia can be related to excessive exercise, heat stroke, toxicities, sepsis, seizures, neoplasia, or immune system-related responses (inflammatory, immune-mediated, infection, transfusion-related reactions).[26] In reptiles, a temperature gradient is important because it allows a reptile to escape from high temperatures by moving to a cooler area of the enclosure. Without this, especially if temperature support in a terrarium is provided via heat rocks or heated glass enclosures, a reptile can succumb to hyperthermia or suffer from burns.[39] Environmental temperatures starting at 38°C (100.4°F) can be lethal in reptiles, and those kept in a glass or plastic enclosures can experience a very rapid death (within 5–15 minutes).[40,43] Small mammals can succumb to high temperatures and hyperthermia very quickly because they do not have an effective way to cool down their body, unlike dogs and cats who can pant to allow evaporation and cooling. Rabbits have a limited system to disperse heat through increasing blood flow to their ears and allowing heat to dissipate into their environment. Birds have a very high tolerance for hyperthermia and can still function at body temperatures of 48 to 49°C (118.4–120.2°F), so they are less prone to the deleterious effects of hyperthermia.[80,81]

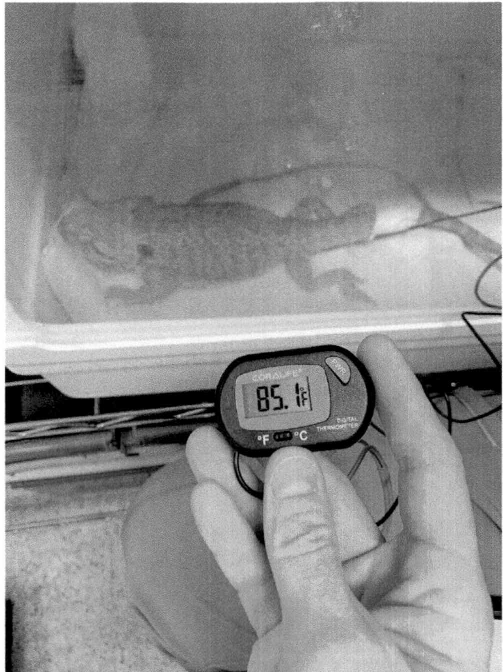

Fig. 7. Continuous cloacal temperature measurement in a bearded dragon (*Pogona vitticeps*) recovering from anesthesia in an incubator.

INDICATIONS FOR COOLING

In small exotic mammals, cooling should be done in any case of suspected heat stroke, or any time a temperature is greater than 40 to 40.5°C (104–105°F), or greater than 38.3°C (101°F) in chinchillas.[82] Lethal temperatures in reptiles are greater than 38°C (100°F) and can manifest by abnormal behavior, open-mouth breathing, gasping, and tachypnea. These signs can be seen just a few degrees above the POTZ of a reptile.[40,41] Birds, especially poultry, are susceptible to heat stroke and hyperthermia which can show symptoms such as weakness or collapse, dyspnea, and abnormal behavior.[83]

OPTIONS FOR COOLING

For small exotic mammals that are hyperthermic, the animal should be immediately moved to a cooler area and a cool wet towel can be wrapped around the body or neck, rewetting and re-wrapping every few minutes to make sure it remains cold. Ice can be packed in a bag and positioned underneath the animal, avoiding direct contact (**Fig. 8**). An IV catheter should be placed to administer room-temperature or cool intravenous fluids. Temperature should be monitored closely to make sure the animal does not cool too quickly, which could result in hypothermia. Cooling measures should be ceased once the animal is at 39°C (102°F).[82]

In birds that are hyperthermic, placement in a cool, oxygenated incubator is usually adequate, but additional measures such as providing subcutaneous or IV fluids, applying alcohol to feet, and minimizing handling can be taken as well.[83] The animal should continue to be cooled until dyspnea has decreased or resolved.

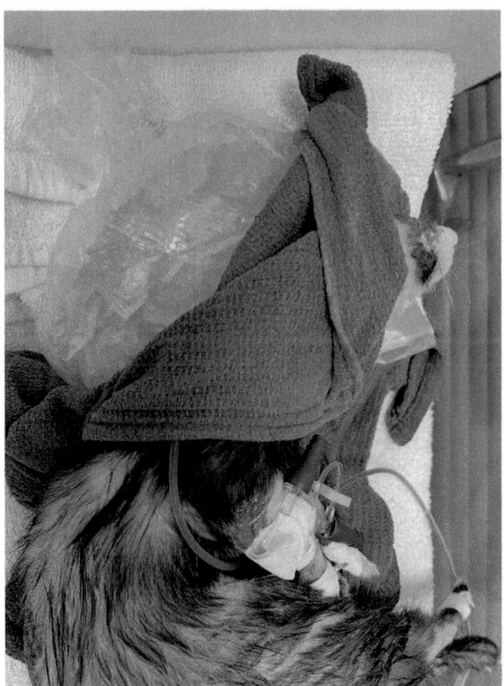

Fig. 8. Active cooling of a hyperthermic (rectal temperature: 107.1°F [41.7°C]) ferret. Ice is packed in a bag and positioned underneath the animal. A towel wet with cold water is wrapped in between the ice pack and the animal to avoid direct contact.

For reptiles, the animal should be placed in cool water to reduce their core temperature along with the administration of subcutaneous fluids. The reptile should then be placed in an incubator or terrarium and the lower end of its POTZ.[40]

CLINICS CARE POINTS

- Body temperature measurement is one of the most important parameters to assess the health of a patient. In multiple species, it has been proven that upon examination, a high or low temperature can help to determine the degree of illness, including the prognosis of a patient.
- Recent studies in rabbits and guinea pigs have shown that on presentation to veterinary hospitals, a low rectal temperature is associated with a higher likelihood of death compared to a normal rectal temperature.
- Temperature measurement is also crucial in the perioperative period to ensure a safe anesthetic event and a smooth recovery for the patient.
- In reptiles, the measurement of cloacal temperature on admission can provide important information, such as whether the reptile could be acting abnormal or lethargic because of exposure to an excessively low temperature during transport to the hospital.
- In birds, if temperature is measured, care must be taken to not artificially elevate the temperature during the physical exam.

DISCLOSURE

No conflict of interest.

REFERENCES

1. Di Girolamo N, Toth G, Selleri P. Prognostic value of rectal temperature at hospital admission in client-owned rabbits. J Am Vet Med Assoc 2016;248(3):288–97.
2. Levy IH, Di Girolamo N, Keller KA. Rectal temperature is a prognostic indicator in client-owned guinea pigs. J Small Anim Pract 2021;62(10):861–5.
3. Inghammar M, Sunden-Cullberg J. Prognostic significance of body temperature in the emergency department vs the ICU in Patients with severe sepsis or septic shock: A nationwide cohort study. PLoS One 2020;15(12):e0243990.
4. Kushimoto S, Gando S, Saitoh D, et al. The impact of body temperature abnormalities on the disease severity and outcome in patients with severe sepsis: an analysis from a multicenter, prospective study of severe sepsis. Crit Care 2013; 17(6):R271.
5. Ramgopal S, Horvat CM, Adler MD. Association of triage hypothermia with in-hospital mortality among patients in the emergency department with suspected sepsis. J Crit Care 2020;60:27–31.
6. Sunden-Cullberg J, Rylance R, Svefors J, et al. Fever in the Emergency Department Predicts Survival of Patients With Severe Sepsis and Septic Shock Admitted to the ICU. Crit Care Med 2017;45(4):591–9.
7. Keane M. Triad of death: the importance of temperature monitoring in trauma patients. Emerg Nurse. Sep 2016;24(5):19–23.
8. Moffatt SE. Hypothermia in trauma. Emerg Med J 2013;30(12):989–96.
9. Singer AJ, Taira BR, Thode HC Jr, et al. The association between hypothermia, prehospital cooling, and mortality in burn victims. Acad Emerg Med 2010;17(4):456–9.
10. Trentzsch H, Huber-Wagner S, Hildebrand F, et al. Hypothermia for prediction of death in severely injured blunt trauma patients. Shock 2012;37(2):131–9.
11. Wang HE, Callaway CW, Peitzman AB, et al. Admission hypothermia and outcome after major trauma. Crit Care Med 2005;33(6):1296–301.
12. Adamsons K, Gandy GM, James LS. The influence of thermal factors upon oxygen consumption of the newborn human infant. J Pediatr 1965;66:495–508.
13. Dahm LS, James LS. Newborn temperature and calculated heat loss in the delivery room. Pediatrics 1972;49(4):504–13.
14. Day RL, Caliguiri L, Kamenski C, et al. Body temperature and survival of premature infants. Pediatrics 1964;34:171–81.
15. Hull D. Oxygen consumption and body temperature of new-born rabbits and kittens expose to cold. J Physiol 1965;177(2):192–202.
16. Oliver TK Jr. Temperature Regulation and Heat Production in the Newborn. Pediatr Clin North Am. Aug 1965;12:765–79.
17. Silverman WA, Fertig JW, Berger AP. The influence of the thermal environment upon the survival of newly born premature infants. Pediatrics 1958;22(5):876–86.
18. Armstrong SR, Roberts BK, Aronsohn M. Perioperative hypothermia. J Vet Emerg Crit Care 2005;15(1):32–7.
19. Cabell LW, Perkowski SZ, Gregor T, et al. The effects of active peripheral skin warming on perioperative hypothermia in dogs. Vet Surg 1997;26:79–85.
20. Clark-Price S. Inadvertent Perianesthetic Hypothermia in Small Animal Patients. Vet Clin North Am Small Anim Pract 2015;45(5):983–94.
21. Herlich A. Perioperative temperature elevation: not all hyperthermia is malignant hyperthermia. Paediatr Anaesth 2013;23(9):842–50.

22. Murison P. Prevention and treatment of perioperative hypothermia in animals under 5kg bodyweight. Practice 2001;23(7):412–8.
23. Pottie RG, Dart CM, Perkins NR, et al. Effect of hypothermia on recovery from general anaesthesia in the dog. Aust Vet J 2007;85(4):158–62.
24. Rodriguez-Diaz JM, Hayes GM, Boesch J, et al. Decreased incidence of perioperative inadvertent hypothermia and faster anesthesia recovery with increased environmental temperature: A nonrandomized controlled study. Vet Surg 2020; 49(2):256–64.
25. Greer RJ, Cohn LA, Dodam JR, et al. Comparison of three methods of temperature measurement in hypothermic, euthermic, and hyperthermic dogs. Journal of the American Veterinary Medical Association 2007;230(12):1841–8.
26. Konietschke U, Kruse BD, Müller R, et al. Comparison of auricular and rectal temperature measurement in normohermic, hypothermic, and hyperthermic dogs. Tierarztl Prax Ausg K Kleintiere Heimtiere 2014;42(1):13–9.
27. Sousa MG, Carareto R, Pereira-Junior VA, et al. Agreement between auricular and rectal measurements of body temperature in healthy cats. J Feline Med Surg 2013;15(4):275–9.
28. Stephens Devalle JM. Comparison of tympanic, transponder, and noncontact infrared laser thermometry with rectal thermometry in strain 13 guinea pigs (Cavia porcellus). Contemp Top Lab Anim Sci 2005;44(5):35–8.
29. Chen PH, White CE. Comparison of rectal, microchip transponder, and infrared thermometry techniques for obtaining body temperature in the laboratory rabbit (*Oryctolagus cuniculus*). Journal of the Americal Association for Laboratory Animal Science 2006;45(1):57–63.
30. Levy I, Allender MC, Keller KA. Comparison of axillary and inguinal body temperature to rectal temperature in healthy guinea pigs (Cavia porcellus). J Exot Pet Med 2020;34:1–5.
31. Hepps Keeney CM, Hung CS, Harrison TM. Comparison of body temperature using digital, infrared, and tympanic thermometry in healthy ferrets (Mustela putorius furo). J Exot Pet Med 2021;36:16–21.
32. Ozawa S, Mans C, Beaufrère H. Comparison of rectal and tympanic thermometry in chinchillas (Chinchilla lanigera). Journal of the American Veterinary Medical Association 2017;25(1):552–8.
33. Paal P, Pasquier M, Darocha T, et al. Accidental Hypothermia: 2021 Update. Int J Environ Res Public Health 3 2022;19(1). https://doi.org/10.3390/ijerph19010501.
34. Levesque DL, Nowack J, Stawski C. Modelling mammalian energetics: the heterothermy problem. Climate Change Responses 2016;3(1). https://doi.org/10.1186/s40665-016-0022-3.
35. Bertelsen MF, Mohammed O, Manger P, et al. The Hairy Lizard: Factoring in Heterothermy in Anesthetic Managment of Arabian Oryx (Oryx leucoryx). Vet Anaesth Analg 2017;44(4):899–904.
36. Ewart SL. Thermoregulation. In: Klein BG, editor. Cunningham's textbook of veterinary physiology. 6 edition. St. Louis, MO: Elsevier; 2020. p. 596–607, chap 53.
37. Seebacher F, Franklin CE. Physiological mechanisms of thermoregulation in reptiles: a review. J Comp Physiol B 2005;175(8):533–41.
38. Dawson WR. *On the physiological Significance of the preferred body Temperatures of reptiles*. Perspectives of biophysical ecology. Berlin, Heidelberg: Springer; 1975.
39. McBride M, Hernandez-Divers SJ. Nursing care of lizards. Vet Clin North Am Exot Anim Pract. May 2004;7(2):375–96, vii.

40. Boyer TH. Emergency care of reptiles. Vet Clin North Am Exot Anim Pract 1998; 1(1):191–206, vii.
41. Martinez-Jimenez D, Hernandez-Divers SJ. Emergency Care of Reptiles. Vet Clin Exot Anim Pract 2007;10(2):557–85.
42. Music MK, Strunk A. Reptile Critical Care and Common Emergencies. Vet Clin North Am Exot Anim Pract 2016;19(2):591–612.
43. Norton TM. Chelonian Emergency and Critical Care. Seminars Avian Exot Pet Med 2005;14(2):106–30.
44. McMaster MK, Downs CT. Thermal variability in body temperature in an ectotherm: Are cloacal temperatures good indicators of tortoise body temperature? J Therm Biol 2013;38(4):163–8.
45. Wellehan JFX, Lierz M, Phalen D, et al. Infecious Disease. In: Speer BL, editor. Current therapy in avian medicine and surgery. 1 edition. St. Louis, MO: Elsevier; 2016. p. 23–106, chap 2.
46. Prinzinger R, PreBmar A, Schleucher E. Mini Review: Body Temperature in Birds. Comparative Biochemistry and Physiology 1991;99A(4):499–506.
47. Ruf T, Geiser F. Daily torpor and hibernation in birds and mammals. Biol Rev Camb Philos Soc 2015;90(3):891–926.
48. Doss GA, Mans C. The Effect of Manual Restraint on Physiological Parameters in Barred Owls (Strix varia). J Avian Med Surg 2017;31(1):1–5.
49. Doss GA, Mans C. Changes in physiologic parameters and effects of hooding in red-tailed hawks (Buteo jamaicensis) during manual restraint. J Avian Med Surg 2016;30(2):127–32.
50. Mans C, Guzman DS, Lahner LL, et al. Sedation and physiologic response to manual restraint after intranasal administration of midazolam in Hispaniolan Amazon parrots (Amazona ventralis). J Avian Med Surg. Sep 2012;26(3):130–9.
51. Greenacre CB, Lusby AL. Physiologic Responses of Amazon Parrots (Amazona species) to Manual Restraint. J Avian Med Surg 2004;18(1):19–22.
52. Doss GA, Fink DM, Mans C. Assessment of sedation after intranasal administration of midazolam and midazolam-butorphanol in cockatiels (Nymphicus hollandicus). American Journal of Veterinary Research 2018;79(12):1246–52.
53. Goic JB, Reineke EL, Drobatz KJ. Comparison of rectal and axillary temperatures in dogs and cats. Journal of the American Veterinary Medical Association 2014; 244(10):1170–5.
54. Burfeind O, von Keyserlingk MA, Weary DM, et al. Short communication: repeatability of measures of rectal temperature in dairy cows. J Dairy Sci. Feb 2010; 93(2):624–7.
55. Lee JY, Wakabayashi H, Wijayanto T, et al. Differences in rectal temperatures measured at depths of 4-19 cm from the anal sphincter during exercise and rest. Eur J Appl Physiol. May 2010;109(1):73–80.
56. Thomovsky E, Johnson PA. Shock pathophysiology. *Compendium*. Yardley, PA: Continuing Education for Veterinarians; 2013.
57. Russell JA, Rush B, Boyd J. Pathophysiology of Septic Shock. Crit Care Clin. Jan 2018;34(1):43–61.
58. Ortiz-Dosal A, Kolosovas-Machuca ES, Rivera-Vega R, et al. Use of infrared thermography in children with shock: A case series. SAGE Open Med Case Rep 2014;2. https://doi.org/10.1177/2050313X14561779. 2050313X14561779.
59. Norris AL, Kunz TH. Effects of Solar Radiation on Animal Thermoregulation. Solar Radiation 2012;1:195–220.
60. Leadford AE, Warren JB, Manasyan A, et al. Plastic bags for prevention of hypothermia in preterm and low birth weight infants. Pediatrics 2013;132(1):e128–34.

61. Baumgart S, Engle WD, Fox WW, et al. Effect of heat shielding on convective and evaporative heat losses and on radiant heat transfer in the premature infant. J Pediatr 1981;99(6):948–56.
62. Brodeur A, Wright A, Cortes Y. Hypothermia and targeted temperature management in cats and dogs. J Vet Emerg Crit Care 2017;27(2):151–63.
63. Hildebrand F, Giannoudis PV, van Griensven M, et al. Pathophysiologic changes and effects of hypothermia on outcome in elective surgery and trauma patients. Am J Surg. Mar 2004;187(3):363–71.
64. Oncken AK, Kirby R, Rudloff E. Hypothermia in critically ill dogs and cats. Compendium on Continuing Education for the Practising Veterinarian 2001;23(6): 506–20.
65. Polderman KH. Mechanisms of action, physiological effects, and complications of hypothermia. Crit Care Med. Jul 2009;37(7 Suppl):S186–202.
66. Esposito RA, Spencer FC. The Effect of Pericardial Insulation on Hypothermic Phrenic Nerve Injury During Open-Heart Surgery. Ann Thorac Surg 1987;43(3): 303–8.
67. Long SY. Approach to Reptile Emergency Medicine. Vet Clin North Am Exot Anim Pract. May 2016;19(2):567–90.
68. Aarnes TK, Bednarsky RM, Lerche P, et al. Effect of pre-warming on perioperative hypothermia and anesthetic recovery in small breed dogs undergoing ovariohysterectomy. Can Vet J 2017;58:175–9.
69. Arrich J, Holzer M, Havel C, et al. Hypothermia for neuroprotection in adults after cardiopulmonary resuscitation. Cochrane Database Syst Rev. Feb 15 2016;2(2): CD004128.
70. Callaway CW, Donnino MW, Fink EL, et al. Part 8: Post-Cardiac Arrest Care: 2015 American Heart Association Guidelines Update for Cardiopulmonary Resuscitation and Emergency Cardiovascular Care. Circulation. Nov 3 2015;132(18 Suppl 2):S465–82.
71. Polderman KH. Application of therapeutic hypothermia in the intensive care unit. Opportunities and pitfalls of a promising treatment modality–Part 2: Practical aspects and side effects. Intensive Care Med 2004;30(5):757–69.
72. Sydenham E, Roberts I, Alderson P. Hypothermia for traumatic head injury. Cochrane Database Syst Rev 2009;2:1–55.
73. Chiu WT, Lin KC, Tsai MS, et al. Post-cardiac arrest care and targeted temperature management: A consensus of scientific statement from the Taiwan Society of Emergency & Critical Care Medicine, Taiwan Society of Critical Care Medicine and Taiwan Society of Emergency Medicine. J Formos Med Assoc. Jan 2021; 120(1 Pt 3):569–87.
74. Hayes GM. Severe seizures associated with traumatic brain injury managed by controlled hypothermia, pharmacologic coma, and mechanical ventilation in a dog. J Vet Emerg Crit Care 2009;19(6):629–34.
75. Moon PF, Ilkiw JE. Surface-induced hypothermia in dogs: 19 cases (1987–1989). Journal of the American Veterinary Medical Association 1993;202(3):437–44.
76. Šulla I, Horňák S, Balik V. Hypothermia as a potential remedy for canine and feline acute spinal cord injury: a review. Acta Vet 2022;91(2):189–99.
77. Paal P, Gordon L, Strapazzon G, et al. Accidental hypothermia-an update : The content of this review is endorsed by the International Commission for Mountain Emergency Medicine (ICAR MEDCOM). Scand J Trauma Resusc Emerg Med 2016;24(1):111.

78. Phalen DN, Mitchell ME, Cavazol-Martinez ML. Evaluation of three heat sources for their ability to maintain core body temperature in the anesthetized patient. J Avian Med Surg 1996;10(3):174–8.
79. Brady RB, Poppell WT. Effect of intravenous fluid warming on core body temperature during elective orthopedic procedures. Can Vet J 2020;61(10):1080–4.
80. Freeman MT, Czenze ZJ, Schoeman K, et al. Extreme hyperthermia tolerance in the world's most abundant wild bird. Sci Rep 2020;10(1):13098.
81. Freeman MT, Czenze ZJ, Schoeman K, et al. Adaptive variation in the upper limits of avian body temperature. Proc Natl Acad Sci U S A 2022;119(26). https://doi.org/10.1073/pnas.2116645119. e2116645119.
82. Schoemaker NJ. History and clinical examination. *Exotic animal Emergency and critical care medicine*. Hoboken, NJ: Wiley Blackwell; 2022. chap 1.
83. Grunkemeyer V, Swisher S. Backyard poultry and waterfowl. *Exotic animal Emergency and critical care medicine*. 1 edition. Hoboken, NJ: Wiley Blackwell; 2022. chap 38.
84. Varga MS. Textbook of rabbit medicine. 2 edition. Butterworth-Heinemann; 2014.
85. Powers LV, Perpiñán D. Basic Anatomy, Physiology, and Husbandry of Ferrets. In: Quesenberry KE, Orcutt CJ, Mans C, et al, editors. Ferrets, rabbits, and rodents clinical medicine and surgery. 4 edition. St. Louis, MO: Elsevier; 2021. p. 1–12, chap 1.
86. Pignon C, Mayer J. Guinea Pigs. In: Quesenberry KE, Orcutt CJ, Mans C, et al, editors. Ferrets, rabbits, and rodents clinical medicine and surgery. 4 edition. St. Louis, MO: Elsevier; 2021. p. 270–97, chap 21.
87. Mans C, Donnelly TM. Chinchillas. In: Quesenberry KE, Orcutt CJ, Mans C, et al, editors. Ferrets, rabbits, and rodents clinical medicine and surgery. 4 edition. St. Louis, MO: Elsevier; 2021. p. 298–322, chap 22.
88. Brattstrom BH. Body Temperatures of Reptiles. Am Midl Nat 1965;73(2):376–422.

Neurologic Assessment and Critical Care of Exotic Animals

Approach to the Neurologic Exam, Species Differences, Prognostic Scales, Commonly Encountered Conditions, Ancillary Diagnostic Tests, and Caring for Neurologically Impaired Patients

Juliet F. Armstrong, DVM, DACVIM (Neurology)*

KEYWORDS

- Exotic animal neurology • Neuroanatomy • Mentation • Coma scale

KEY POINTS

- The approach to the neurologic examination is maintained across species with key differences based on variations in neuroanatomy
- Performing the neurologic examination should be methodical and logical for all patients and the order and extent of the examination may depend upon the patient's clinical condition and cooperation
- Ancillary diagnostics may complement clinicopathologic evaluation and physical examination in critically ill neurologic patients

INTRODUCTION

As exotic animal species, including birds, reptiles, and small mammals, are becoming more popular household companions, they are increasingly being presented for veterinary care to small animal practitioners and specialists. Many disorders of other body systems have been well characterized in these species; however, the characterization of neurologic conditions is limited. Across some of these species, correlates between feline and canine neurology can be made, but variations in the nervous system

Small Animal Specialty Medicine, NorthStar VETS Robbinsville
* NorthStar VETS 315 Robbinsville-Allentown Road, Robbinsville, NJ 08691.
E-mail address: juliet.f.armstrong@gmail.com

Vet Clin Exot Anim 26 (2023) 545–566
https://doi.org/10.1016/j.cvex.2023.05.007
vetexotic.theclinics.com
1094-9194/23/

anatomy make evaluating exotic animal species more challenging in addition to the paucity of information on their neurologic systems and diseases.

When performing a neurologic examination on any species, the aim is to accurately identify the anatomic structures the responsibility for the abnormalities identified. This neurolocalization approach, coupled with appropriate history taking, allows for the development of a focused list of differential diagnoses in order to guide a diagnostic approach and development of treatment options. Performing the neurologic examination should be methodical for all patients and the order and extent of examination may depend upon the patient's clinical condition and cooperation. Once the neurolocalization and treatment plan have been identified, serial neurologic examinations and other general neurologic supportive care measures should be instituted for the care of the patient.

COMPONENTS OF THE NEUROLOGIC EXAMINATION

Classically, the components of the neurologic examination evaluated in veterinary medicine include mentation, cranial nerve assessment, gait/posture, postural reactions/proprioception, tone and reflexes, pain via palpation, and sensation/nociception (**Fig. 1**).

- Mentation: appropriate (BAR/QAR, dull) versus inappropriate (obtunded, stuporous, coma)
- Cranial Nerves: II (Optic), III (oculomotor), IV (trochlear), V (trigeminal), VI (abducens), VII (facial), VIII (vestibulocochlear), IX (glossopharyngeal), X (vagus), XI (accessory), XII (hypoglossal)
- Gait/Posture:
  - Ataxia: Proprioceptive, Cerebellar, Vestibular
  - Head tilt
  - Head turn
- Postural Reactions/Proprioception
- Segmental tone/reflexes: patellar reflexes, withdrawal reflexes, cutaneous trunci reflex, perineal reflex, anal tone, tail tone
- Pain/Palpation
- Nociception – only to be tested in the absence of voluntary motor

In exotic animal species, modifications to these components, however, are made based on varying neuroanatomy, clinical condition, and patient cooperation.

Obtaining a History

As many exotic species are prey animals, and generally more sensitive to handling and stress, obtaining a thorough history is essential in guiding a neurologic assessment. A clinical history, with attention paid to details regarding husbandry, housing, behavior, diet, and other in-contact/co-housed animals is critical. The observation of behavior and mentation may be difficult in a hospital setting, and history taking should be guided to directly address these items. Information with regards to nutrition (which may contribute to the development of neuropathies), trauma, and toxin exposure may help to narrow a differential list even before a neurologic localization is obtained. The onset of clinical signs and progression, as well as information on other animals within the same enclosure/habitat, are also essential to developing a differential list.

MENTATION ASSESSMENT

When assessing a patient's mentation, observation in the examination room before performing a hands-on examination is helpful. Nearly all exotic pet species are prey

NEUROLOGICAL EXAMINATION

MENTATION						
Appropriate:				Inappropriate:		
BAR	QAR	Dull		Obtunded	Stuporous	Comatose

GAIT					
Ambulatory/Nonambulatory (circle one)					
Normal	Paraparetic		Paraplegic	Tetraparetic	Tetraplegic
	Proprioceptive ataxia	Vestibular ataxia	Cerebellar ataxia	Circling L/R	Falling L/R

POSTURE					
Normal	Head tilt L/R	Head turn L/R	Wide-based	Kyphosis	Other:

POSTURAL REACTIONS				
	Hopping		Placing	
	Left	Right	Left	Right
Thoracic limbs				
Pelvic limbs				

LIMB/TRUNK REFLEXES, RESPONSES, ETC					
Thoracic limbs	Left	Right	Pelvic limbs	Left	Right
Withdrawal			Withdrawal		
Tone			Patellar		
Muscle mass			Tone		
+/- Nociception			+/- Nociception		
Tail tone and movement:		TL palpation:		Cervical palpation/ROM:	

CRANIAL NERVE EVALUATION				
PLR OS OD	Menace OS OD	Palpebral OS OD	Physiologic nystagmus OS OD	Nasal sensation L R

Neuroanatomic localization:	Differentials:	Plan

Fig. 1. Key components of the neurologic exam for use in tracking patient assessments and creating differential diagnoses. Table adapted from worksheet developed by Susan Arnold, DVM, Diplomate of the American College of Internal Medicine (Neurology).

species or are naturally curious by nature, so they should be quite alert and aware of the hospital environment surrounding them. In caged animals, or those that cannot freely move about a room, asking directed questions about at home behaviors and interactions may allow for better characterization of abnormalities, especially as defining a mental status can sometimes be nuanced.

Mentation is described as one of the following:

- Appropriate: Bright, quiet, alert, responsive, dull
- Inappropriate
  - Obtunded: reduced response to the environment
    - Mild obtundation can be mistaken for lethargy or to be secondary to systemic illness. This is best noticed by an owner most familiar with the pet. In these cases, there may be some decrease in response to auditory stimulus.
    - Moderate obtundation results in animals that are responsive to sound, but stronger stimuli are required for a response to be obtained.
    - In severe cases of obtundation, patients are usually non-ambulatory but responsive to loud noises or stimuli.
  - Stuporous: asleep, requires stimulation to elicit a reaction, near unconscious
  - Comatose: unconscious, a patient cannot be aroused despite noxious stimulus

Other aspects of mentation that may be described may include compulsive behaviors, agitation, anxiety, aggression, confusion, loss of learned behaviors, or dementia.

Ultimately a patient's level of consciousness (despite being a spectrum) can give the clearest picture of the mental state. Consciousness is produced by a functioning forebrain and reticular activating system in the brainstem. For those patients that are awake, the quality of their consciousness should also be assessed with things such as confusion and disorientation being considered.

Mental state and level of consciousness may also wax and wane, so serial neurologic assessment of patients, especially those that are critically ill, is essential. For hospitalized patients, adding a line or "treatment" for the notation of the patient's mentation/level of consciousness can help track the patient's improvement or decline in order to help determine the next best steps in patient care.

CRANIAL NERVE EVALUATION

Each cranial nerve carries specific functions and can be evaluated through a series of standard tests.

- Menace response (Evaluation of CN II, CN VII, prosencephalon)
- Pupillary Light Reflex (Evaluation of CN II and CN III)
- Oculocephalic reflex/physiologic nystagmus/doll's eye reflex (Evaluation of CN III, CN IV, CN VI, CN VIII)
- Palpebral Reflex (Evaluation of CN V and CN VII)
- Nasal stimulation response (Evaluation of CN V and prosencephalon)
- Gag reflex (Evaluation of CN IX and X)

Additional key observations to assess cranial nerve function include the assessment of eye movement (such as nystagmus), facial symmetry, muscle tone, and eye position (strabismus). The tongue and jaw should also be assessed for symmetry and tone.

Small Mammal Cranial Nerves

Like dogs and domestic cats, there are 12 pairs of cranial nerves that encompass both sensory and motor functions. The entirely sensory cranial nerves are I, II, and VIII. The entirely motor cranial nerves are III, IV, VI, and XII. The remainder (V, VII, IX, X, and XI) have mixed sensory and motor function.

Avian cranial nerves

Birds, such as mammals, have 12 pairs of cranial nerves that encompass both sensory and motor functions. The entirely sensory cranial nerves are I, II, and VIII and the entirely motor cranial nerves are III, IV, VI, and XII. The remainder (V, VII, IX, X, and XI) have mixed sensory and motor function.

The menace response is a learned response and not a reflex, but birds that are stoic or excited may not demonstrate a response even though nerve function is intact.

Avian pupil movements are poor in response to light and there is no consensual response as birds have complete decussation of the optic nerves at the chiasm. The pupillary light reflexes may not be as robust as observed in mammals due to the iris being striated muscle in birds giving them some voluntary control over pupil size independent of the response to light.

The control of eye and head movements is stimulated by the vestibular centers; with branches of the oculomotor, trochlear, and abducens nerves innervating the extrinsic eye muscles. When assessing the palpebral reflex, it is important to remember that the eyelids of birds are innervated by CN V. Eyelid sensation is provided by the ophthalmic branch (upper lid) and maxillary branch (both lids), while eyelid closure is controlled by the mandibular branch.

Prehension assessment via tongue movement and beak strength assesses CN V, and IX-XII. CN VII contributes to prehension by the partial innervation of the muscles opening the jaw while the mandibular branch of CN V provides motor function to the jaw. In parrots, their kinetic skull means that not only the lower jaw but also the upper jaw is required for opening the beak.

Reptile cranial nerves

In reptiles, the only moveable portions of the face are the eyelids. This makes the assessment of the muscles of facial expression limited. However, reptiles with eyelids can menace.

The anatomy of the visual system of reptiles is like that of mammals except that the nerve tracts in the optic chiasm project contralaterally and with only limited ipsilateral projection in turtles, snakes, and lizards as is needed for binocular vision. Snakes, in contrast, have a much less complex to even absent visual nerve tracts.

Olfactory nerves that travel to the cortex relaying chemical information from the nares exist, and the vomeronasal organ, in lizards and snakes, projects information to the cerebrum via the accessory olfactory tract.

Reptiles only hear low frequencies compared to mammals and only a few species use air conducted sound. Instead, most reptiles detect vibrations through the columella and other inner ear structures from which information is carried to the midbrain through CN VIII.

Other key cranial nerve differences include:

- CN II – The iris is composed of skeletal muscles therefore PLRs cannot be reliably evaluated in reptiles and their irises are not traditionally responsive to mydriatic agents
- CN III – In species that can move globes independently, evaluation of extraocular muscle movement occurs independently for each globe
- CN III, IV and VI supply the extraocular muscles
- CN IV supplies the nictitans
- CN V is sensory to infrared receptors with other sensory and motor functions retained as in mammals

- CN VIII – need low-frequency evaluation if BAER (brainstem auditory evoked response) testing is performed in some species given vibration-oriented hearing as opposed to air-conducted hearing
- CN XI – absent in some snakes and lizards

MODIFICATIONS FOR THE SMALL MAMMAL NEUROLOGIC EXAMINATION

The key components of the neurologic examination in small mammals are like that in dogs and domestic cats, recognizing that, as prey animals, some subtle features may be more challenging to assess. Additionally, sedatives or tranquilizers should be avoided prior to neurologic assessment in order to avoid confounding interpretation of examination findings.

In nervous prey animals, such as the rabbit, the order of examination may need to be modified to minimize stress and reduce handling/manipulation required; starting with those portions that are unlikely to induce pain and ending with those that require close handling or are more likely to cause discomfort or pain.

Modifications to the neurologic examination for these small mammals include:

1. General observation or mental status and gait – noting specifically head posture due to their predisposition towards vestibular conditions
2. Palpation of bones, joints, and muscles (noting tone and strength)
3. Postural reactions
4. Spinal reflex evaluation
5. Cranial nerve evaluation
6. Testing nociception (indicated only when there is absence of voluntary motor)

MODIFICATIONS FOR THE AVIAN NEUROLOGIC EXAMINATION

The avian nervous system is divided into the central (brain and spinal cord) and peripheral nervous system. The avian brain, however, is lissencephalic (lacking gyri and sulci) and fills the skull completely. In some species, such as cockatiels and budgerigars, the skull thinness lends to more fragile structures which may allow for easier damage to the brain. The avian brain also has an underdeveloped cerebral cortex, but a large corpora striata (the main centers for sensory motor correlation), large optic lobes (responsible for the well-developed optic and sensory systems), midbrain (with an oculomotor center that is involved in locomotion and flight), and a large cerebellum that lacks the lateral lobes found in mammalian brains.

The avian spinal cord runs the entire length of the spinal canal and there is no cauda equina present in birds. Like mammals, the cervical and lumbosacral areas are enlarged and given rise to the regions that form the brachial and lumbosacral plexus. Spinal nerves exit from the intervertebral foramen laterally at each vertebral segment with the number of spinal nerves varying with the vertebral formula of each species.

The components of the neurologic examination vary with birds in the following ways:

1. Mentation – assess from a distance at first and then ascertain patient is appropriately attuned to hospital environment
2. Cranial nerves
3. Flight – may need to occur at the end of the examination, as recapture after the test can be traumatic/stressful
4. Gait/Posture
   a. Torticollis – CN XI (cervical muscle contractions)
   b. Perching ability – be sure to have appropriately shaped, sized, and textured perches for the species being evaluated

5. Reflexes
   a. Wing withdrawals evaluate cervicothoracic segments
   b. Leg withdrawals evaluate thoracolumbar segments
   c. Vent Sphincter Reflex – touch mucosa with a fine object and observe closure; coordinated by the lumbosacral segments (pudendal plexus and caudal segments of the spinal cord)
   d. Pedal Flexor Reflex – apply a pinch stimulus to the skin of each foot and evaluate the response of the ipsilateral and contralateral limb
      i. Withdrawal requires an intact ischiatic nerve and intact spinal segment at the sacral plexus (can be altered by space occupying lesions affecting the kidney or pelvic canal)
   e. Patellar reflexes: some birds do not have a patella, but do still have a patellar ligament, or similar structure
6. Postural Reactions
   a. Resting wing posture
   b. Wing fanning

Some practitioners may simplify this approach and instead group changes on a neurologic examination according to head signs, wing signs, leg signs, and vent signs. With this approach, cervical spinal cord lesions are suspected when wing, leg and vent signs are observed. Thoracolumbar lesions suspected when leg and vent signs are seen, and lumbosacral lesions are suspected when only vents signs are documented.

MODIFICATIONS FOR THE REPTILE NEUROLOGIC EXAMINATION

The reptilian brain has no cortical gyri or sulci in the cerebral hemispheres and there is no neocortex. As a result, the reptilian nervous system functions more from spinal reflexes than cerebral stimulation; meaning that there are more autonomous reflexes to evaluate.

The spinal cord in reptiles extends the whole length of the vertebral column to the tail as there is no cauda equina. As with the canine and feline intumescences, there are brachial or sacral enlargements of the spinal cord in turtles, lizards, and crocodiles that correspond to appendicular sensorimotor processing. The locomotor centers reside within the spinal cord making the prognosis for recovery from spinal cord injury better than in other species.

As a result of their varying anatomy, the key differences in the neurologic examination of reptiles include:

- Much of the reptilian neurologic examination can be performed via observation and with minimal physical manipulation
- The observing clinician should know the normal behavior for a species to avoid the misinterpretation of potentially normal findings. For example, a vasovagal maneuver (ocular pressure application) causing stupor, or a tonic immobility occurs in some species when turned over and stroked – as is the case in some lizards and crocodiles.
- Evaluation of the righting reflex in snakes can help to delineate lesion localization as they will be able to right themselves cranial to a lesion but not caudal

Therefore, the overall neurologic assessment in reptiles is according to the following:

1. Mentation
2. Gait/Posture: Should be assessed by providing the appropriate surfaces (branch, water, floor)

3. Tone/Reflexes:
   a. The myotatic reflexes (eg, patellar reflex) are unreliable in reptiles
   b. Temperature differences may alter withdrawal reflexes as nerve conduction velocity is temperature dependent
   c. The cloacal reflex involves the contraction of the cloaca, ventral tail movement, and clasping of the pelvic limb in turtles after touching the cloaca.
   d. There is a “scratch reflex” noted in many reptiles where the spinal cord locally produces complex movements through what are called central pattern generators. This is not a voluntary action.
   e. The panniculus reflex can be assessed in reptiles by pricking the skin and observing for a skin twitch.
   f. Normally, snakes can maintain their body position, climb vertically, and possess a normal continuous smooth movement in all of the body
   g. Snake muscle tone may be evaluated by the gripping of the skin
   h. Turtles should be able to retract their head/limbs and keep the limb positioned correctly when standing/moving
   i. In chelonians the ability to withdraw limbs into their shell allows for the evaluation of tone and muscle strength
   j. Aquatic reptiles might swim in one direction only with CNS diseases, but other differentials for that movement pattern are more common such as pneumonia, the presence of coelomic air, and gastroenteritis.
4. Cranial nerves – as mentioned earlier, extensive evaluation is not possible in reptile patients
5. Posture and Postural Reactions:
   a. Reptiles should be able to raise and lower their head with no uncontrolled head bobbing.
   b. Boas can demonstrate a stargazing behavior as a sign of CNS disease
   c. Active postural tests such as hopping, “wheelbarrowing,” and placing have very limited utility in reptiles
   d. The righting reflex is useful in many species as the drive to regain a normal dorsal-ventral orientation is preserved. Lizards and chelonians will use their neck and limbs to help with the rollover. Snakes will roll their heads first and then the rest of body. Any delay in the roll is likely a sign of some neurologic impairment. In snakes they will be able to right cranial to the lesion but not caudal.
6. Pain and Tone

HEAD TRAUMA AND COMA SCALES

Traumatic injuries via vehicular trauma, fall injuries, bite wounds, or crush/compressive injuries are frequently encountered in veterinary medicine, and within that category, head trauma and traumatic brain injuries are common. As primary and secondary brain injuries compound to affect prognosis, coma scales have been adapted from human medicine to serially track patient factors, guide prognosis and predict the probability of survival to discharge.

Coma Scales

The modified Glasgow Coma Scale (MGCS) is used as a tool in small animal companion medicine to prognosticate outcomes initially and serially in dogs and cats with traumatic brain injuries.[1–3] The MGCS has three categories for evaluation: motor activity, brainstem reflexes, and level of consciousness; with each category having a score between 1 and 6. This may yield a total score up to 18 for a single patient at any point in time, with lower scores indicating more severe and significant neurologic deficits (**Fig. 2**). In dogs, significant association between admission MGCS and survival to the 48-h mark has been documented; with dogs receiving a score less than or equal to 8 at admission having only a 50% probability of survival.[1] Moreover, MGCS is a useful way of serially tracking patient status for prognostication, but the literature suggests that individual measures should not be used to determine patient prognosis in the absence of other information.[3] Recognizing that some exotic animal behavior may be altered by physical examination and hospitalization, the same measures may be applied to help predict their prognosis.

The FOUR score (Full Outline of UnResponsiveness Score) is used in human medicine to evaluate eye responses, motor responses, brainstem reflexes, and respiration patterns in comatose or stuporous patients. This scale is more useful in humans with metabolic derangements, sepsis, and shock, or with other nonstructural brain injuries as it is designed to identify changes in consciousness earlier than other scales.[4] This scale, however, requires response to verbal instruction from the patient and is not readily applicable to veterinary patients. One study, however, combined this scale with the MGCS scale and another coma recovery scale used in human medicine to

Modified Glasgow Coma Scale (MGCS)		
Motor Activity	Normal gait, normal reflexes	6
	Hemiparesis, tetraparesis, decerebrate rigidity	5
	Recumbent, intermittent extensor rigidity	4
	Recumbent, constant extensor rigidity	3
	Recumbent, constant extensor rigidity with opisthotonus	2
	Recumbent, hypotonia, depressed or absent spinal reflexes	1
Brainstem Reflexes	Normal PLR and oculocephalic reflexes	6
	Slow PLR and normal to reduced oculocephalic reflexes	5
	Bilateral unresponsive miosis, normal/reduced oculocephalic reflexes	4
	Pinpoint pupils with reduced to best oculocephalic reflexes	3
	Unilateral, unresponsive mydriasis, reduced/absent oculocephalic reflexes	2
	Bilateral, unresponsive mydriasis, reduced/absent oculocephalic reflexes	1
Level of Consciousness	Occasional periods of alertness and responsive to environment	6
	Depression or delirium, capable of responding but may be inappropriate	5
	Semicomatose, responsive to visual stimuli	4
	Semicomatose, responsive to auditory stimuli	3
	Semicomatose, responsive only to repeated noxious stimuli	2
	Comatose, unresponsive to repeated noxious stimuli	1

	Total sum of individual scores from motor activity, brainstem reflexes, and level of consciousness	**Prognosis**
MGCS Score	3-8	Grave
	9-14	Guarded
	15-18	Good

Fig. 2. Modified Glasgow Coma scale. Categories of assessment include motor activity, brainstem reflexes, and level of consciousness. Serial tracking recommended to prognosticate on patients with intracranial conditions.

characterize behavior in rats during coma induction and recovery – the Tübingen-Boston Rat Coma Scale.[5] This scale assessed eye blink, motor function (reflexive and purposeful), brainstem reflexes (including pupillary, corneal and pinna reflexes), respiration patterns, righting reflex, auditory responses, and whisker movement to track recovery from traumatic injury.

Point of Care Testing and Prognoses in Head Trauma

Amongst point of care testing, hyperglycemia in head trauma patients has been associated with decreased survival in dogs but not cats due to the propensity for cats to become hyperglycemic in times of stress.[3] Similar information is not readily available for exotic species; however, one study in rats indicated that hyperglycemia will worsen outcomes in models of ischemic brain injury.[6] A rabbit model of traumatic brain injury found that insulin use to maintain normoglycemia prevented the weight loss, lactic acidosis, and monocyte dysfunction that occurred in hyperglycemic animals with induced brain injuries – suggesting again that hyperglycemia carries a negative prognosis for patients of many species affected by ischemic brain injury.[7]

Considerations for Wildlife

In many wildlife cases, due to the limited ability for hands on examination, a specific neurologic localization is difficult to ascertain and may be only of academic value. This is in part due to species-related behaviors that can conceal normal responses or make altered mental and physical states hard to evaluate in times of stress. In most cases, this may not have a significant impact on treatment choices. Documenting changes in neurologic abnormalities over time, however, may be of more value where marked deterioration, or failure to improve, as noted over several days may carry a poor prognosis for recovery and eventual release.

Specific to wildlife release potential, ocular evaluation, and auricular examination in cases of head trauma is important. Altered cranial nerve function in association with a traumatic brain injury may limit the normal protective mechanisms of the eye and increase the risks of ocular pathology that may make an animal (such as a raptor) unable to be released.[8] Examination of the external ear canals for hemorrhage can increase the suspicion of a traumatic brain injury. In nocturnal hunting species this may be a better prognostic indictor with regards to potential release.[8] As hearing is difficult to assess in birds, ancillary testing such as brainstem auditory evoked response testing (BAER testing) may be beneficial.

COMMONLY ENCOUNTERED NEUROLOGIC DISEASES

Although correlates between neurologic disease can be made with dog and domestic cat conditions, some exotic species may be more predisposed to certain conditions based upon dietary needs, endemic infections, and cohabitation/husbandry practices. To that end, given the difficulties in assessing all components of the nervous system in several species, prior to directed diagnostics for specific conditions, a systemic workup including a complete blood count and chemistry profile is essential to ensure metabolic conditions are not confounding the interpretation of a neurologic assessment.

Small Mammals (Rabbits, Guinea Pigs, Ferrets)

Hypoglycemia

Seizures in ferrets are most caused by hypoglycemia secondary to an insulinoma – especially in middle-aged or older ferrets. Aside from stabilizing the blood glucose and targeted treatment toward the insulinoma, seizures may be managed with diazepam or midazolam (IV, IM, IN or per rectum) with doses between 0.25 and 1 mg/kg.[9] Longer term anticonvulsants have also been used in ferret to include phenobarbital (3 mg/kg BID), and Levetiracetam (20–60 mg/kg PO TID).[9] There are however, no pharmacokinetic studies on the use of phenobarbital, gabapentin, zonisamide, or levetiracetam in ferrets.

***Encephalitozoon cuniculi* infection in rabbits**

With its worldwide distribution, *Encephalitozoon cuniculi* is a microsporidian pathogen that can infect various mammals. It has a direct lifecycle with both horizontal and vertical (transplacental) transmission. In rabbits, postnatal transmission usually occurs within 6 weeks from the infected dam or from having had contact with other infected animals.[10] The infective spores may either be ingested or inhaled, with oral ingestion from infected rabbit urine being the most common source; infective spores can be found in the urine 1 month after infection and can be excreted up to 2 months after infection with intermittent shedding possible thereafter.[11,12]

Infection seems to be widespread, being found in 50% to 75% of rabbit colonies.[13] As the infected host animal becomes less immune competent with age, *E cuniculi* is associated with clinical disease and central neurologic signs are the most common manifestation. Other clinical signs associated with *E cuniculi* infection may include renal insufficiency (chronic interstitial nephritis), ocular disorders (phacoclastic uveitis with cataract development and intraocular masses); this is due to the target organs for infection being those with high blood flow[14–16] The neurologic signs typically have sudden onset and may be associated with stressful events including changes in the environment. The vast majority, however, do not exhibit other clinical signs concurrent with neurologic infection.

Central disease should be accompanied by mentation change, multiple cranial nerve deficits, and postural reactions deficits, but at times signs may mimic peripheral disorders. Due to the anxious/nervous nature of the affected species, it can be challenging to differentiate peripheral from central vestibular disease – making differentiation between otitis interna and encephalitozoonosis complicated. According to one study, evaluation of the presence and degree of a head tilt may serve as a prognostic indicator, such that animals demonstrating frequent rolling and lateral recumbency carrying a poorer prognosis.[15]

The diagnostic work up for encephalitozoonosis includes IgG and IgM antibody testing. However, due to the large number of asymptomatic seropositive rabbits, the presence of antibodies may only confirm pathogen exposure but does not necessarily confirm *E cuniculi* as cause of the clinical signs.[14,15] Measures of IgM appear to be helpful for the determination of early stages of infection as they have been shown to decline to zero by day 35 after infection; but IgM alone is not a definitive diagnostic tool due to the likelihood of latent infections.[17]

Otitis interna

Apart from encephalitozoonosis, otitis interna is the other major differential for vestibular dysfunction in small mammals. In some cases, signs of an upper respiratory infection and facial nerve lesions may be helpful in determining the presence of otitis. If possible, pursuing a CT scan on patients can provide invaluable information on whether otitis media/interna is present.

Disseminated idiopathic myofasciitis in ferrets

This condition, also known as myofasciitis or polymyositis, continues to have no known cause and affects young ferrets (ages 5–24 months).[18] It presents with diverse and nonspecific signs including lethargy, decreased appetite, lymphadenopathy, green diarrhea, oculonasal discharge, coughing, and seizures.[18,19] It is often painful and associated with a persistently elevated temperature.[18]

Intervertebral disc disease in ferrets

There are several reports of intervertebral disc disease affecting ferrets with the most affected site being L2-3.[20–22] Predisposing factors such as vertebral abnormalities (wedge/hemivertebrae) are reported, and affected ferrets have been between 7 months and 6 years of age.[22] The diagnosis can be obtained via CT evaluation (with myelography) or via MRI.

Myasthenia Gravis in Ferrets

This condition, caused by a defect in the neuromuscular junction secondary to immune-mediated disease or to a congenital defect in the acetylcholine receptor, causes diffuse lower motor neuron weakness in ferrets. It has been reported in three ferrets whose diagnosis was made via electrodiagnostic testing exhibiting a decremental response of the compound muscle action potential with repetitive nerve stimulation, in addition to elevated anti-acetylcholine receptor antibodies.[23–25] Like in other species, this condition is treated with pyridostigmine bromide.

Avian Neurologic Disease

Many birds present as emergency cases when affected with clinical signs that may be attributable to neurologic disease. Some conditions may be associated with a good prognosis, but others carry an infectious potential with guarded or terminal prognoses. As a result, early intervention, appropriate neurologic localization, and subsequent diagnosis are key. This, however, is made more difficult by the likelihood that birds tend to present late during their condition and are therefore at higher risks of rapidly deteriorating. As there are varying causes for neurologic signs – related to husbandry, nutrition, and infectious possibilities - appropriate history taking and examination is key.

Hypocalcemia

Birds consuming a seed diet and those with the lack of exposure to natural or artificial UV light leads to a Vitamin D deficiency and a reduced dietary absorption of available calcium. Rarely renal conditions can result in similar processes.[26]

The neurologic signs manifested in the face of hypocalcemia include ataxia, tremors, and seizures. Bone deformities, delaying clotting times, and dystocia may also result. Treatment involves controlling neurologic signs and stabilizing calcium levels via the administration of oral or injectable calcium salts. Additional sedatives or anticonvulsants may be required.

Hypoglycemia

Hypoglycemia may be associated with septicemia, chronic stress, dietary insufficiency, or exertion in an underweight bird. Affected patients may present weak, collapsed of having signs of incoordination or seizure activity. A full systemic work up to identify causes for the hypoglycemia – closely investigating endocrine dysfunction and hepatic disease – is important to target therapy beyond just glucose supplementation.

Hyperglycemia

Stress-induced hyperglycemia leading to seizures has been reported in goshawks but not in other birds.[27]

Vitamin E deficiency (nutritional encephalomalacia)

The recommended dietary level of vitamin E in domestic poultry is 10 to 25 IU/kg feed dry matter.[28] In deficient birds (often between 2 and 6 weeks of age), clinical signs include ataxia and head retraction. Ischemic necrosis of the cerebellar cortex and white matter occurs as a result of deficiency.

Thiamine (B1) deficiency

Clinical signs of thiamine deficiency include ataxia, ascending paralysis, and opisthotonos.[29] Affected birds generally respond to oral or parenteral administration of vitamin B1.

Riboflavin (B2) deficiency

Birds with this deficiency have weakness, limb atrophy, and a plantigrade posture with the toes curled inward although sudden death may also occur because of a demyelinating peripheral neuritis.[29,30] Since riboflavin has been added to commercial poultry feed, it rarely occurs.

Botulism (limberneck)

In birds, this infection usually is the result of the ingestion of botulinum type C, but occasionally types A and E are involved.[29] Although uncommon in companion birds, it is a frequent infection seen in waterfowl.[29,31,32] The pathognomonic sign of infection is a limber neck resulting from paralysis of the cervical muscles. Most birds, however, exhibit pelvic limb paresis initially which then progresses to affect the wings and neck.[29]

Avian paramyxovirus type 1 (newcastle disease)

Infection with this virus, often reported in young wild birds, pigeons, and domestic poultry, results in motor dysfunction and a nonsuppurative encephalomyelitis causing head shaking, tremors, head tilt, circling, and torticollis.[33,34]

West nile virus

This mosquito-borne flavivirus causes a diffuse encephalitis. Live and inactivated vaccines against this virus have been evaluated in young domestic geese with positive effects.[35]

Psittacosis (chlamydophila psittaci)

This obligate intracellular bacterium is widespread in parrots and has a zoonotic potential. The inhaled or ingested organisms can affect the liver and respiratory systems to most commonly cause clinical signs such as lethargy, anorexia, diarrhea, opisthotonos, ataxia, seizures, and tremors. Diagnosis includes PCR performed on fecal matter or detection of serum antibodies.

Treatment requires supportive care, sedatives, and/or anticonvulsants as well as appropriate antibiotic therapy – with tetracyclines (most commonly doxycycline) being used for a 6-week course.[36]

Proventricular dilation syndrome (avian bornavirus)

This syndrome causes neuropathies and intestinal signs (namely weight loss, the presence of undigested food in feces, and delayed crop emptying). The progressive neuronal damage that occurs from infection disrupts neurotransmitter activity and affects the nerves associated with intestinal tract function. Additionally, the viral coat proteins resemble neurotransmitters and antibodies against these proteins can result in autoimmune destruction to worsen neurologic signs. The most noted changes occur in the proventriculus by way of a flaccid paralysis.[37]

Diagnosis is achieved via crop biopsy, which demonstrates a lymphoplasmacytic ganglioneuritis. Additionally, since the identification of the suspected causative agent (avian bornavirus) PCR and serology have allowed for targeted testing.

Treatment is limited to anti-inflammatory administration (celecoxib or meloxicam), but no treatment regimen resolves the condition and clinical proventricular dilation syndrome is usually fatal.

Gallid herpesvirus 1 (Marek's disease)

This highly contagious retroviral infection induces a lymphoproliferative disease in poultry with clinical disease characterized by leg weakness, lameness, dropped wings, opisthotonos, and paralysis. Young birds, often at the point of laying, are affected with the onset of lymphomas and paralysis occurring 4 to 12 weeks after infection.[38] Prevention is via the vaccination of eggs or chicks at 1 day of age prior to potential exposure.

Avian influenza virus

This infection causes 75% to 100% mortality within 10 days of infection with clinical signs including paresis, paralysis, vestibular dysfunction, and behavior changes.[39]

Heavy metal intoxication

A very common cause of neurologic signs in pet and wild birds is heavy metal toxicity; with lead being the most identified. Affected birds may present with central or peripheral neurologic signs including leg weakness, a plantigrade stance, abnormal posture, reduced flight, or cluster seizures.

Radiographs may identify metallic particles in the proventriculus, and bloodwork may show a mild leukocytosis, elevation in liver values, and a hypochromic anemia. A definitive diagnosis required the measurement of lead levels.

When possible, any identified metallic foreign bodies should be removed via proventricular flushing or endoscopic removal. Heavy metal chelation should also be initiated in cases with clinical signs, even if foreign material is successfully removed. Fluid therapy is also important to minimize renal injury.

Organophosphates, carbamates, and pesticides

Delayed neurotoxicity caused by these toxins, results in a neurologic condition characterized by progressive pelvic limb ataxia and paralysis.[40,41] There are over 80 different registered organophosphates and carbamates in the United States with birds being 10 to 20 times more susceptible to these acetylcholinesterase inhibitors than mammals.

Toxicity being classified into 2 types (Type I and Type II) depending on the time delay to the onset of signs. Type I toxicity has a longer delay period (10–21 days) to sign and affects the spinal cord and brainstem, whereas Type II toxicity has a shorter delay period (4–7 days) and can affect the midbrain and prosencephalon.[41]

Atherosclerosis

Clinical signs associated with atherosclerosis include cerebrovascular events, sudden onset blindness, ataxia, paresis, and seizures.[29]

Fibrocartilaginous embolism

Fibrocartilaginous embolic myelopathy and ischemic myelopathies have been described in turkeys with peracute onset of paresis and ataxia.[42] The articular cartilage of the vertebral body endplates is suggested to be the source of the emboli based on necropsies performed in affected birds.[42]

Intracranial neoplasia

In a retrospective evaluation of budgerigars 1% had intracranial tumors identified.[43]

Idiopathic epilepsy

Seizures without any other structural or metabolic cause have been characterized in chickens in which presumed epilepsy has a genetic basis.[44] Control of seizure activity in birds can be achieved with diazepam (0.1–1 mg/kg IV or IO). Long-term anti-convulsant medications such as phenobarbital (1–2 mg/kg IV or IO or IM q6-12 to effect) can be used with an ultimate maintenance dose of 1 to 10 mg/kg PO BID.[45]

Lysosomal storage diseases

Gangliosidoses are most caused by deficiencies with *B*-galactosidase (GM1 gangliosidosis) or *B*-hexosaminidases (GM2 gangliosidosis).[46] These enzymatic deficiencies lead to accumulations of GM1 or GM2 within neurons.

Avian vacuolar myelinopathy

In the southeastern US, wild birds (namely Bald Eagles and American Coots) have been diagnosed with AVM - caused by a cyanobacterial neurotoxin. On neurologic examination, most affected birds exhibit ataxia, decreased withdrawals reflexes, postural reaction deficits, and decreased vent responses. Other clinical signs may include beak and tongue weakness, head tremors, absent PLRs, anisocoria, blindness, and nystagmus.[47,48]

Reptilian Neurologic Disease

As with the other exotic species discussed, neurologic disorders in reptiles are often associated with husbandry, environmental, and nutritional causes. Some chelonians will circle, have a head tilt, and display behaviors consistent with blindness as they emerge from hibernation; this is believed to be secondary to brain microabscessation or fatty liver syndrome.[49]

Hypothiaminosis/Leukoencephalopathy

Freezing fish consumed by reptile species will increase thiaminase activity and deplete thiamine levels in the fish consumed. In reptiles consuming these fish, signs of deficiency may include muscle twitching, incoordination, blindness, seizure activity, torticollis, spiral locomotion, jaw gaping, dysphagia, and death. In chelonians enophthalmos may be noted.

Biotin Deficiency

When raw, non-fertile eggs are chronically ingested, signs of biotin deficiency including muscle tremors, generalized weakness.

Toxins

Reptiles are very sensitive to insecticides (organophosphates, carbamates, and nicotine). Ivermectin is toxic to chelonians with no known safe dosing rate. Metronidazole has a long pharmacokinetic half-life in reptiles and vestibular signs and death have been reported in snakes given high doses of the medication (100 mg/kg); therefore, the current recommendation is to avoid doses greater than 25 to 50 mg/kg, especially in snakes.[50]

Spinal Osteopathy

Proliferative osteoarthritis, or spinal osteopathy, is a condition documented to affect snakes following a suspected bacterial infection in the vertebrae that results in abnormal bone growth. .[51] Other similar conditions have no association with infection or trauma and are thought to be related to metabolic or nutritional causes.[52]

ANCILLARY DIAGNOSTICS

As the popularity of exotic species has increased, several studies have developed imaging protocols that correlate with the improved access to CT and MRI. This access has allowed for improving diagnostic accuracy, guiding prognoses, and developing targeted treatment protocols. Differences in anatomy means that modification to the traditional companion small animal techniques is required. Most notably, the protocols that are often utilized in dogs and cats result in a length of anesthesia for imaging that is prolonged for exotic species: putting them at risk for complications such as hypothermia, subclinical respiratory disorders, and death.[53]

Radiographs

As an inexpensive and noninvasive form of patient evaluation, radiographs completed under sedation or general anesthesia to facilitate positioning may help to identify the cause of neurologic disease. Survey radiographs in a stable patient may help to identify skull fractures, but the avian skull anatomy makes these radiographs difficult to interpret.

Computed Tomography

In small animal companion medicine, computed tomography imaging is the recommended trauma diagnostic for assessed traumatic brain injuries especially in that it requires less time, is less expensive and allows for better imaging of bone and acute hemorrhage.[8,54] Computed tomography has been used with some success to locate other intracranial lesions in birds as well, although it was only 80% sensitive.[55,56]

The difficulties in CT imaging, include the often-small size of the patient (especially in avian species) and the pneumatic structure of some bones make it difficult for imaging algorithms to differentiate between soft tissue and bone. In contrast, for other species such as the rabbit, the use of CT scanning has allowed for better characterization of middle ear disease as well as joint and spinal abnormalities.

Magnetic Resonance Imaging

Although the use of MRI has increased in small animal companion medicine, protocols for use are not widely established in exotic species. The small patient size is a technical limitation of most studies, and it can be difficult to establish a balance between imaging small lesions with appropriate image resolution for diagnostic purposes and extended anesthetic times which increase patient complication risks.[57]

MRI does not always allow for a satisfactory depiction of aerated bones in some avian skulls and motion artifacts in small reptiles make MRI imaging difficult to interpret.[58] Some protocols have, however, been developed to minimize anesthesia time to approximately 35 minutes under anesthesia with intubation which allows for intermittent positive pressure ventilation.[59] In some circumstances, as in reptiles, MRI may be more advantageous for intra-abdominal organ evaluation rather than CT.[60–62]

Cerebrospinal Fluid Analysis

As in small animal companion medicine, the analysis of CSF is of most use in infectious, inflammatory, and neoplastic disorders. Just as the neurologic examination principles are modified for species based on their neuroanatomy and behaviors, the same is true for options regarding the collection of spinal fluid samples.

The synsacrum of birds, composed of fused lumbar and sacral vertebrae and pelvis, means that lumbar puncture is near impossible. Instead, collection is via thoracolumbar sampling or through the foramen magnum between the cerebellum and dorsal surface of the medulla.[57] For this cerebellomedullary cistern sampling, the patient is placed in lateral recumbency and the caudodorsal skull region is aseptically prepared. The atlanto-occipital joint is flexed at a thirty-to-forty-degree angle, and a 27-gauge hypodermic needle is placed at dorsal midline. The needle is inserted slightly caudal to the occipital protuberance and is directed rostrally at a forty-five-degree angle to the horizontal axis of the head, advancing through the skin slowly at 1-mm intervals until a slight change in resistance is felt. Using a hypodermic needle with a translucent hub, rather than a spinal needle with a stylet, allows for a "flash" of fluid to be easily identified once the dura has been penetrated and limits the risk of advancing the needle into the parenchyma. In small mammals, 1 mL of CSF per 5 kg body weight may be removed safely, although this volume has not been confirmed in birds.

Electrodiagnostics

The use of electrodiagnostic techniques (EMG, electroencephalography, and nerve conduction studies) may aid in the diagnosis of neurologic dysfunction.

Electromyography (EMG study) evaluating the electrical activity of muscles via insertion of a recording electrode into the muscle helps to examine the integrity of the motor unit – which consists of the lower motor neuron and the innervated muscle fibers. Contraindications to performing this diagnostic include bleeding disorders and/or recurrent infections. Anesthesia is required for evaluation, but the assessment of prognosis for return to function has been suggested for use in wild birds.[63]

Nerve conduction studies are simple and reliable tests to evaluate peripheral nerve function. A technique has been well described in birds (rheas and owls) such that reference ranges for motor nerve conduction velocities of the ulnar and tibial nerves have been established for normal animals.[63] In cases of axonal damage or dysfunction, there will be a documented loss of measured amplitudes. In contrast, cases of demyelination will lead to prolonged conduction times. Temperature and age predictably affected measured values in companion animals and the same is presumed to be true for exotic species.

Electroencephalography (EEG) is the evaluation of electrical events in the cerebral cortex. In poultry normal EEG responses to stimuli have been documented, but due to variation between species, results of this testing can be difficult to interpret.[57]

Brainstem Auditory Evoked Response Testing

This form of testing is a qualitative test that determines if a patient can hear in one or both ears but doesn't characterize the degree of hearing nor differentiate the exact cause of hearing loss. Methods for testing have been developed in ferrets as young as 8 weeks of age[64] and owls.[65]

Muscle Biopsies

Biopsy techniques are well-established in several mammalian species but are not well-documented for avian patients. The muscle selected for biopsy should be one that is clinically affected with the disease process with commonly acquired muscles including the vastus lateralis, cranial tibial, triceps brachii, temporalis, and biceps femoris muscles.

NURSING CARE AND MONITORING OF HOSPITALIZED NEUROLOGIC PATIENTS

Once a neurolocalization and likely diagnosis has been determined, the development of a treatment and care plan tailored to the patient's neurologic status is key.

Standard monitoring and treatment plans for neurologic patients should include the following:

- Serial assessment of mentation and level of consciousness (hourly evaluation for the most affected patients is recommended)
- Minimize stress as stress may exacerbate neurologic signs - especially in patients with vestibular disease.
  - Use sedatives; taking care to avoid over sedation which may make serial assessment of mentation and level of consciousness challenging.
  - Where possible, bundle treatments (handling, monitoring, medication administration) to minimize patient stress
- Maintain appropriate temperature (some species reflex assessments are temperature dependent)
- Although most hospitalized prey species will benefit from a hiding space, it is very important to balance the patient's needs for privacy with the need to serially assess the patient
- For patients that are immobile or nonvisual associated with their neurologic status, develop a targeted nutritional plan (syringe or tube feeding, parenteral fluid therapy, weight checks, etc.)
- Continuity of care with the same nurse monitoring a hospitalized patient within and across shifts, will allow for subtle changes in a patient's status being detected sooner
- Animals that are paralyzed or recumbent are unable to move away from their urine or feces and this may predispose them to urine scald/fecal build up. Provision of clean bedding, grooming the patient as necessary, and the application of Vaseline to limbs may limit the development of skin irritation.
- Recumbency care (including rotating patient recumbency, provision of plenty of padded bedding, and limb range of motion exercises) will help with the prevention of joint contracture and pressure sores.

SUMMARY

With accurate neurologic localization, a focused list of differential diagnoses can be created. Performing the neurologic examination should be methodical and logical for all patients and the order of extent of examination may depend upon the patient's clinical condition and cooperation. Applications of objective scale measures (such as coma scales), and ancillary diagnostics (electrodiagnostics, advanced imaging, biopsy techniques, and BAER testing) complement physical assessment and clinicopathologic assessment in these neurologic patients. Correlates between canine and domestic feline examinations may be made with specific detail taken to adapting examination approaches and differential lists to each species.

CLINICS CARE POINTS

- When performing a neurologic examination, remember to evaluate mentation and behavior first as part of the hands-off assessment. In some cases, this assessment can only be accurately obtained in talking directly with owners or caretakers.

- For patients with intracranial lesions, serial mentation monitoring (using coma scales) will help determine prognosis for recovery.
- When creating differential diagnoses for neurologic conditions in exotic species, remember that they may be more predisposed to metabolic/nutritional conditions based on dietary needs, cohabitation, and husbandry practices.
- Remember to obtain a thorough nutritional and husbandry history for all exotic species
- Whenever possible, bundle treatments for neurologic patients to minimize stress associated with their care.

DISCLOSURE

The author has nothing to disclose.

REFERENCES

1. Platt SR, Radaelli ST, McDonnell JJ. The prognostic value of the modified Glasgow Coma Scale in head trauma in dogs. J Vet Intern Med 2001;15(6):581–4.
2. Sharma D, Holowaychuk MK. Retrospective evaluation of prognostic indicators in dogs with head trauma: 72 cases (January – March 2011): prognostics indicators in canine head trauma. J Vet Emerg Crit Care 2015;25(5):631–9.
3. Cameron S, Weltman J, Fletcher DJ. The prognostic value of admission point-of-care testing and modified Glasgow Coma Scale score in dogs and cats with traumatic brain injuries (2007-2010): 212 cases. J Vet Emerg Crit Care 2022;32: 75–82.
4. Iyer V, Mandrekar J, Danielson R, et al. Validity of the FOUR score coma scale in the medical intensive care unit. Mayo Clin Proc 2009;84(8):694–701.
5. Pais-Roldán P, Edlow B, Jiang Y, et al. Multimodal assessment of recovery from coma in a rat model of diffuse brainstem tegmentum injury. Neuroimage 2019; 189:615–30.
6. Hoffman WE, Braucher E, Pelligrino DA, et al. Brain lactate and neurologic outcome following incomplete ischemia in fasted, nonfasted, and glucose-loaded rats. Anesthesiology 1990;72:1045–50.
7. Furnary AP, Wu Y, Bookin SO. Effect of hyperglycemia and continuous intravenous insulin infusions on outcomes of cardiac surgical procedures: The Portland Diabetic Project. Endocr Pract 2004;10(S2):21–33.
8. Jolly Megan. Treatment of traumatic brain injury in Morepork owls: a review of diagnostic and treatment options. In: Association of Avian Veterinarians Australasian Committee Ltd. Annual Conference 2015;23:31–9.
9. Huynh M, Piazza S. Musculoskeletal and Neurologic Diseases. Ferrets, Rabbits, and Rodents 2021;117–30.
10. Hunt C. Radiographic interpretation of the vertebral column. In: Harcourt-Brown F, Chitty J, editors. BSAVA manual of rabbit surgery, dentistry and imaging. Gloucester (United Kingdom): BSAVA Publications; 2013. p. 76–83.
11. Künzel F, Fisher PG. Clinical Signs, Diagnosis, and Treatment of Encephalitozoon cuniculi Infection in Rabbits. The Veterinary Clinics of North America. Exotic Animal Practice 2018;21(1):69–82.
12. Franssen FF, Lumeij JT, van Knapen F. Susceptibility of Encephalitozoon cuniculi to several drugs in vitro. Antimicrob Agents Chemother 1995;39:1265–8.
13. Lyngset A. A survey of serum antibodies to Encephalitozoon cuniculi in breeding rabbits and their young. Lab Anim Sci 1980;30:558–61.

14. Harcourt-Brown FM, Holloway HK. Encephalitozoon cuniculi in pet rabbits. Vet Rec 2003;152(14):427–31.
15. Künzel F, Gruber A, Tichy A, et al. Clinical symptoms and diagnosis of encephalitozoonosis in pet rabbits. Vet Parasitol 2008;151:115–24.
16. Jass A, Matiasek K, Henke J, et al. Analysis of cerebrospinal fluid in healthy rabbits and rabbits with clinically suspected encephalitozoonosis. Vet Rec 2008;162: 618–22.
17. Jeklova E, Jekl V, Kovarcik K, et al. Usefulness of detection of specific IgM and IgG antibodies for diagnosis of clinical encephalitozoonosis in pet rabbits. Vet Parasitol 2010;170(1–2):143–8.
18. Garner MM, Ramsell K, Schoemaker NJ, et al. Myofasciitis in the domestic ferret. Vet Pathol 2007;44:25–38.
19. Garner MM, Ramsell K, Morera N, et al. Clinicopathologic features of a systemic coronavirus-associated disease resembling feline infectious peritonitis in the domestic ferret (Mustela putorius). Vet Pathol 2008;45:236–46.
20. Lu D, Lamb CR, Patterson-Kane JC, et al. Treatment of a prolapsed lumbar intervertebral disc in a ferret. J Small Anim Pract 2004;45:501–3.
21. Morera N, Valls X, Mascort J. Intervertebral disk prolapse in a ferret. Vet Clin North Am Exot Anim Pract 2006;9:667–71.
22. Srugo I, Chai O, Yaakov D, et al. Successful medical management of lumbar intervertebral disc prolapse in a ferret. J Small Anim Pract 2010;51:447–50.
23. Antinoff N. Diagnosis and successful treatment of myasthenia gravis in a ferret. San Antonio, TX: Proc Annu Conf Assoc Exot Mamm Vet; 2015.
24. Couturier J, Huynh M, Boussarie D, et al. Autoimmune myasthenia gravis in a ferret. J Am Vet Med Assoc 2009;235:1462–6.
25. Papageorgiou S, Gnirs K, Quinton JF, et al. Clinical and serologic remission of acquired myasthenia gravis in a domestic ferret (Mustela putorius furo). J Am Vet Med Assoc 2019;254(10):1192–5.
26. Stanford M. Clinical pathology of hypocalcaemia in adult grey parrots (Psittacus e erithacus). Vet Rec 2007;161(13):456–7.
27. Forbes NA. Differential diagnosis and treatment of fitting in raptors, with particular attention to the previously unreported condition of stress induced hyperglycemia in northern goshawks (*Accipiter gentilis*). Isr J Vet Med 1996;51(3–4):183–8.
28. Aye PP, Morishita TY, Grimes S, et al. Encephalomalacia associated with vitamin E deficiency in commercially raised emus. Avian Dis 1998;42(3):600–5.
29. Bennet RA, Neurology. In: Ritchie BW, Harrison GJ, Harrison LR, editors. Avian medicine: principles and application. Lake Worth, FL: Wingers Publishing; 1994. p. 728–47.
30. Wada Y, Kondo H, Itakura C. Peripheral neuropathy of dietary riboflavin deficiency in racing pigeons. J Vet Med Sci 1996;58(2):161–3.
31. Goulden S. Botulism in water birds. Vet Rec 1995;137(13):328.
32. Kurtdede A, Sancak AA. Botulism in a long-legged buzzard (Buteo rutinus). Vet Rec 2002;151(2):64.
33. Bailey TA, Nicholls PK, Wernery U, et al. Avian paramyxovirus type 1 infection in houbara bustards (Chlamydotis undulata macqueenii): clinical and pathologic findings. J Zoo Wildl Med 1997;28(3):325–30.
34. Kuiken T, Wobeser G, Leighton FA, et al. Pathology of Newcastle disease in double-crested cormorants from Saskatchewan, with comparison of diagnostic methods. J Wildl Dis 1999;35(1):8–23.
35. Malkinson M, Banet C, Khinich Y, et al. Use of live and inactivated vaccines in the control of West Nile fever in domestic geese. Ann N Y Acad Sci 2001;951:255–61.

36. Guzman DS, Diaz-Figueroa O, Tully T Jr, et al. Evaluating 21-day doxycycline and azithromycin treatments for experimental Chlamydophila psittaci infection in cockatiels (Nymphicus hollandicus). J Avian Med Surg 2010;24(1):35–45.
37. Dennison SE, Paul-Murphy JR, Adams WM. Radiographic determination of proventricular diameter in psittacine birds. J Am Vet Med Assoc 2008;232(5):709–14.
38. Gimeno IM, Witter RL, Reed WM. Four distinct neurologic syndromes in Marek's disease: effect of viral strain and pathotype. Avian Dis 1999;43(4):721–37.
39. Perkins LEL, Swayne DE. Pathobiology of A/Chicken/Hong Kong/220/97 (H5N1) avian influenza virus in seven Gallinaceous species. Vet Pathol 2001;38:149–64.
40. Pennycott TW. Diazinon poisoning in pigeons. Vet Rec 1996;138(4):96.
41. Varghese RG, Bursian SJ, Tobias C, et al. Organophosphorus-induced delayed neurotoxicity: a comparative study of the effects of tri-ortho-tolyl phosphate and triphenyl phosphite on the central nervous system of the Japanese quail. Neurotoxicology 1995;16(1):45–54.
42. Stedman NL, Brown TP, Rowland GN. Intravascular cartilaginous emboli in the spinal cord of turkeys. Avian Dis 1998;42(2):423–8.
43. Suchy A, Weissenböck H, Schmidt P. Intracranial tumours in budgerigars. Avian Pathol 1999;28(2):125–30.
44. Rosenthal K. Disorders of the avian nervous system. In: *Avian medicine and surgery*. Philadelphia: WB Saunders Co; 1996. p. 461–74.
45. Clippinger TL, Platt SR. Seizures. In: Olsen GH, Orosz SE, editors. Manual of avian medicine. St. Louis, MO: Mosby Inc; 2000. p. 170–82.
46. Bermudez AJ, Johnson GC, Vanier MT, et al. Gangliosidosis in emus (Dromaius novaehollandiae). Avian Dis 1995;39(2):292–303.
47. Larsen RS, Nutter FB, Augspurger T, et al. Clinical features of avian vacuolar myelinopathy in American coots. J Am Vet Med Assoc 2002;221(1):80–5.
48. Thomas NJ, Meteyer CU, Sileo L. Epizootic vacuolar myelinopathy of the central nervous system of bald eagles (Haliaeetus leucocephalus) and American coots (Fulica americana). Vet Pathol 1998;35(6):479–87.
49. Ferrell, Shannon Thomas. In Proceedings NAVC Conference 2013 Exotics Small Animal. Help, My Reptile Can't Get up! Neurology for the Reptile Clinician. January 21, 2013. Orlando, Florida.
50. Gibbons PM. Advances in reptile clinical therapeutics – topics in medicine and surgery. J Exot Pet Med 2014;23:21–8.
51. Isaza R, Garner M, Jacobson E. Proliferative osteoarthritis and osteoarthrosis in 15 snakes. J Zoo Wildl Med 2000;31(1):20–7.
52. Altan E, Kubiski SV, Burchell J, et al. The first reptilian circovirus identified infects gut and liver tissues of black-headed pythons. Vet Rec 2019;50:35.
53. Głodek J, Adamiak Z, Przeworski A. Magnetic Resonance Imaging of Reptiles, Rodents, and Lagomorphs for Clinical Diagnosis and Animal Research. Comp Med 2016;66(3):216–9.
54. Sande A, West C. Traumatic brain injury: a review of pathophysiology and management. J Vet Emerg Crit Care 2010;20(2):177–90.
55. Rosenthal K, Stefanacci J, Quesenberry K, et al. Computerized tomography in 10 cases of avian intracranial disease. Proc Assoc Avian Vet 1995;16:305.
56. Jenkins JR. Use of computed tomography (CT) in pet bird practice. Proc Assoc Avian Vet 1991;276–9.
57. Clippinger TL, Bennett RA, Platt SR. The avian neurologic examination and ancillary neurodiagnostic techniques: A review update. Vet Clin Exot Anim Pract 2007;803–36.

58. Bartels T, Krautwald-Junghanns ME, Portmann S, et al. The use of conventional radiography and computer-assisted tomography as instruments for demonstration of gross pathological lesions in the cranium and cerebrum in the crested breed of the domestic duck (Anas platyrhynchos f.dom.). Avian Pathol 2000; 29(2):101–8.
59. Foss KD, Keller KA, Kehoe SP, et al. Establishing an MRI-Based Protocol and Atlas of the Bearded Dragon (*Pogona vitticeps*) Brain. Front Vet Sci 2022;9: 886333.
60. Pees M. Modern Imaging Techniques in Reptiles (CT/MRI). In: NAVC Conference proceedings, Exotcics small animal. January 21, 2013. Orlando, Florida.
61. Straub J, Jurina C. Magnetic resonance imaging in chelonians. Sem Avian Exot Pet Med 2001;10:181–6.
62. Holland M, Jennings D. Use of electromyography in seven injured wild birds. J Am Vet Med Assoc 1997;211(5):607–9.
63. Clippinger TL, Platt SR, Bennett RA, et al. Electro- diagnostic evaluation of peripheral nerve function in rheas and barred owls. Amer J Vet Res 2000;61(4): 469–72.
64. Piazza S, Huynh M, Cauzinille L. Brainstem auditory-evoked response (BAER) in client-owned pet ferrets with normal hearing. Vet Rec 2014;174(23):581.
65. Brittan-Powell EF. Auditory brainstem responses in the Eastern Screech Owl: An estimate of auditory thresholds. J Acoust Soc Am 2005;118(1):314–21.

Point of Care Ultrasound in Exotic Animal Emergency and Critical Care

Sara Gardhouse, DVM, DABVP (ECM), DACZM

KEYWORDS

• Exotic animal • Non-invasive • Point of care ultrasound • POCUS

KEY POINTS

- POCUS examination of exotic companion animals can aid in the diagnosis of a variety of conditions both unique to reptiles, birds, and small mammals as well as those seen in both exotic pets and domestic small animal patients.
- Many exotic companion animals are prey species, and the use of a rapid, noninvasive, and highly informative diagnostic can provide invaluable, critical information for the patient.
- POCUS can aid in the diagnosis of free fluid in the abdomen, pleural effusion, and pericardial effusion, and can also aid in ultrasound-guided abdominocentesis, thoracocentesis, and pericardiocentesis. POCUS can also aid in ultrasound-guided cystocentesis.
- POCUS also has utility in identification of obvious cardiac chamber enlargement, subjectively assessing cardiac contractility, estimating intravascular volume status, and tracking GI motility and urine production.

INTRODUCTION

The use of point of care ultrasound in the emergency setting can provide rapid, important, non-invasive, bedside clinical information. POCUS in the emergency room can have a multitude of uses including identification of a diagnosis in an unstable patient, identification of the presence or absence of free fluid in the pleural, pericardial, peritoneal, or coelomic space, as well as allowing for assessment of the thorax and abdomen to help understand why a patient may be declining.[1,2]

Exotic animal patients frequently present with acute on chronic illnesses due to their excellent ability to mask signs of illness; this makes the rapid POCUS assessment obtained at triage invaluable for initial stabilization, but also for continued progress tracking throughout hospitalization. The recent advances in ultrasound technology have provided improved image quality with smaller sized probes, making the use of these instruments more practical in smaller patients.[3]

Evolution Veterinary Specialists, 34 Van Gordon Street, Ste. 160, Lakewood, CO 80228, USA
E-mail address: saramgardhouse@gmail.com

Vet Clin Exot Anim 26 (2023) 567–589
https://doi.org/10.1016/j.cvex.2023.05.002 vetexotic.theclinics.com

The indications and principles in exotic animals are similar to domestic small animal patients, although some unique conditions and abnormalities exist, which will be described in this article.

THE USE OF POCUS IN THE EXOTIC ANIMAL EMERGENCY SETTING

Use of POCUS in Reptilian Patients

Unique reptile anatomy

To successfully perform POCUS assessment in reptiles, a strong understanding of their normal anatomy is required.[1] There is a large amount of anatomic heterogeneity amongst the reptile groups, which can make extrapolation from one species to the next challenging.[4]

In general, reptiles typically have simple organ structures. The liver has two lobes, and in snakes, the gall bladder is caudal to the elongated liver.[4] The heart of most reptiles has three chambers (the crocodilian heart is an exception with four chambers).[4] Most lizard and chelonian hearts are located cranially at the level of the pectoral girdle, with the exception of the varanids where the heart is positioned more caudally.[5] The unique heart location in many lizards as well as the shell in chelonians can make echocardiography difficult. In snakes, the heart is typically located one-third to one-fourth of the body's length, caudal to the head, which is usually more easily accessed for imaging.[5]

Moving caudal to the heart, most reptiles will have a combined thoracoabdominal cavity, which is commonly referred to as the coelom, and so a diaphragm will not be encountered.[4] In some reptile species, the coelom is divided by the presence of septa.[6] Tegus have a post-hepatic septum that is located in the middle of the coelom, while monitor lizards and chelonians have a post-pulmonary septum that divides the pleural cavities from the remainder of the coelom.[6] Crocodilians are similar in their septa and subdivisions to avian species (described below).[7] Knowledge of the presence of these septa has clinical relevance when determining the presence or absence of free fluid and the location of the fluid in the different coelomic spaces.

Assessment of the rest of the coelom can be difficult in some reptile species, including chameleons, skinks, and snakes, as these species have air sacs within the coelom (similar to birds), which can present challenges during POCUS.[4] In many lizard species, the kidneys are located in a caudal, retroperitoneal location, being positioned between the base of the tail and just ventral to the cranial acetabular area.[4] The urinary bladder is only present in some species of reptiles, including chelonians (turtles and tortoises), and many lizards.[4] Snakes and crocodilians do not possess a urinary bladder.[4] Most reptile species are egg-bearing (oviparous), so the ovary, follicles, oviduct, and developing eggs can be imaged with POCUS, but some reptiles produce live young including boas, viperids, and some chameleon and skink species.[4] Most reptile species have two large fat pads in the caudoventral coelom adjacent to the kidney and gonads, with absence of other foci of intracoelomic fat.[4]

Reptile positioning

Prior to any handling or diagnostics, the stability of the reptile patient should be assessed. If assessed to be stable, most reptile patients can be initially imaged under manual restraint. Chemical restraint can be utilized further in a diagnostic work up, when a more detailed assessment is necessary, in specific situations, such as an aggressive patient, or for performance of ultrasound-guided procedures (**Fig. 1**).[1,8] If the reptilian patient is noted to be in respiratory distress, pain, or any other condition compromising stability, stabilization and sedation prior to imaging may be

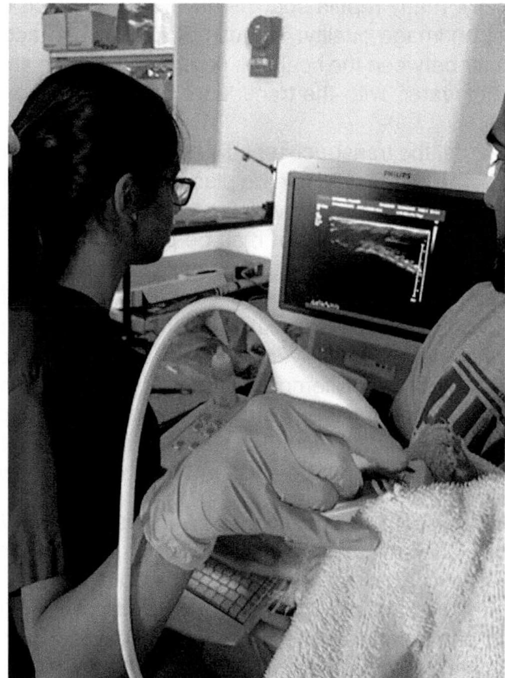

Fig. 1. Coelomic ultrasound of a bearded dragon (*Pogona vitticeps*). This patient was stable and the ultrasound was performed awake with manual restraint. (From: Dr. Trinita Barboza, DVM, DVSc.)

indicated. Most lizards, snakes, and chelonians can be appropriately imaged in dorsal recumbency.[8]

Ultrasound probe selection

There is a wide variety in size and shape of reptile patients, with many anatomic variations and considerations, and therefore, it is not possible to recommend a single transducer for their ultrasound evaluations.[3] In general, for smaller snakes and lizards, a linear transducer is recommended; for chelonians, a sector or phased array transducer or curvilinear (microconvex) transducer that has a small footprint is used.[3] The small footprint is essential in chelonian patients due to the small acoustic windows that exist between the shell and the limbs (cranial and caudal to the thoracic limbs, and cranial to the pelvic limbs (prefemoral fossa).[3] The frequency of the transducer selected depends on the size of the patient with higher frequency transducers providing excellent spatial resolution and detail, but being unable to penetrate to deep depths.[3] As a result, higher frequency transducers are typically recommended for smaller patients.[3]

Imaging the normal reptile coelom

The success of a POCUS exam in reptiles, in part, will depend on the accessible acoustic windows, especially in chelonian patients. Regardless of the species being examined, it is very important to approach the POCUS exam systematically to ensure that all anatomy is evaluated and, thus, all abnormalities are detected. It is also very important to consider that there is a vast amount of sonographic variation amongst reptile species, which can result in the misinterpretation of normal structures as abnormal. Additionally, many reptile species have scales, which trap air, which can have a large impact on image quality. The use of alcohol and acoustic coupling gel to fully displace the air between the scales is recommended. As an alternative, placement of the patient in water, with the transducer protected will also help to provide good quality images.[1]

For snakes and lizards, the transducer should be placed in a longitudinal orientation. In chelonian patients, the transducer can be placed cranial and caudal to the thoracic limbs and cranial to the pelvic limbs, providing a total of three accessible acoustic windows.[3] If the chelonian is soft-shelled, it may be possible to scan through the plastron.[3] The first acoustic window in chelonians is located between the neck and the cranial forelimb and allows for assessment of the heart and liver.[3] The second chelonian acoustic window in chelonians is located behind the caudal forelimb and also allows for assessment of the heart and liver.[3] The third acoustic window in chelonians is located in a region termed the prefemoral fossa and is located cranial to the pelvic limb, allowing for assessment of the gastrointestinal tract, the urogenital tract, and the bladder.[3] The size of acoustic windows can be limiting in chelonians, especially those that are more terrestrial in nature and tend to have smaller windows.[3]

Diseases of the reptile patient that can benefit from POCUS examinations

Coelomic distension. Coelomic distension can result from a variety of etiologies, including a mass, free fluid, abscess, granuloma, infectious disease, such as parasites, and enlargement/increased activity of the reproductive tract.[9] POCUS assessment of coelomic distension can identify ascites, neoplasia, abscesses or granulomas, hernias, organomegaly, and reproductive upregulation.[3] The presence of ascites is easily detected in reptile patients due to the anechoic appearance and free-floating appearance of intracoelomic structures (**Fig. 2**). Organomegaly and intracoelomic masses may be detected on POCUS, especially in species like snakes, where there is a focal body swelling. The use of color Doppler can also help to identify the presence or absence of blood flow to that structure. Hepatic enlargement and lipidosis are very common in a wide range of reptile species and may be detectable on POCUS with the presence of a hyperechoic (bright) liver (**Fig. 3**).[10,11]

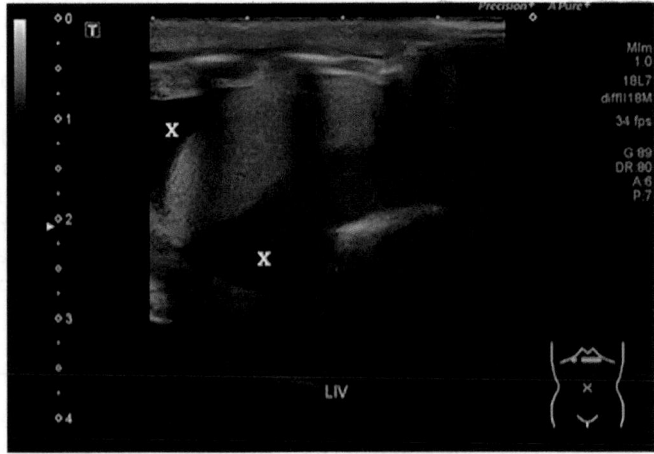

Fig. 2. 6 year old female intact bearded dragon (*Pogona vitticeps*) that presented for coelomic distension. On POCUS, a large volume of coelomic effusion of uncertain etiology was detected. The areas of coelomic effusion are denoted by the two white "x".

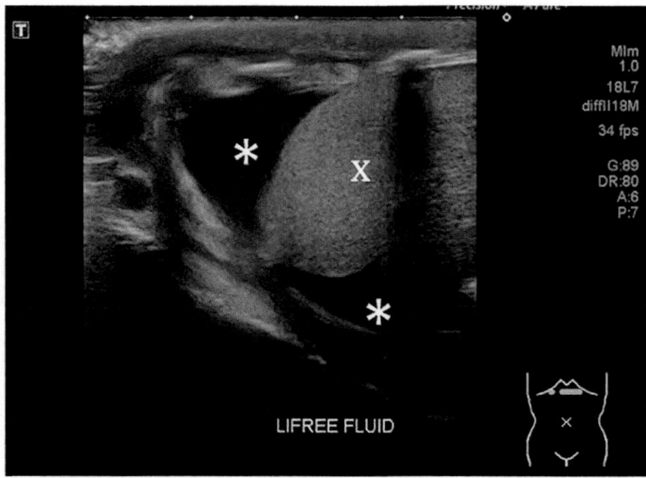

Fig. 3. 1 year old female intact bearded dragon (*Pogona vitticeps*) that presented for anorexia and decreased frequency of defecation for greater than four weeks duration. Physical examination was largely unremarkable. On FAST scan, the liver appeared moderately enlarged and uniformly hyperechoic (near-isoechoic to the fat bodies) (x). Additionally, a large volume of mildly echogenic free coelomic fluid was identified of unknown etiology (*).

Specific organ POCUS in reptiles

The renal system The unique location of the kidney in most reptile species makes ultrasonographic evaluation of the renal system challenging.[8] Diseases such as urolithiasis in high-risk species may be detectable as a hyperechoic abnormality with clean acoustic shadowing, however. Species considered high-risk for urolithiasis typically are the desert species, such as uromastyx and chuckwalla, as well as many of the larger tortoise species.[12]

The reproductive system. POCUS can be a useful technique to determine the sex in many reptile species.[13] The ovaries in females and the testicles in males are intracoelomic. If the gonads are visualized, in snakes they are located in the last third of the body.[4] If the ovaries are active in the female patient, they are often easily visualized as a large number of follicles (**Fig. 4**).[1] Normal follicles will appear as multiple round, anechoic structures with a 2 layered wall that has an inner echoic layer and an outer anechoic later.[14] Additionally, eggs can be identified as shadowing structures.[1] If the gonads are inactive, in either the male or female reptile patient, though, they will be very difficult to identify.[1] The hemipenes can also be visualized in male reptile patients, and may be normally calcified in some species such as monitor lizards.[8,14–16]

In addition to the identification of the sex of the patient, and normal reproductive structures, POCUS can also be very useful to identify abnormalities of the reproductive tract. Reproductive disease is common in reptiles, especially in the female that commonly presents with pre- or post-ovulatory stasis. Preovulatory follicles appear differently than postovulatory follicles with a hypoechoic appearance compared to the hyperechoic calcified shell of the postovulatory follicles.[1] Ultrasound can also be useful to determine if the follicles seen are abnormal; follicles that are unovulated in stasis will present with a heterogeneous pattern and an irregular surface compared to the smooth, well-demarcated surface of normal follicles.[14,17,18] Additionally, as follicular stasis progresses, anechoic fluid may be detected around the follicles with

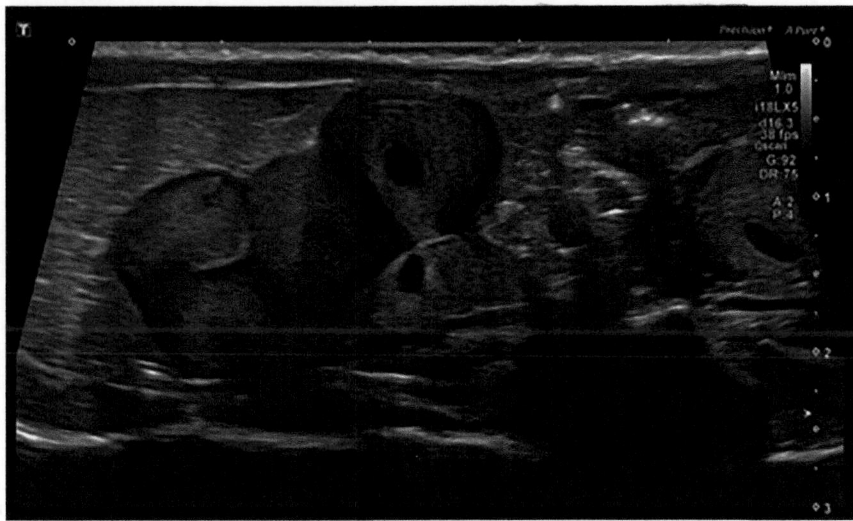

Fig. 4. 1 year old female intact bearded dragon (*Pogona vitticeps*) that presented after being stepped on by the owner and became acutely lethargic following the incident. On POCUS for evaluation of large amounts of free fluid in the coelom, a large number of normal follicles were discovered. The follicles represented multiple, conglomerated, oval 9-11 mm structures with an anechoic center.

echogenic free-floating particles that represent inflammatory debris. Allowing the ultrasound probe to sit stationary on the follicles for a short time can also be useful to rule out the presence of peristalsis which would indicate they are intestinal loops versus follicles (**Figs. 5-12**).

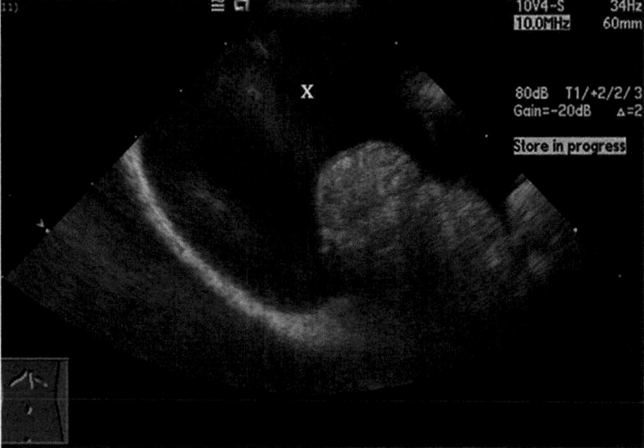

Fig. 5. 10 year old double yellow fronted Amazon parrot (*Amazona oratrix*) that presented for coelomic distension. Full evaluation of the patient revealed a heart murmur, right sided heart failure and free coelomic effusion on FAST scan (pictured below). The 'x' represents the large volume of free coelomic effusion in this patient.

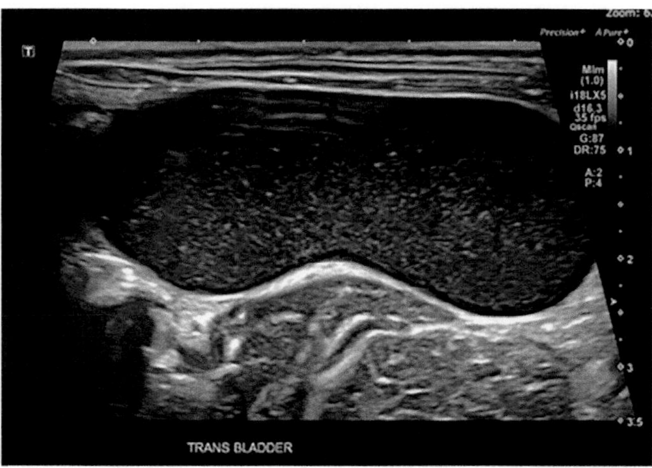

Fig. 6. Ultrasound image of normal rabbit (*Oryctolagus cuniculus*) bladder demonstrating the large amount of sediment that can be present.

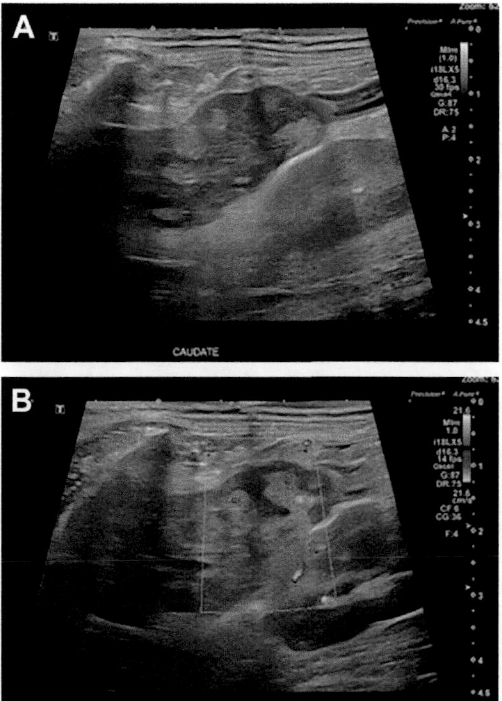

Fig. 7. Ultrasound image from a 5 year old male neutered rabbit (*Oryctolagus cuniculus*) that presented for a 1 day history of anorexia and lethargy. On physical examination, the rabbit demonstrated cranial abdominal pain and hypothermia. POCUS of the abdomen demonstrated a torsion of the caudate liver lobe (*A*) with lack of blood flow noted to the affected lobe when Doppler ultrasound was utilized (*B*).

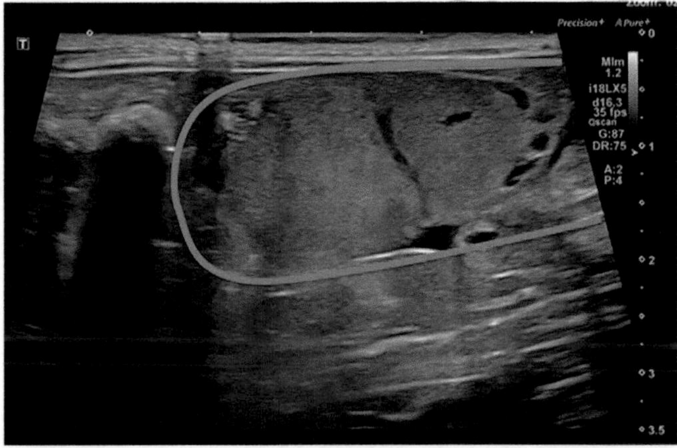

Fig. 8. 6 year old female intact rabbit (*Oryctolagus cuniculus*) that presented with a history of decreased appetite, lethargy, and decreased stool production. On physical examination, a large mass was palpable in the caudal abdomen. On POCUS of the abdomen, severe uterine nodular enlargement was noted with differentials of neoplasia, or severe endometrial hyperplasia with cystic regions. Following normal chest radiographs, ovariohysterectomy of the rabbit was performed and histopathology of the uterus was consistent with adenocarcinoma. The large, nodular uterus is delineated by the blue outline.

The Gastrointestinal System

Liver

The normal reptilian liver should have a homogeneous echogenicity and is typically easy to locate, except in chelonians.[1] The liver should be evaluated for the presence of masses that could be indicative of neoplasia, abscesses, granulomas, or cysts, as well as for a change in echogenicity, with hepatic lipidosis causing a hyperechoic liver

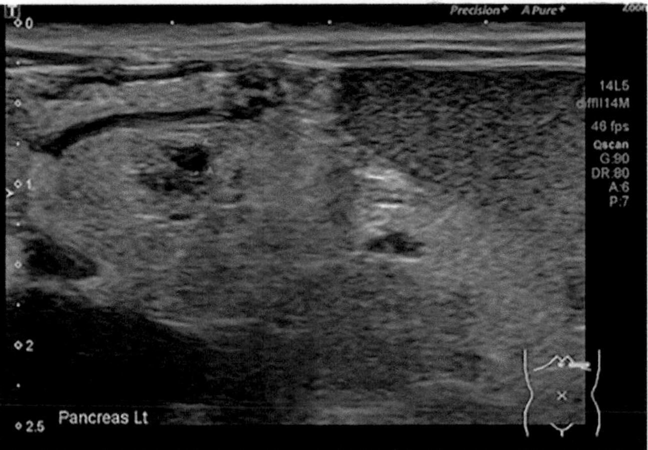

Fig. 9. 6 year old male neutered ferret (*Mustela putorius furo*) that presented for an annual wellness examination and screening for disease. Physical examination revealed mild splenomegaly. On POCUS of the abdomen, a nodule was noted in the pancreas (noted by A on figure).

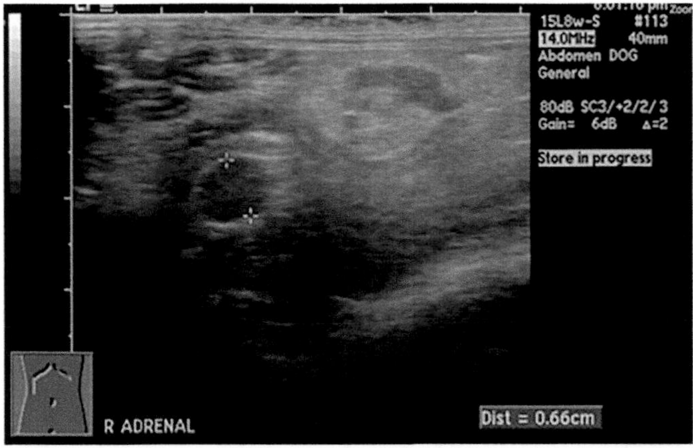

Fig. 10. 5 year old male neutered ferret (*Mustela putorius furo*) that presented with a history of progressive alopecia and behavioral changes. FAST scan of the abdomen revealed left adrenomegaly. The width of the left adrenal gland (denoted by crosses) was 6.6 mm (reference range for the left adrenal gland: width 2.8 ± 0.5 mm (mean ± SD)[96]).

appearance.[10] Hepatic lipidosis is common in a number of captive reptile species, particularly bearded dragons.[10,11]

The Cardiovascular System

Although the echocardiographic examination in reptiles may be more challenging, and present difficulties due to a lack of normal values, it is still possible to obtain baseline information and evaluate for the presence of cardiac chamber enlargement, contractility, and the presence of pericardial effusion. Echocardiographic examination values

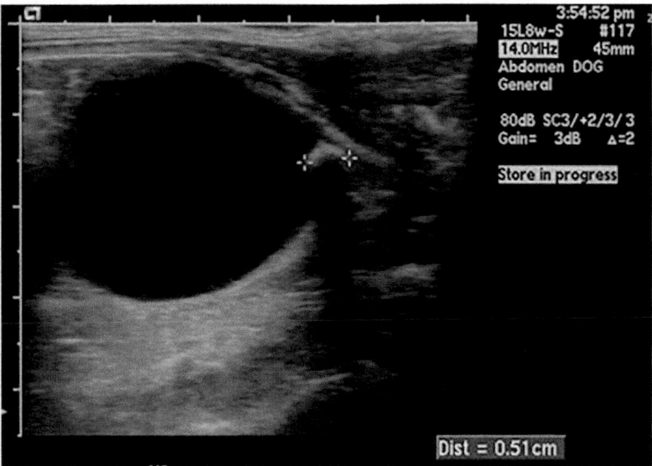

Fig. 11. 3 year old male intact guinea pig (*Cavia porcellus*) that presented with a history of stranguria and change in urine color. On physical examination, there was pain detected in the caudal abdomen and a firm bladder. FAST scan of the abdomen demonstrated a calculus at the level of the trigone of the bladder (denoted by crosses). Note the shadowing present from the stone.

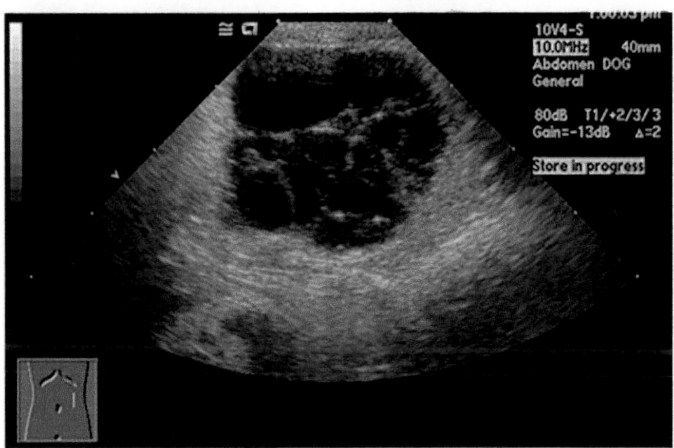

Fig. 12. 4 year old female intact guinea pig (*Cavia porcellus*) that presented for progressive abdominal distension. On physical examination, the guinea pig had bilateral palpable masses at the level of the kidneys and ovaries. FAST scan of the abdomen revealed bilateral ovarian cysts.

have been reported in bearded dragons (*Pogona vitticeps*), Boid snakes, green sea turtles (*Chelonia mydas*), and Aldabra tortoises (*Aldabrachelys gigantea*).[19–24]

In bearded dragons, there are numerous reports of the presence of aneurysms arising from the internal carotid or the aorta.[25,26] Clinically, these patients present with a large swelling, ranging from fluctuant to firm on the dorsolateral neck.[26,27] POCUS of this swelling would demonstrate a fluid-filled cavity with the presence of color blood flow on Doppler.

Use of POCUS in avian patients

Avian anatomy dramatically differs from mammalian anatomy and this presents many unique challenges when it comes to ultrasonography in these patients.

Unique avian anatomy. The respiratory system of avian patients is not accessible via ultrasonography. The lungs in avian species are located in a dorsal position and are overall not able to be compressed.[28] The air exchange is also unique in birds, where gas is exchanged at the parabronchial tissue and air capillaries, not the alveoli as it is in mammals.[29] Avian species also have a complex air sac system, typically with a total of nine air sacs located throughout their entire body and between their organs.[28] As a result of this dispersion of a large amount of air throughout their body, ultrasonography and the available acoustic window to examine the coelom is often limited in these patients to a single window located just caudal to the sternum. Additionally, it is relatively uncommon for birds to have pleural effusion which reduces the utility of TFAST examination in these species.

The avian coelom consists of a number of divisions that create subcavities, with most birds having a total of seven.[7] The subcavities are divided by various septa which are highlighted on ultrasound in the presence of effusion within each of the subcavities.[7] Many of the organs in the avian coelom may appear different, with a bilobed liver with variable presence of a gallbladder (present in cockatoos and raptors, but absent in other parrots and pigeons).[7] The stomach is divided into two anatomic regions called the proventriculus (glandular stomach) and the ventriculus (muscular stomach).[7] The kidneys are inaccessible by ultrasound in birds, with each kidney having three lobes (cranial, middle, caudal).[7] The kidneys lie in the ventral (renal) fossa of the synsacrum.[7] The majority of female birds only have a left reproductive system (ovary and oviduct) and are oviparous.[7] The right ovary is occasionally retained in some birds of prey, although rarely do they have a functional right oviduct.[7]

Each bird has different anatomy and accessibility with respect to the size of the keel.[7] Chickens have a smaller and fenestrated keel making ultrasound more feasible compared to passerines that are small and have a larger and elongated keel.[7]

Avian positioning. Prior to any handling or diagnostics, the stability of the avian patient should be assessed.[30] Many avian patients will benefit from some degree of sedation prior to ultrasonography, especially those with respiratory concerns. Dyspnea is common in any avian patient that presents with coelomic distension.[30] Whenever possible, stabilization of the patient should be performed before performing diagnostics.[30] In addition to assessment for stability, it is also critical to have a veterinary nurse or support staff that are comfortable restraining a wide range of avian species safely. Many avian patients can be assessed in dorsal recumbency, some in lateral recumbency, and in some scenarios, even a standing avian patient can undergo ultrasonography effectively. In avian patients that present with dyspnea or coelomic distension, it is best to examine the patient in an upright position.

There are two commonly utilized acoustic windows in avian patients. The first window is located just caudal to the sternum at the level of the ventromedial coelom.[30] The second window can be used in certain species such as pigeons and chickens, and is located just behind the last rib, laterally on the right side.

Ultrasound probe selection. Typically, a high frequency transducer is recommended, ranging from 7.5-18 MHz with a small footprint, usually a pediatric transducer.[2]

Imaging the normal avian coelom. The initial assessment of the coelom should start with the ventromedial acoustic window with the transducer positioned in a longitudinal fashion on the ventral coelom. In avian patients, there are natural featherless regions termed apterylae that can be located by gently parting the feathers.[30] These areas are very useful when performing POCUS in birds. The feathers should be parted to allow for maximum probe to skin contact. The use of 70% isopropyl alcohol and acoustic coupling gel in combination will allow for excellent images in birds; however, it is important to take into consideration the size of the patient and the amount used, as hypothermia can occur rapidly in these small patients.[30] In most avian patients, the ventromedial acoustic window will allow for visualization of the liver, ventriculus, gonads (when active), and heart; however, in very small patients, even visualization of these organs may be limited.[2,31] The spleen, normal kidneys, and inactive gonads are extremely difficult to identify in avian patients.[32] Additional utility of POCUS in avian patients include identification of masses or other coelomic abnormalities.

Diseases of the avian patient that can benefit from POCUS

Coelomic distention Coelomic distention is a common presentation in the avian patient and a common cause is the presence of ascites.[30] Ascites is typically recognizable based on the anechoic and triangular appearance combined with the presence of structures wafting within the effusion. When evaluating for ascites in the avian patient, it is useful to hold the bird in an upright position to ensure that the fluid settles in a gravity-dependent ventral region. Additionally, this positioning can aid with breathing in a patient that contains a large amount of effusion and has compromised breathing. Additionally, when easily accessible, the use of POCUS can allow for collection of effusions for analysis via coelomocentesis. All birds with free coelomic effusion should also be evaluated for the presence of pericardial effusion, as the two conditions commonly occur concurrently.

Coelomic distension can also occur as a result of the presence of organomegaly or a mass within the coelom. A common organ that is enlarged in the avian patient is the liver. Hepatomegaly can be strongly suspected based on radiographs demonstrating liver extension beyond the margins of the sternum caudally and beyond the acetabula laterally.[32] The use of POCUS can confirm this suspicion. A normal avian liver will appear similar in echotexture to that of a mammal, being coarse and homogeneous.[32] The presence of a mass within the coelom can also be determined with the use of POCUS. These masses often have a complex echotexture and can be differentiated from abscesses and granulomas with the use of color flow Doppler.[33,34] Typically, masses will have complex blood flow patterns compared to granulomas and abscesses that are often of poor vascularity.[33,34]

Reproductive disease is common in avian patients, and identification of normal, active reproductive organs, as well as diseased reproductive organs is possible with the use of POCUS.[35,36] The visualization of ovaries is only possible when the female bird is sexually upregulated and there are follicles of varying sizes present, representing different stages of development.[37] It is also possible to recognize an active oviduct in a female avian patient due to the presence of eggs, and the absence of contractility that would be seen in the similarly shaped intestines.[37] Diseases of the female reproductive system that can be detected with POCUS include cysts, neoplasia, salpingitis, and laminated eggs.[37]

Specific Organ POCUS in Avian Patients

Cardiac disease

Cardiac disease is a common presentation in the avian patient.[38] History and physical examination findings often result in a high suspicion of cardiac disease, in combination with radiographs.[38] Affected birds commonly have a history of dyspnea, episodes of weakness or syncope, coughing, exercise intolerance, distension of the coelom, and lethargy.[39] Cardiac size is well described in many species of birds, and suspicion of cardiomegaly on radiographs should prompt POCUS of the heart prior to a complete echocardiogram.[40–44] The location of the heart is cranial to the liver, and is most easily identified through the ventromedial acoustic window.[31] POCUS of the heart can identify cardiac chamber enlargement, pericardial effusion, and poor contractility of the heart. Common cardiac abnormalities that are identified in the avian patient include pericardial effusion and right ventricular dilation, commonly as a result of right-sided congestive heart failure.[45]

Small mammal patients

Unique exotic companion mammal anatomy. The gastrointestinal system of the herbivorous exotic companion mammals including rabbits and hystricomorph rodents (guinea pigs, chinchillas, degus) is unique compared to a typical carnivorous patient.[46] These herbivorous exotic companion mammals have an exceptionally large gastrointestinal tract.[46] Commonly, the gastrointestinal tract of these species becomes air-filled with ileus, and additionally is almost never empty of ingesta presenting challenges with ultrasound imaging.[35] Another portion of the gastrointestinal tract in these species, the cecum can also present challenges with the presence of gas obscuring the view of other abdominal organs.[46] The cecum in rabbits is located in the right abdomen, with the cecum in guinea pigs located in the central left abdomen. Rabbits also have a large amount of gastro-intestinal lymphoid tissue (GALT) located in the abdomen, specifically a sacculus rotundus at the ileocecal junction, which can be confused for a mass as a novel ultrasonographer.[46] Additionally, in rabbits, the vermiform appendix is located at the blind end of the cecum and appears thickened with finger-like projections.[46] Ferrets do not have a cecum.[47]

The spleen in rabbits is very small and is not always visualized on POCUS but may be more easily located on a complete abdominal ultrasound.[48] In contrast, ferrets have a very large spleen that is easily detected on POCUS examination.[49] Ferrets also have a single large jejunal lymph node that may be mistaken for a mass or lesion.[49]

In male guinea pigs, the presence of large paired seminal vesicles or vesicular glands are often confused with female uterine horns.[50]

Exotic companion mammal positioning. Prior to any ultrasound examination of an exotic companion mammal patient, the stability of the patient should be assessed. If there is concern for respiratory distress or high levels of stress, sedation and/or anesthesia may be useful prior to diagnostic evaluation. Additionally, if respiratory distress is a concern, supplemental flow by oxygen can be provided throughout the examination. It is extremely important with exotic companion mammals to have an individual who is comfortable with restraint and handling of the species. Depending on the status of the patient, positioning can range from the traditional dorsal recumbency, to lateral recumbency, to standing.

Ultrasound probe selection. Depending on the size of the exotic companion mammal, the probe selection may vary. For larger patients such as rabbits and ferrets, a curvilinear (microconvex) probe, or linear probe with a range of 5-10 MHz can be utilized. For smaller exotic companion mammals, a higher frequency probe (7.5–18 MHz) can be useful and has a much smaller footprint. The limitations of the higher frequency probe include the decreased depth penetration of the probe which is contrasted with the improved spatial resolution.[51]

Imaging the normal exotic companion mammal. The indications for POCUS examination of exotic companion mammals are similar to those of dogs and cats. In ferrets, the utility of a gastrointestinal ultrasound often has much greater utility than the herbivorous exotic companion mammals which have large amounts of gastrointestinal gas.[51]

POCUS in the exotic companion mammal has high sensitivity and specificity to detect the presence of effusion and can provide excellent information regarding the presence or absence of free fluid.

POCUS in ferrets

Urogenital system A common emergent presentation of the domestic ferret is stranguria, with primary rule outs of urolithiasis and prostatic disease secondary to adrenal disease.[52] POCUS can be useful to rapidly rule in or out the presence of a cystolith that could be the cause of the ferret's clinical signs.[52] Additionally, the use of an ultrasound can provide for a safer option to obtain a urine sample compared to a blind approach. Prostatic disease, typically cyst or abscess formation, is a complication of adrenocortical disease in ferrets and can also result in urinary obstruction and stranguria.[52] POCUS can demonstrate the presence of prostatic cysts, which often appear with hypoechoic to anechoic fluid, or abscesses, which often contain more heterogeneous fluid.[52] Additionally, POCUS may also identify enlarged or irregular adrenal glands.[53]

Gastrointestinal and hepatobiliary systems Another common ferret emergency presentation is gastrointestinal foreign bodies. Ferret foreign bodies are not always radiodense and thus may not be as obvious as when routine radiographs are performed in other species.[54] The use of ultrasound is often extremely important to confirm a foreign body obstruction in a ferret, but the ultrasound examination often left to a skilled sonographer. POCUS can still confirm the presence of effusion, suspected obstruction evidenced by distended bowel loops, or plication, however.[54] Fluid sampling can also be performed if fluid is detected, which may help to rule in or out a septic abdomen.

Spleen Splenomegaly is extremely common in the domestic ferret in North America over one year of age.[55] The most common cause of splenomegaly in ferrets is extramedullary hematopoiesis (EMH), although other reported causes include neoplasia (most commonly lymphoma), hypersplenism, and splenic congestion.[55] In cases of EMH, the spleen typically has a uniform echogenicity versus the mottled, often "Swiss cheese" appearance of splenic neoplasia; however, it is not uncommon to detect small hypoechoic regions of the spleen in cases of EMH that could be confused with neoplastic nodules.[55] Definitive diagnosis requires cytologic or histologic sampling.[55] Other rare splenic disorders in the ferret include splenic torsion, splenic abscesses, and splenic rupture.[55,56]

Pancreas Ferrets commonly present on emergency for hypoglycemia due to pancreatic β-islet cell tumors (insulinomas).[57] These tumors typically consist of small nodules, sometimes microscopic in size.[58] Detection of pancreatic nodules is possible but may only be recognized by skilled sonographers.[59]

Neoplasia Lymphoma is a common neoplastic presentation of ferrets. There are many varied presentations of lymphoma in ferrets including thoracic disease with a mediastinal mass, thoracic lymphadenopathy, and/or pleural effusion, abdominal disease with splenic, hepatic, or renal involvement, or many others.[57] In these cases, the use of POCUS can provide utility in assessing for the presence of pleural effusion and obtaining a sample for both therapeutic and diagnostic purposes. Additionally, ultrasound-guided aspiration of an enlarged lymph node or abdominal mass may yield a diagnosis of lymphoma in a patient.[60]

Cardiac disease Cardiac disease is a common presentation in ferrets, especially with increasing age.[61] The use of POCUS to evaluate the heart may provide a quick diagnostic assessment to the underlying cause of the patient's presenting signs with common cardiac diseases being dilated cardiomyopathy, cardiac arrhythmias, and acquired valvular disease.[61] Normal echocardiographic measurements have been published for ferrets.[62] In unstable patients with respiratory signs, this quick POCUS assessment can provide a large amount of information rapidly.

POCUS in rabbits

Urogenital system. Urolithiasis is a common disease detected in the domestic rabbit population. A multitude of factors are suspected to contribute to this disease including their unique calcium metabolism, genetic and husbandry related factors, among others.[63] In rabbits, there is unregulated absorption of dietary calcium, and thus excess calcium that is not required is excreted in the urine.[64] This results in urinary sludge which appears as slightly hyperechoic urine in the bladder on ultrasonographic assessment.[63] Ultrasound can also be useful for detection of urolithiasis in the form of discrete urinary calculi, or as an aid in obtaining a sample of urine via cystocentesis. In rabbits, cystocentesis can prove more challenging than other species as a result of a flaccid bladder wall that often indents but does not easily allow the needle to enter. Ideally, rabbits should be sedated prior to cystocentesis as they often react when the needle enters, which can result in iatrogenic damage.

Intact female rabbits commonly develop uterine adenocarcinoma by the age of three to four.[63] When the history of the animal combined with physical examination findings of a caudal abdominal mass suggests uterine adenocarcinoma, POCUS can aid in a diagnosis.[63] When the neoplastic disease becomes advanced, enlarged abdominal lymph nodes and intrabdominal metastasis may be detected, in addition to free abdominal fluid. Calcification of the uterus and the intrabdominal masses is common.[65]

Gastrointestinal and hepatobiliary systems. Liver lobe torsion is a common diagnosis in rabbits. Rabbits typically present with non-specific signs such as lethargy, anorexia, and reduced fecal output to lack of defecation.[66–73] The most sensitive diagnostic test for diagnosis involves a combination of bloodwork and ultrasound performed by a skilled sonographer.[69] The condition is typically treated with surgery, though medical management and supportive care of these cases has been successful as well.[69] The affected liver lobe will be identified by the absence of blood flow with Doppler, often with a mild to moderate amount of modified transudate fluid, often localized around the liver.[74]

Hepatic coccidiosis is diagnosed in young rabbits and causes the liver to appear with a characteristic heterogeneous appearance, with a hyperechoic parenchyma, hyperechoic bile ducts, and hyperechoic gall bladder wall.[75]

Other Findings

Abscesses

Rabbits have thick, caseous exudate contained within their abscesses that may not appear liquid on ultrasound.[76] Thoracic and abdominal abscesses occur with some frequency in rabbits and can be detected with the use of POCUS.[77,78] The addition of color flow Doppler can have utility in distinguishing between an abscess, which should have minimal blood flow, and a soft tissue mass which can have substantial blood flow.[33]

Rabbits that present with unilateral exophthalmos lacking a history of trauma, and evidence of dental disease on oral examination, may be suspected to have a retrobulbar abscess.[79] Retrobulbar abscesses can occur as a result of periapical infection of the maxillary cheek teeth in rabbits.[80] The use of POCUS in the ocular region can aid in the diagnosis, especially in cases where computed tomography may not be an option for the owner or the patient.[79]

POCUS in Guinea pigs

Urogenital system Urolithiasis is also a common presentation in guinea pigs.[81] Most commonly, guinea pigs have a single, large calculus, but multiple calculi are possible. Ultrasonography can aid in the detection of single or multiple calculi, urinary sludge, and aid in the collection of a urine sample via cystocentesis.

Ovarian cysts are common in intact female guinea pigs over the age of three.[81] Guinea pigs with ovarian cysts can present with a range of clinical signs from none to evidence of abdominal enlargement, pain, anorexia, and lethargy.[81] Ovarian cysts can be diagnosed via ultrasound assessment, located dorsal to the kidney, continuous with the ovary.[82] Ovarian cysts will appear anechoic, fluid-filled and demonstrate acoustic enhancement, making them easily differentiated from a mass through the use of color flow Doppler, which demonstrates no intra-cystic blood flow in comparison to masses, which often have significant blood flow.[82] Ultrasound-guided aspiration and drainage can be utilized from both a diagnostic and therapeutic stand point, though recurrence of cystic fluid is common following drainage.

POCUS in chinchillas

Urogenital system Intact female chinchillas may present with a caudal abdominal mass effect on physical examination, representing uterine enlargement. Pyometra is well-documented in this species. The use of POCUS can demonstrate an enlarged, fluid-filled uterus, containing fluid with varying degrees of echogenicity, from anechoic to hyperechoic.[83]

POCUS in hamsters

Gastrointestinal and hepatobiliary systems Hamsters commonly develop hepatic cystic disease.[84] The hepatic cyst can usually be diagnosed initially via palpation and confirmed with the use of POCUS.[84] The cysts can be present in varying shapes and sizes.[84]

POCUS in hedgehogs

Urogenital system Uterine disease is common in intact female hedgehogs, with one of the most common diseases being neoplasia.[85] The most common neoplastic diseases of the uterus in hedgehogs include uterine adenosarcoma, endometrial stromal sarcomas, adenoleiomyosarcoma and adenoleiomyoma.[85] Other uterine diseases that have been reported in this species include endometrial polyps, pyometra, and metritis.[85,86]

Neoplasia Overall, neoplasia is a common disease in African pygmy hedgehogs, with a wide range of discrete and disseminated neoplasms described.[86] POCUS may be useful for the detection of thoracic and abdominal masses in this species.

Additional Uses for POCUS in all Species in the Emergency Setting

POCUS during cardiopulmonary resuscitation (CPR)

While very little literature exists regarding the utility of POCUS during CPR in animals, it has been suggested to improve outcomes in the human medical field.[87] In a large multi-institutional study in humans, cardiac activity on ultrasound was the variable demonstrated to be most associated with survival following cardiac arrest.[87] Directly visualizing the heart to determine if coordinated contraction is occurring in the heart, or whether the chambers are acting in concert can be invaluable in any patient. In patients where auscultation or ECG can be difficult, such as reptiles, POCUS can prove even more essential to CPR.

POCUS for assessment of fluid status

Along similar lines, POCUS can be useful in assessing the type of shock that an animal may be experiencing, as well as provide utility regarding the fluid status of the animal. In dogs, the caudal vena cava collapsibility index (CVCCI) has been demonstrated to accurately predict fluid responsiveness in critically ill dogs with perfusion abnormalities.[88] Similarly, the caudal vena cava (CVC) diameter, and collapsibility index (CV) have been used to demonstrate the intravascular volume status in dogs.[89]

A large number of other parameters have been assessed in humans, particularly the diameter and collapsibility of various other large vessels to help assess fluid resuscitation status, as well as signs of fluid overload in patients.[90] Some of these include the inferior vena cava, common carotid artery, subclavian vein, internal jugular vein, and femoral vein.[90] While at this time, these values are largely unknown in exotic companion animals, future research and experience are likely to demonstrate that they are equally useful in these species.

Thoracic POCUS

While there has been significant advancement in the use of POCUS for abdominal assessment, it is also important to discuss the utility of this modality in the assessment of the thorax as well. In particular, POCUS has become increasingly used when assessing the lungs. A-lines refer to echogenic, gradually fading horizontal lines that are spaced equally below the pleural line and are a representation of air/gas that is below the pleura. A-lines can be normal, or can be indicative of a pneumothorax.[91] Thus, additional factors, such as a glide sign or a curtain sign, should be evaluated to determine if a pneumothorax is present.[92] When evaluating a thorax for A-lines, the linear transducer is best. B-lines can also be visualized on a thoracic POCUS, and represent discrete vertical reverberation artefacts that originate from the pleural line and obscure A-lines.[91] Unlike A-lines, B-lines are not observed in pneumothorax and are only seen when there is a pleura/tissue interface.[91] Numerous B-lines indicate an interstitial-alveolar lung abnormality, such as pulmonary contusions, lung consolidation from pneumonia, or fluid build-up from congestive heart failure.[92] There are many other 'signs' that have been described with thoracic POCUS that can be useful for detection of lung consolidation and other significant abnormalities as well.[91] Again, while not described in exotic companion animals, the lung anatomy of exotic mammals does not differ substantially from dogs and cats, so these same principles can be applied. It is important to note that B lines are considered a normal finding in reptiles and should therefore, not be interpreted as pathology. The use of T-FAST in a critical care setting can provide a rapid, point-of-care assessment in respiratory and cardiac patients (and most especially in differentiating between these two organ systems as the cause of respiratory distress).

THE USE OF POCUS IN A CRITICAL CARE SETTING

When an exotic patient is hospitalized, several sequelae of hospitalization and critical illness, such as ileus and acute kidney injury, can be better monitored with the use of POCUS as well. Clinicians can monitor patients for new or resolving pleural, pericardial, peritoneal, and retroperitoneal effusions, which may indicate fluid overload and heart failure, gastrointestinal rupture/dehiscence, or new onset bleeding when blood pressure and perfusion is re-established. As previously described, effusions will typically be recognized as triangular or "sharp-edged" hypo- or anechoic fluid rather than rounded edged fluid that is typically found within a visceral organ (although pericardial effusion is the exception to this rule). A patient's fluid status (volume under- or overloaded) can also be assessed throughout hospitalization as described previously to adjust the patient's fluid therapy prescription.

A patient's gastrointestinal tract can also be assessed for its general motility. Gastrointestinal ileus is very common in many hospitalized patients and determining if the gastrointestinal system is experiencing peristalsis or is experiencing complete paresis can help drive the intensity of supportive care measures and steer GI supportive therapies. There has been preliminary work on peristalsis baselines in rabbits.[93] POCUS has also been utilized to assessed gastric residual volume (a critical factor in avoiding aspiration pneumonia in critically ill patients) and ascertaining appropriate positioning of feeding tubes in human medicine, and utilizing ultrasound in hospitalized exotic patients in a similar fashion is likely achievable and worthwhile.[94]

Another concerning complication of hospitalization, anesthesia, and critical illness is acute kidney injury (AKI), with patients with AKI and anuria or oliguria having significantly worse prognoses. There are several formulas and methods published and described in small domestic animal medicine to determine urinary bladder volume.[95] With the secretive and easily stressed nature of many hospitalized exotic patients, tracking urine production via ultrasound can be essential in determining if a patient is experiencing anuria or oliguria.

Overall, even though there is a paucity of studies on these techniques in exotic veterinary patients, there appears to be no contraindication to applying these techniques to critically ill exotic patients in order to provide them the highest level of care.

SUMMARY

Exotic companion animals are frequently presented for a variety of problems ranging from routine to severely life-threatening. Owners frequently expect high-level diagnostic and treatment care for these patients, which can and should include the use of point of care ultrasound. Given that many exotic companion animals are prey species, point of care ultrasound provides a rapid, efficient diagnostic tool that provides a lot of information rapidly, especially in unstable patients. The diagnostic, treatment, and prognostic information afforded by POCUS allows for the provision of high standard of care to exotic companion animals.

CLINICS CARE POINTS

- POCUS in exotic companion animals is a rapid, efficient, and high yield diagnostic tool that carries great potential to provide useful information with minimal patient stress.
- In the reptile and avian patient, the biggest challenge associated with POCUS is the marked anatomical differences and variations that exist. Additionally, the presence of air sacs in birds and some reptiles also dramatically reduces the availability of acoustic windows for ultrasonography.
- POCUS can aid in the diagnosis of free fluid in the abdomen, pleural effusion, and pericardial effusion, and can also aid in ultrasound-guided abdominocentesis, thoracocentesis, and pericardiocentesis. POCUS can also aid in ultrasound-guided cystocentesis.
- POCUS also has utility in identification of obvious cardiac chamber enlargement, subjectively assessing cardiac contractility, estimating intravascular volume status, and tracking GI motility and urine production.

DISCLOSURE

The authors declare that they have no relevant or material financial interests that relate to the research described in this article.

REFERENCES

1. Schumacher T, Toal R. Advanced radiography and ultrasonography in reptiles. Seminars Avian Exot Pet Med 2001;10(4):162–8.
2. Doneley B. Ultrasound. In: Doneley B, editor. Avian medicine and surgery in practice companion and aviary birds. FL, USA: Mason Publishing; 2010. p. 104–5.
3. Hochleithner C, Holland M. Ultrasonography. In: Mader D, editor. Current therapy in reptile medicine and surgery. Philadelphia, USA: Saunders; 2014. p. 107–27.
4. O'Malley B. General anatomy and physiology of reptiles. In: O'Malley B, editor. Clinical anatomy and physiology of exotic species: structure and function of mammals, birds, reptiles, and amphibians. Philadelphia, USA: Elsevier Saunders; 2005. p. 17–39.
5. Kik M, Mitchell M. Reptile cardiology: a review of anatomy and physiology, diagnostic approaches, and clinical disease. Seminars Avian Exot Pet Med 2005; 14(1):52–60.
6. Dunker H. Coelom-gliederung der wirbeltiere - funktionelle aspekte. Verh Anat Ges 1978;72:91–112.
7. Taylor W. Pleura, pericardium, and peritoneum: the coelomic cavities of birds and their relationship to the lung-air sac system. In: Speer B, editor. Current therapy in avian medicine and surgery. Philadelphia, USA: Elsevier, Inc.; 2016. p. 345–62.

8. Bucy D, Guzman D, Zwingenberger AL. Ultrasonographic anatomy of bearded dragons (Pogona vitticeps). J Am Vet Med Assoc 2015;246(8):868–76.
9. Barten S, Simpson S. Differential diagnosis by clinical signs: lizards. In: Divers S, Stahl S, Mader M, editors. Mader's reptile and Amphibian medicine and surgery. Philadelphia, USA: Elsevier; 2017. p. 1257–65.
10. Hernandez-Divers SJ, Cooper JE. Reptile hepatic lipidosis. In: Association of Reptilian and. Amphibian Veterinarians 2001;8:193–200.
11. Barboza T. Hepatic lipidosis in the bearded dragon (Pogona vitticeps): diagnostics and therapeutic investigations. Ontario, Canada: University of Guelph; 2012.
12. Reavill D, Schmidt R. Urinary tract diseases of reptiles. J Exot Pet Med 2010;19: 280–9.
13. Bertocchi M, Bigliardi E, Pelizzone I, et al. Monitoring of the reproductive cycle in captive-bred female Boa constrictor: preliminary ultrasound observations. Animals 2021;3069:1–16.
14. Banzato T, Russo E, Finotti L, et al. Ultrasonographic anatomy of the coelomic organs of boid snakes (Boa constrictor imperator, Python regius, Python molurus molurus, and Python curtus). Am J Vet Res 2012;73(5):634–45.
15. di Ianni F, Volta A, Pelizzone I, et al. Diagnostic sensitivity of ultrasound, radiography and computer tomography for gender determination in four species of lizards. Vet Radiol Ultrasound 2015;56(1):40–5.
16. Gnudi G, Volta A, di Ianni F, et al. Use of ultrasonography and contrast radiography for snake gender determination. Vet Radiol Ultrasound 2009;50(3):309–11.
17. Bertocchi M, Pelizzone I, Parmigiani E, et al. Monitoring the reproductive activity in captive bred female ball pythons (P. regius) by ultrasound evaluation and noninvasive analysis of faecal reproductive hormone (progesterone and 17β-estradiol) metabolites trends. PLoS One 2018;13(6):e0199377.
18. Nielsen EL, Hespel AM, Kottwitz JJ, et al. Evaluation of the follicular cycle in ball pythons (Python regius). J Herpetol Med Surg 2016;26(3–4):108–16.
19. Silverman S, Sanchez-Migallon Guzman D, Stern J, et al. Standardization of the two-dimensional transcoelomic echocardiographic examination in the central bearded dragon (Pogona vitticeps). J Vet Cardiol 2016;18(2):168–78.
20. Schroff S, Starck JM, Krautwald-Junghanns ME, et al. Echocardiography in Boid snakes: demonstration and blood flow measurements. Tierarztl Prax Ausg K Kleintiere Heimtiere 2012;40(3):180–90.
21. Bagardi M, Bardi E, Manfredi M, et al. Two-dimensional and doppler echocardiographic evaluation in twenty-one healthy *Python regius*. Vet Med Sci 2021;7(3): 1006–14.
22. Snyder PS, Shaw NG, Heard DJ. Two-dimensional echocardiographic anatomy of the snake heart (Python molurus bivittatus). Vet Radiol Ultrasound 1999;40(1): 66–72.
23. March DT, Marshall K, Swan G, et al. The use of echocardiography as a health assessment tool in green sea turtles (Chelonia mydas). Aust Vet J 2021;99(1–2): 46–54.
24. Campolo M, Oricco S, Cavicchio P, et al. Echocardiographic evaluation of four giant Aldabra tortoises (Aldabrachelys gigantea). Vet Rec Open 2019;6(1):e000274.
25. Barten S, Wyneken J, Mader D. Aneurysm in the dorsolateral neck of two bearded dragons (Pogona vitticeps). In: 13th Annual Conference of the Association of Reptiles and Amphibians. ; 2006:43-44.
26. Finneburgh BM, Eshar D. Diagnostic challenge. J Exot Pet Med 2019;30:85–7.

27. Barten S, Wyneken J, Mader D, et al. Aneurysm in the dorsolateral neck of two bearded dragons (Pogona vitticeps). In: Proceedings of the association of reptilian and amphibian veterinarians. Reptilian Amphib Vet; 2006. p. 43–4.
28. O'Malley B. Avian anatomy and physiology. In: O'Malley B, editor. Clinical anatomy and physiology of exotic species: structure and function of mammals, birds, reptiles, and amphibians. Philadelphia, USA: Elsevier Limited; 2005. p. 97–161.
29. Fedde MR. Relationship of structure and function of the avian respiratory system to disease susceptibility. Poult Sci 1998;77(8):1130–8.
30. Bowles H, Lichtenberger M, Lennox A. Emergency and critical care of pet birds. Vet Clin Exot Anim Pract 2007;10(2):345–94.
31. Helmer P. Advances in diagnostic imaging. In: Harrison G, Lightfoot T, editors. Clinical avian medicine. FL, USA: Spix Publishing; 2006. p. 653–8.
32. Krautwald-Junghanns ME, Riedei U, Neumann W. Diagnostic use of ultrasonography in birds. Proc Assoc Avian Vet 1991;269–75.
33. Ballard DH, Mazaheri P, Oppenheimer DC, et al. Imaging of abdominal wall masses, masslike lesions, and diffuse processes. Radiographics 2020;40(3): 684–706.
34. Toprak H, Kiliç E, Serter A, et al. Ultrasound and Doppler US in evaluation of superficial soft-tissue lesions. J Clin Imaging Sci 2014;4:12.
35. Oglesbee B. Gastrointestinal hypomotility and gastrointestinal stasis in rabbits. In: Oglesbee B, editor. Blackwell's five-minute veterinary consult: small mammal. 2nd ed. NJ, USA: Wiley-Blackwell; 2011. p. 425–8.
36. Gros L, Cococcetta C, Coutant T, et al. Ultrasonographic evaluation of the coelomic cavity in Rhode Island Red hybrid hens (*Gallus gallus* domesticus). Vet Radiol Ultrasound 2022;63(5):620–32.
37. Krautwald-Junghanns ME. Aids to diagnosis. In: Coles B, editor. Essentials of avian medicine and surgery. NJ, USA: John Wiley and Sons; 2008. p. 98–101.
38. de Wit M, Schoemaker NJ. Clinical approach to avian cardiac disease. Seminars Avian Exot Pet Med 2005;14(1):6–13.
39. Strunk A, Wilson GH. Avian cardiology. Vet Clin Exot Anim Pract 2003;6(1):1–28.
40. Straub J, Pees M, Krautwald-Junghanns ME. Measurement of the cardiac silhouette in psittacines. J Am Vet Med Assoc 2002;221(1):76–9.
41. Velayati M, Mirshahi A, Razmyar J, et al. Radiographic reference limits for cardiac width of budgerigars (Melopsittacus undulatus). J Zoo Wildl Med 2015; 46(1):34–8.
42. Schnitzer P, Sawmy S, Crosta L. Radiographic measurements of the cardiac silhouette and comparison with other radiographic landmarks in wild galahs (Eolophus roseicapilla). Animals 2021;11(3):587.
43. Murray H, Torrey S, Pokras M, et al. Establishing cardiac measurement standards in three avian species. J Avian Med Surg 1997;11:15–9.
44. Silva JP, Castiglioni MCR, Doiche DP, et al. Radiographic measurements of the cardiac silhouette in healthy blue-fronted Amazon parrots (Amazona aestiva). J Avian Med Surg 2020;34(1):26–31.
45. Krautwald-Junghanns ME. Radiography and ultrasonography in the backyard poultry and waterfowl patient. J Avian Med Surg 2017;31(3):189–97.
46. Kohles M. Gastrointestinal anatomy and physiology of select exotic companion mammals. Vet Clin Exot Anim Pract 2014;17(2):165–78.
47. Pignon C, Huynh M, Husnik R, et al. Flexible gastrointestinal endoscopy in ferrets (Mustela putorius furo). Vet Clin Exot Anim Pract 2015;18(3):369–400.
48. Banzato T, Bellini L, Contiero B, et al. Abdominal ultrasound features and reference values in 21 healthy rabbits. Vet Rec 2015;176(4):101.

49. Suran JN, Latney L v, Wyre NR. Radiographic and ultrasonographic findings of the spleen and abdominal lymph nodes in healthy domestic ferrets. J Small Anim Pract 2017;58(8):444–53.
50. Stan F. Anatomical particularities of male reproductive system of guinea pigs (Cavia porcellus). Bulletin UASVM Veterinary Medicine 2015;72(2):288–95.
51. Fischetti A. Diagnostic imaging. In: Quesenberry KE, Carpenter JW, editors. Ferrets, rabbits and rodents - clinical medicine and surgery. Philadelphia, USA: Saunders; 2012. p. 502–10.
52. Pollock C. Disorders of the urinary and reproductive systems. In: Quesenberry KE, Carpenter JW, editors. Ferrets, rabbits and rodents - clinical medicine and surgery. Philadelphia, USA: Saunders; 2012. p. 46–61.
53. Barthez PY, Nyland TG, Feldman EC. Ultrasonography of the adrenal glands in the dog, cat, and ferret. Vet Clin Small Anim Pract 1998;28(4):869–85.
54. Sharma A, Thompson M, Scrivani P. Comparison of radiography and ultrasound for diagnosing small-intestinal obstruction in vomiting dogs. Vet Radiol Ultrasound 2011;52(3):248–55.
55. Morrisey J, Draus M. Cardiovascular and other diseases. In: Quesenberry KE, Carpenter JW, editors. Ferrets, rabbits and rodents - clinical medicine and surgery. Philadelphia, USA: Saunders; 2012. p. 62–77.
56. Rooney T, Gardhouse S, Berke K, et al. Diagnosis and surgical treatment of a primary splenic torsion in a domestic ferret (Mustela putorius furo). J Small Anim Pract 2021;62(11):1026–9.
57. Antinoff N, Williams B. Neoplasia. In: Quesenberry KE, Carpenter J, editors. Ferrets, rabbits and rodents - clinical medicine and surgery. Philadelphia, USA: Saunders; 2012. p. 103–21.
58. Rosenthal K, Wyre N. Endocrine diseases. In: Quesenberry KE, Carpenter J, editors. Ferrets, rabbits and rodents - clinical medicine and surgery. Philadelphia, USA: Saunders; 2012. p. 86–102.
59. Wu RS, Liu YJ, Chu CC, et al. Ultrasonographic features of insulinoma in six ferrets. Vet Radiol Ultrasound 2017;58(5):607–12.
60. Suran JN, Wyre NR. Imaging findings in 14 domestic ferrets (Mustela putorius furo) with lymphoma. Vet Radiol Ultrasound 2013;54(5):522–31.
61. Wagner RA. Ferret cardiology. Vet Clin Exot Anim Pract 2009;12(1):115–34.
62. Vastenburg M, Boroffka S, Shoemaker N. Echocardiographic measurements in clinically normal ferrets anesthetized with isoflurane. Vet Radiol Ultrasound 2004;45(3):228–32.
63. Klaphake E, Paul-Murphy J. Disorders of the reproductive and urinary systems. In: Quesenberry KE, Carpenter JW, editors. Ferrets, rabbits and rodents - clinical medicine and surgery. Philadelphia, USA: Saunders; 2012. p. 217–31.
64. Redrobe S. Calcium metabolism in rabbits. Seminars Avian Exot Pet Med 2002; 11(2):94–101.
65. Kunzel F, Grinninger P, Shibly S. Uterine disorders in 50 pet rabbits. J Am Anim Hosp Assoc 2015;51(1):8–14.
66. Graham JE, Orcutt CJ, Casale SA, et al. Liver lobe torsion in rabbits: 16 cases (2007 to 2012). J Exot Pet Med 2014;23(3):258–65.
67. Sheen JC, Vella D, Hung L. Retrospective analysis of liver lobe torsion in pet rabbits: 40 cases (2016-2021). Vet Rec 2022;191(7):e1971.
68. Graham J, Basseches J. Liver lobe torsion in pet rabbits. Clinical consequences, diagnosis, and treatment. Vet Clin Exot Anim Pract 2014;17(2):195–202.

69. Ozawa SM, Graham JE, Guzman DSM, et al. Clinicopathological findings in and prognostic factors for domestic rabbits with liver lobe torsion: 82 cases (2010–2020). J Am Vet Med Assoc 2022;260(11):1–9.
70. Taylor HR, Staff CD. Clinical techniques: Successful management of liver lobe torsion in a domestic rabbit (*Oryctolagus cuniculus*) by surgical lobectomy. J Exot Pet Med 2007;16(3):175–8.
71. Saunders R, Redrobe S, Barr F, et al. Liver lobe torsion in rabbits. J Small Anim Pract 2009;50(10):562.
72. Wilson RB, Holscher MA, Sly DL. Liver lobe torsion in a rabbit. Lab Anim Sci 1987; 37(4):506–7.
73. Wenger S, Barrett EL, Pearson GR, et al. Liver lobe torsion in three adult rabbits. J Small Anim Pract 2009;50(6):301–5.
74. Graham J, Orcutt C, Casale S. Liver lobe torsion in rabbits: 16 cases (2007-2012). J Exot Pet Med 2014;23(3):258–65.
75. Cam Y, Atasever A, Eraslan G. Eimeria stiedae: Experimental infection in rabbits and the effect of treatment with toltrazuril and ivermectin. Exp Parasitol 2004;119: 164–72.
76. Millward L. Rabbit. In: Sharkey LC, Radin MJ, Seelig D, editors. Veterinary cytology. NJ, USA: Wiley-Blackwell; 2020. p. 766–81.
77. Varga M. Abscesses. In: Varga M, editor. Textbook of rabbit medicine. 2nd ed. Elsevier; 2014. p. 249–70.
78. Perpinan D. Abdominal abscess in a rabbit. Exot Dvm 2009;11(1):13–5.
79. Holmberg BJ. Ophthalmology of exotic pets. In: Maggs DJ, Miller PE, Ofri R, editors. Slatter's fundamentals of veterinary ophthalmology. Philadelphia, USA: Saunders Elsevier; 2017. p. 427–41.
80. Capello V, Lennox A. Small mammal dentistry. In: Quesenberry KE, Carpenter JW, editors. Ferrets, rabbits and rodents - clinical medicine and surgery. Philadelphia, USA: Saunders; 2012. p. 452–71.
81. Hawkins M, Bishop C. Disease problems of guinea pigs. In: Quesenberry KE, Carpenter JW, editors. Ferrets, rabbits and rodents - clinical medicine and surgery. Philadelphia, USA: Saunders; 2012. p. 295–310.
82. Beregi A, Zorn S, Felkai F. Ultrasonic diagnosis of ovarian cysts in 10 guinea pigs. Vet Radiol Ultrasound 1999;40(1):74–6.
83. Mans C, Donnelly T. Disease problems of chinchillas. In: Quesenberry KE, Carpenter JW, editors. Ferrets, rabbits and rodents - clinical medicine and surgery. Philadelphia, USA: Saunders; 2012. p. 311–25.
84. Brown C, Donnelly T. Disease problems of small rodents. In: Quesenberry K, Carpenter JW, editors. Ferrets, rabbits and rodents - clinical medicine and surgery. Philadelphia, USA: Saunders; 2012. p. 354–72.
85. Mikaelian I, Reavill D. Spontaneous proliferative lesions and tumors of the uterus of captive African hedgehogs. J Zoo Wildl Med 2004;35(2):216–20.
86. Ivy E, Carpenter J. African hedgehogs. In: Quesenberry KE, Carpenter JW, editors. Ferrets, rabbits and rodents - clinical medicine and surgery. Philadelphia, USA: Saunders; 2012. p. 411–27.
87. Gaspari R, Weekes A, Adhikari S, et al. Emergency department point-of-care ultrasound in out-of-hospital and in-ED cardiac arrest. Resuscitation 2016; 109:33–9.
88. Donati PA, Guevara JM, Ardiles V, et al. Caudal vena cava collapsibility index as a tool to predict fluid responsiveness in dogs. J Vet Emerg Crit Care 2020;30(6): 677–86.

89. Giraud L, Fernandes Rodrigues N, Lekane M, et al. Caudal vena cava point-of-care ultrasound in dogs with degenerative mitral valve disease without clinically important right heart disease. J Vet Cardiol 2022;41:18–29.
90. Pourmand A, Pyle M, Yamane D, et al. The utility of point-of-care ultrasound in the assessment of volume status in acute and critically ill patients. World J Emerg Med 2019;10(4):232.
91. Bhoil R, Ahluwalia A, Chopra R, et al. Signs and lines in lung ultrasound. J Ultrason 2021;21(86):e225.
92. Boysen S., AFAST and TFAST in the Intensive Care Unit, In: Silverstein D.C. and Hopper K., *Small, Animal Critical Care Medicine*, Second Edition, 2015, W.B. Saunders; Philadelphia, USA, 988–994
93. Oura TJ, Graham JE, Knafo SE, et al. Evaluation of gastrointestinal activity in healthy rabbits by means of duplex Doppler ultrasonography. Am J Vet Res 2019;80(7):657–62.
94. Brotfain E, Erblat A, Luft P, et al. Nurse-performed ultrasound assessment of gastric residual volume and enteral nasogastric tube placement in the general intensive care unit. Intensive Crit Care Nurs 2022;69. https://doi.org/10.1016/J.ICCN.2021.103183.
95. Kendall A, Keenihan E, Kern ZT, et al. Three-dimensional bladder ultrasound for estimation of urine volume in dogs compared with traditional 2-dimensional ultrasound methods. J Vet Intern Med 2020;34(6):2460–7.
96. O'Brien RT, Paul-Murphy J, Dubielzig RR. Ultrasonography of adrenal glands in normal ferrets. Vet Radiol Ultrasound 1996;37(6):445–8.

Sedation and Anesthesia in Exotic Animal Critical Care

H. Nicole Trenholme, DVM, MS, DACVECC (SA), DACVAA*

KEYWORDS

• Avian • Critically ill • Immobilization • Minor species • Reptiles • Small mammal

KEY POINTS

- To perform diagnostics and therapeutic care for exotic patients that are sick or injured, sedation and/or anesthesia is frequently required.
- It is important for the clinician to consider drug choice, route of administration, and dose based on each patient's unique characteristics as well as potential comorbidities.
- Appropriate preparation of equipment and supplies, including in the event of an emergency, is necessary prior to administration of anesthetics to compromised exotic patients.
- When possible, utilization of drugs with a wide safety margin and/or those that are reversible may aid in the successful anesthesia of these patients.

INTRODUCTION

Medical management of exotic animal species is inherently challenging due to the diversity within these groups. Sedation and anesthesia are often required for diagnostics and therapeutics. As these patients are often much smaller, more critical management is necessary to ensure optimal environmental conditions, enable accurate monitoring, and allow for appropriate response to complications, even in health. When these patients present with illness, a layer of complexity is added, making an already challenging management even more difficult. Through this review, the highlights of the current literature with regards to many of these patient subsets, including small mammals, avian, and reptiles are covered, including a focus on how to apply these findings in an ill or injured patient.

PRE-SEDATION AND PRE-ANESTHETIC CONSIDERATIONS

Each type of animal has their own anatomical features, normal vital parameters, and fluid requirements. Additionally, each species has its own fasting recommendations,

Department of Veterinary Clinical Medicine, University of Illinois College of Veterinary Medicine, 1008 West Hazelwood Drive, LAC 251, Urbana, IL 61802, USA
* Corresponding author. Department of the Veterinary Teaching Hospital, University of Illinois College of Veterinary Medicine, 1008 West Hazelwood Drive, LAC 251, Urbana, IL 61802.
E-mail address: N.Trenholme@evolutionvet.com

Vet Clin Exot Anim 26 (2023) 591–622
https://doi.org/10.1016/j.cvex.2023.05.003 vetexotic.theclinics.com

environmental preferred optimum temperature zones (POTZ), and unique pharmacokinetics and pharmacodynamics (**Table 1**). Being familiar with these normal values and management practices aids in the recognition of abnormal findings when ill or injured. These patients present challenges at all stages of sedation and anesthesia. Whether performing invasive or non-invasive procedures, the circulating blood volume and amount of acceptable loss should be determined. If blood loss is an anticipated complication (eg, trauma has occurred, surgery being performed), then it may behoove the clinician to evaluate and recruit an appropriate blood donor to be on standby. Supplementation of oxygen for three to 5 minutes via a tight-fitting oxygen mask is also highly recommended to reduce the risk of desaturation in the process of intubation. This is recommended even in healthy animals, as it can greatly extend the period between induction and desaturation.[1] This becomes more important with more challenging intubation scenarios or in patients that lack the physiologic reserve due to illness.

EQUIPMENT AND SUPPLIES

The same principles apply for sedation and anesthesia as are used with other veterinary species; however, some of the equipment may need to be altered. Pre-planning regarding appropriate monitoring equipment and supplies, including the best modalities for each patient, is important. When any drug is given for sedation or anesthesia, a higher likelihood of complications exists in critically ill minor species, which could prove to be detrimental to the patient.

Table 1
Environmental considerations for exotic companion animals, including preferred optimum temperature zone (POTZ), core temperature, normal heart rate (HR), and pre-anesthetic fasting recommendations for common exotic animals

Patient Type	POTZ (°F)	Body Temperature (°F)	HR (Beats min^{-1})	Fasting (hours)
Small mammals				
Chinchilla	60–75	98–100.4	150–350	2–3
Ferret	59–70	100–104	200–300	3–4
Guinea pig	65–75	101.5–102.2	200–250	2–3
Mouse	68–79	97.8–100.4	310–840	0–3
Rat	64–79	99.5–100	330–400	0–3
Rabbit	60–65	102–103	140–180	1–4
Avian				
Parrot	65–85	102–109	250–600	1–3 (<300G)
Chicken (adult)	70–75	105–107	200–300	3–6
Duck (adult)	55	102–107.5	80–140	3–6
Reptiles				One feeding cycle
Chelonian	68–86	78.8–89.6	10–40	6–24
Lizard	75.2–91.4	82.4–95	10–80	24–72
Snake	77–93.2	84.2–91.4	45–85	72–360

These are approximations based on the evaluation of data from multiple species within each category that are healthy. There are outliers in each group and physiologic changes with different behaviors (eg, diving, altered temperature), so investigation into normal values of each individual species that a veterinarian is working with is recommended to optimize care. Additionally debilitated animals may have values that are very different from those listed above.

Doppler allows continuous monitoring of heart rate and allows the anesthetist to glean the strength of each cardiac contraction, as the Doppler "woosh" of life will vary in intensity, depending on the cardiac output. In some patients, it may also be utilized to obtain a non-invasive blood pressure, if a cuff can be placed proximal to the crystal. This is not feasible in all patients, and some adaptations may be necessary to allow for continuous monitoring, such as taping of the crystal to the patient for small rodents, utilization of tongue depressors to maintain the crystal in the appropriate location on the wing of a bird, or a modified pen-like Doppler for chelonians (**Fig. 1**).

Electrocardiography (ECG) can also be utilized in exotic companion animals, with some modifications. By trimming the ECG pad down to the size of just the metal component, an ECG can be easily placed on the paws of small mammals or the defeathered skin of avian species, with the electrodes being connected in the same fashion as is typical of other species. An esophageal probe can be placed to the level of the heart, which is then attached with an adapter to a monitor (**Fig. 2**).

When a patient is immobilized, *respiratory rate and effort* should be monitored manually. *Mainstream capnography* (**Fig. 3**), which requires a lower air sampling rate than sidestream capnography, can allow the anesthetist to monitor end tidal carbon dioxide ($ETCO_2$) levels as well; however, this is typically an underestimate of the actual $ETCO_2$.[2] A non-rebreathing circuit allows for quicker manipulation of anesthetic depth, though it requires higher oxygen flow rates and therefore higher disposables

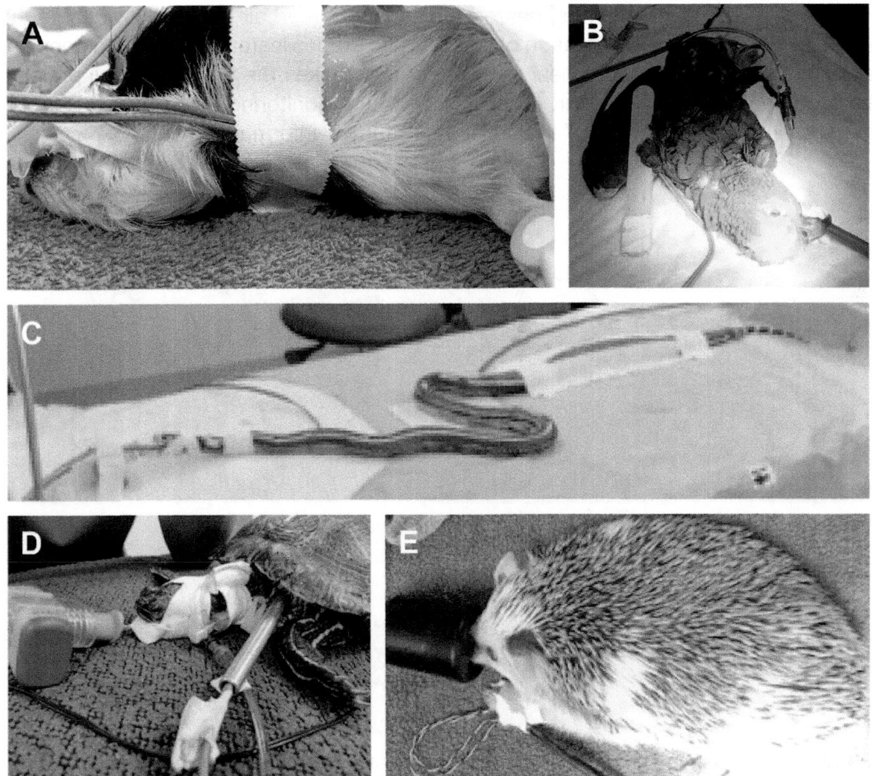

Fig. 1. Utilization of Doppler for heart rate monitoring on various species, including: (*A*) guinea pig; (*B*) parrot; (*C*) snake; (*D*) chelonian; (*E*) hedgehog.

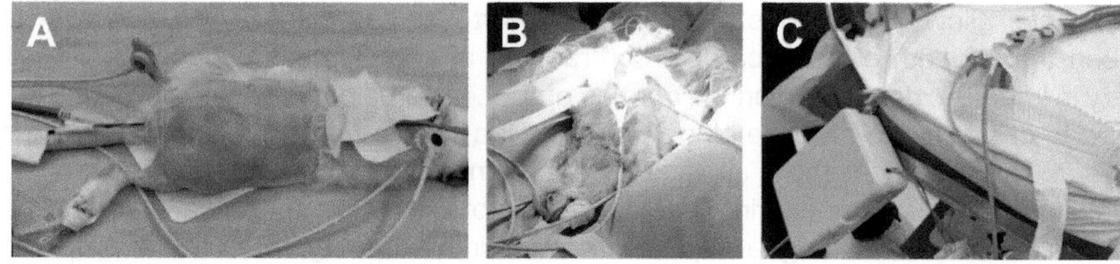

Fig. 2. Electrocardiography electrode placement in various species, including: (*A*) rat; (*B*), parrot; (*C*) snake.

costs.[3,4] Different species require different types of endotracheal tubes to reduce the risk of damage to the proximal airway. These species specifics are discussed within individual sections. Specialized ventilators enable the administration of smaller tidal volumes or may be pressure limited. Oxygenation can often be easily monitored with the utilization of a pulse oximeter. This is more challenging on individuals with scales, thickened or pigmented skin, often overestimating the level of oxygenation.[5] In these instances, esophageal pulse oximeters may be utilized.[6]

It is also important to monitor the patient's body temperature closely to maintain near normal core temperature, which can be measured via *thermometer* in the esophagus, cloaca, or rectum. Maintenance of body temperature is vital to exotic companion species, and this typically requires one or more active heating devices, which can include ambient heating lamps, heated tables, and forced air heating devices. In the author's experience, the utilization of clear plastic drapes instead of the cloth ones enables more trapping of heat near the patient and makes the typically small patients easier to visualize and monitor. (See "Temperature Monitoring and Thermal Support in Exotic Animal Critical Care" in this issue for further information.)

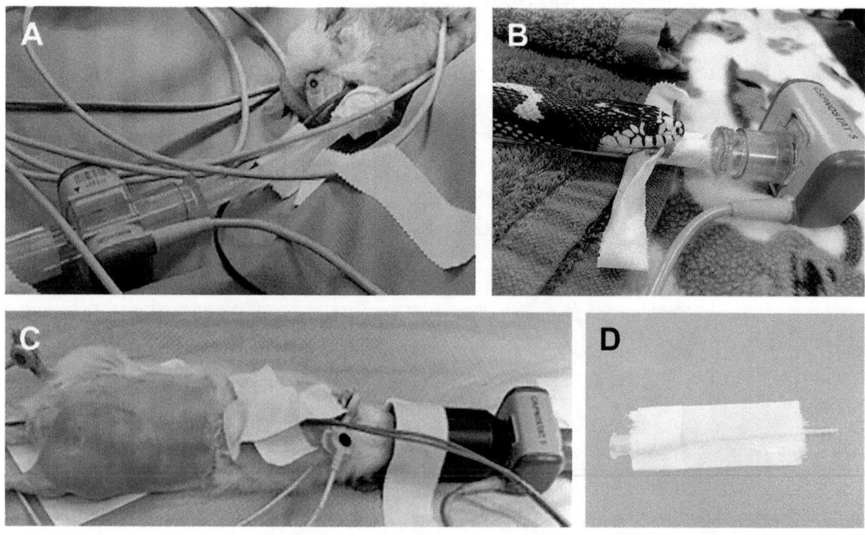

Fig. 3. Airway management strategies including mainstream capnograph on various intubated and non-intubated species, including: (*A*) intubated parrot; (*B*), intubated snake; (*C*) non-intubated rat; (*D*) 20G intravenous catheter utilized as an endotracheal tube for a 50g chameleon.

THERAPEUTIC OPTIONS

When choosing a sedation and/or anesthetic regimen for exotic companion animals, care should be taken to tailor the drug choice to the patient needs and pathophysiology. One protocol is not going to be appropriate for utilization in every species and every level of health. Exotic companion species that present for being ill are more fragile than their healthy counterparts, and this may make them more prone to complications than healthy subjects. As an example, a combination of ketamine and xylazine has been investigated in geriatric mice, and it was found to have an increased mortality, even when utilized at low standard doses.[7] Although age is not a disease, this was a study performed in older rodents with no known comorbidities; the increased risk of sedation and anesthesia would be compounded by the presence of one or more comorbidities.

There are numerous routes of administration of drugs. Intramuscular (IM), intraperitoneal (IP), intracoelomic (IC), intravenous (IV), and subcutaneous (SC) routes of administration are all possibilities, and the decision on the route of administration may be determined by logistical challenges or particular drug reactions. A study in rats given a combination of ketamine-xylazine found that muscle necrosis occurred in a majority of rats, which did not occur with the IP route of administration.[8] Avoiding drugs that may cause local vasoconstriction may also be beneficial. Intramuscular administration is also associated with a greater challenge when administering large volumes of injectate. However, IP injections have been associated with a high level of failure.[9] In an ideal world, anesthetics would only be given IV to ensure efficient uptake of the drug and less risk of tissue trauma. Ill or injured companion exotics may require sedation or anesthesia for the placement of an intravenous catheter safely, however. Therefore, despite the risk of tissue damage from IM injection, initial sedation is often given via this route. If the injectate volume is deemed too large for that patient, then multiple injection sites can be chosen.

GOALS

To care for an ill or injured exotic companion species, it is important to consider the same tenants of management that would be utilized in traditional species. The end goal for a thriving patient is to maintain oxygen delivery to the tissues. This includes ensuring adequate circulating volume, cardiac contractility, normal heart rate and rhythm, optimization of ventilation and perfusion, and oxygen carrying capacity. This may require oxygen supplementation, intravenous or intraosseous catheter placement, volume resuscitation, and analgesia. Sedation with limited reduction in cardiac output and tissue perfusion should be chosen. Therefore, the administration of alpha 2 agonist medications should be avoided in these patients.[7] Similarly, locoregional anesthesia may be utilized to reduce the depth of anesthesia necessary to perform invasive procedures.

Efforts should be made to reduce stress and allow for swift yet careful handling of the ill exotic, keeping the safety of personnel in mind. Efforts should be made to stabilize the patient prior to handling, diagnostics, or surgical intervention. There will be unique considerations for each subset of patients.

SMALL MAMMALIAN SPECIES

Exotic small mammals allow for the most parallels to be drawn to domestic animals, such as dogs and cats, including similar POTZ and body temperatures. Difference to keep in mind, however, are that small mammals often have shorter limbs, a higher metabolic rate, higher fluid requirement, potential need for dextrose supplementation, and elevated doses to achieve the same level of effect.

Exotic companion animals have a higher risk with sedation and anesthesia as compared to domestic species. Rabbits have an increased risk of anesthetic death, even when healthy (1.39%). In rabbits that were systemically ill, that risk increased dramatically (7.37%), with almost half of those occurring during the anesthetic event.[10] Although this data is not available in other small mammalian subsets, anesthetic mortality rates exist. Ferrets (0.33%) are similar to canids (0.17%) and felids (0.24%), while other small mammals carry a high risk of anesthetic death (1.72%). In that same study, individual anesthetic mortality rates included: rats (2%), hamster (3.66%), chinchillas (3.29%), and guinea pigs (3.80%).[10] Steps should be taken to consider all potential outcomes and concerns in these patients when they present for critical illness, as their risk with sedation and/or anesthesia will be greatly increased. This should include the consideration of the advantages and disadvantages of drugs (**Table 2**).

SEDATION

When given alone to rabbits, alfaxalone IM may produce enough sedation to enable the placement of an intravenous catheter and allow for the induction of anesthesia. In healthy rabbits, 4 to 8 mg/kg produced about 30 to 60 minutes of sedation.[11] Both alfaxalone (2 mg/kg) and ketamine (5 mg/kg) have been evaluated in combination with butorphanol (1 mg/kg) and midazolam (1 mg/kg) for non-invasive procedures, with the alfaxalone protocol achieving longer sedation and the ketamine protocol being associated with reduced food intake following sedation.[12] Alfaxalone (6 mg/kg) has produced satisfactory sedation alone with synergistic effects and prolonged sedation when combined with butorphanol (0.3 mg/kg) or midazolam (1 mg/kg).[13] Rabbits have a good sedative effect from intranasal (IN) sedatives combining butorphanol (0.4 mg/kg), midazolam (2 mg/kg), and dexmedetomidine (0.1 mg/kg) with profound effect. Judicious monitoring of oxygenation and vital parameters recommended, as to hypotension, bradypnea, hypoxemia, and hypercapnia were noted in healthy rabbits.[14] Therefore, IN administration of this multimodal drug combination not recommended in critically ill small mammals. If intramuscular administration is not possible, IN administration of butorphanol and/or midazolam could be considered, avoiding the alpha-2 agonist due to the cardiovascular depressant effects.

Guinea pigs may also be sedated with alfaxalone 5 mg/kg IM for 30 minutes of sedation with no hypoxemia or hypothermia noted in healthy subjects.[15] Alfaxalone at higher doses (10–40 mg/kg) SC alone or combined with buprenorphine or midazolam produces sedation but not immobility for 35 to 120 minutes, though dysphoria was appreciated at recovery.[16,17] As a solo agent in healthy guinea pigs, ketamine 30 mg/kg and alfaxalone 5 mg/kg have been found to produce sedation IM.[18] In the author's experience, when a painful procedure is being anticipated, hydromorphone may be utilized with other sedatives (ketamine, midazolam) for sedation in guinea pigs. However, current studies available only elucidate the pharmacokinetics and do not directly assess for sedation or analgesia.[19] Ferrets administered alfaxalone at 5 mg/kg with butorphanol 0.2 mg/kg are sedated ~30 minutes but have mild transient hypotension and hypoxemia.[20]

As with any anesthetic, when administered alone or in combination with other sedatives, there is a risk of prolonged recovery or even loss of airway protection.[17] These effects are likely going to be more profound in critically ill subjects, and care should be taken when sedating less thrifty animals. Continuous monitoring should start as soon as sedation is administered.

Table 2
Summary of advantages and disadvantages of sedatives and anesthetics in small mammalian species

Drug Class	Routes of Administration	Advantages	Disadvantages	References
Benzodiazepines	IM, IV, IN, SC	Cardiovascularly sparing Reversible	Not a good sole sedative May cause dysphoria	Rabbit[13,14,24,29]
Opioids (butorphanol, nalbuphine, hydromorphone, buprenorphine)	IM, IV, SC	Safe Cardiovascularly sparing	Limited data on pharmacodynamics	Rabbit[13,14] Guinea pigs[18] Ferrets[20]
Alpha-2 agonists	IM, IV, IN, SC	Reversible	Reduction of cardiac output likely not tolerated in critically ill patients May be associated with hypotension, bradypnea, hypoxemia, and hypercapnia	Rabbit[14,24,28] Rats[7] Guinea pigs[15,31,32]
Neurosteroid (Alfaxalone)	IV, IO, IM, SC	Synergistic sedation when combined with other drugs Minimal apnea if titrated to effect slowly	Large volume Limited sedation period Not reversible May be associated with hypotension and hypoxemia May make intubatable at higher doses or with critical illness Dysphoria	Rabbit[11,13,25–28] Guinea pig[15–18] Ferret[20]
Cyclohexamines (Ketamine, Telazol)	IM, IV, SC	Short lived sedation Good co-induction agent for rabbits Less laryngospasm in rabbits Less cardiovascular and respiratory depressant effects MAC and MIR reducing	Reduced food uptake Inconsistent sedation alone Muscle stiffness if not given with relaxant	Rabbit[12,23,29,50] Guinea pig[18,31,32] Ferret[36]
Propofol	IV only	Reduce smooth muscle contraction in airway Short duration of action Can be used as TIVA	Requires high doses when used alone Apnea Negative ionotroph	Rabbit[21–23,50] Guinea pig[30] Ferret[24]

Abbreviations: IM, intramuscular; IN, intranasal; IV, intravenous; MAC, minimum alveolar concentration; MIR, minimum infusion rate; SC, subcutaneous; TIVA, total intravenous anesthesia.

ANESTHETIC INDUCTION

Once vascular access of obtained, induction with injectable anesthetics is possible. Various induction protocols have been evaluated in rabbits. Propofol has been investigated as a means of inducing anesthesia in rabbits, and both IV and IO routes of administration have been deemed acceptable in healthy animals.[21] In healthy rabbits for routine procedures, propofol has been utilized for the induction of anesthesia without significant complications.[22] However, rabbits, in particular, are prone to subclinical respiratory disease, which can be worsened by exposure to the hospital or the physiological stress of being ill or injured. Utilization of propofol alone in critically ill rabbits is not recommended due to the increased risk of apnea and the need for ventilatory support following the high dose requirement for intubation.

Utilization of co-induction agents, such as ketamine, has been associated with less apnea and more control during the intubation process.[23] Other induction combinations, such as medetomidine-propofol and medetomidine-propofol-midazolam have been evaluated in rabbits and both were safe and effective for the induction of anesthesia in healthy rabbits; however, caution should be exercised in the utilization of these protocols in ill rabbits, as these patients may not be able to tolerate the reduction in cardiac output induced by the administration of an alpha-2 agonist.[24] Alfaxalone administered IV (10 mg/kg) in premedicated rabbits developed clinically significant hypoxemia between two and 4 minutes after induction.[25] Caution is encouraged with the utilization of this as an induction agent in ill rabbits, as studies have shown periods of apnea over 20 minutes in premedicated rabbits given higher doses of alfaxalone.[26] When evaluated at lower doses (2–3 mg/kg) given slowly over 60 seconds, alfaxalone has been shown to be a safe an effective induction agent. Although apnea was noted in this study, it was for a much shorter time period (~45 seconds) and was minimized by adequate pre-oxygenation.[27] Alfaxalone-medetomidine at high doses IM causes the immobilization of wild caught rabbits.[28] Ketamine-midazolam has been associated with less laryngospasm and better maintenance of heart rate as compared to ketamine-medetomidine.[29] This is expected due to the skeletal muscle relaxant and cardiovascular sparing properties of benzodiazepines. Ketamine-midazolam may be reasonable for the induction of anesthesia in a critically ill rabbit.

In an ex-vivo model, propofol was found to reduce tracheal smooth muscle contraction in guinea pigs.[30] However, due to the risk of apnea and the inherent challenges associated with guinea pig intubation (see later in discussion), this is not recommended as a sole induction agent. Ketamine combined with other agents has been shown to have the least cardiovascular and respiratory depressant effects.[31,32] However, these combinations often include an alpha-2 agonist. Although these are reversible, there is still a high risk of cardiovascular depression with their use. For more critically ill patients, a combination of ketamine with a muscle relaxant, such as a benzodiazepine, is recommended.

Compared to other small mammals, ferrets present fewer challenges during the induction period. As has been shown in other species, propofol can act as a negative ionotrope in ferrets.[33] However, if administered slowly to effect, propofol has less of a risk of negative cardiovascular effects and apnea. Ketamine has also been associated with a negative ionotrophic effect in ferrets.[34] However, this is often overridden by the ketamine-induced catecholamine release that occurs with concurrent sympathetic nervous system stimulation.[35] In critically ill animals with the depletion of catecholamine stores, the negative ionotrophic effects may predominate. Ketamine should always be combined with a muscle relaxant, such as midazolam, to reduce muscle tension, tremors and paddling that is associated with ketamine as a sole induction agent.[36]

When possible, induction should be performed with injectable medications, as the amount of inhalant needed to intubate a patient causes significant cardiovascular compromise and unacceptable personnel exposure. Although it is possible to perform inhalant induction, this induction method leads to a physical struggle during the initial phase and a prolonged period of apnea, hypoxemia, hypercapnia, and bradycardia.[37] Therefore, this method is not recommended for utilization in the already ill companion exotic patient.

OROTRACHEAL INTUBATION

Rabbits are challenging to intubate. Some clinicians advocate for a blind intubation technique with a capnograph attachment to the ETT to allow for the confirmation of appropriate intubation, but this method is prone to failure and oropharyngeal trauma. Direct visualization of the rima glottidis can often be difficult, so the utilization of a stylet or scope has been described, with the addition of topical lidocaine to reduce laryngospasm.[38] Rabbits have been managed with cuffed or non-cuffed ETT, and supraglottic airway devices (SGAD).[39] A particular SGAD, the V-gel, has been formulated for utilization in rabbits and allows for assisted ventilation in rabbits without the need to endotracheally intubate. This is associated with less laryngeal trauma.[40] In comparison studies, SGAD placement is faster with less mucosal damage as compared to traditional ETT placement, though the SGAD sealed the airway less.[41] Guinea pigs require scope assistance to allow for endotracheal intubation, as they have a narrow oral commissure and a small airway opening.[42–44] They also store food in their cheek pouches, which can make them prone to aspiration and upper airway obstruction. Cotton-tipped applicators (CTA) can gently scoop retained food particles out of the oropharyngeal region to reduce this risk. Additionally, guinea pigs are prone to oropharyngeal trauma causing hemorrhage due to increased vasculature in the area and the narrow opening created by the palatal ostium, as well as regurgitation with laryngeal stimulation. Care should be taken to minimize trauma to the oropharynx in guinea pigs. For smaller patients, an over-the-needle catheter can be utilized as an ETT if fitted with an appropriate wye piece adapter. Care should be taken to support the patient and the catheter to minimize the risk of extubation and kinking, which could result in subsequent airway obstruction. In the author's experience, a tongue depressor can be used to support the ETT and the patient, allowing for the movement of the patient with the ETT as a single unit (see **Fig. 3**D). At times, it may be beneficial to avoid intubation. In these instances, the utilization of a tight-fitting face mask made specifically for rodents may be utilized (see **Fig. 3**C). Provided that the patient maintains spontaneous ventilation, this may be utilized to maintain anesthesia with volatile anesthetics for more invasive procedures. The biggest drawback is the patient cannot be ventilated and the airway is not protected.

The intubation process for ferrets is very similar to dogs and cats. Their head is very conical in shape, making it difficult to tie behind the ears or over the muzzle to secure the ETT. With ferrets, as well as guinea pigs, hedgehogs, and other conically shaped head patients, it is recommended to secure the ETT by suturing a piece of tape around the ETT and then suturing to the lip of the patient (**Fig. 4**). This will help to reduce the risk of accidental extubation, which could be detrimental and results in arrest if unable to re-intubate during a surgical procedure.

ANESTHETIC MAINTENANCE AND MONITORING

Volatile anesthetics, such as isoflurane or sevoflurane can be used. With a rebreathing circuit, sevoflurane may be preferred due to the physiochemical properties that hasten

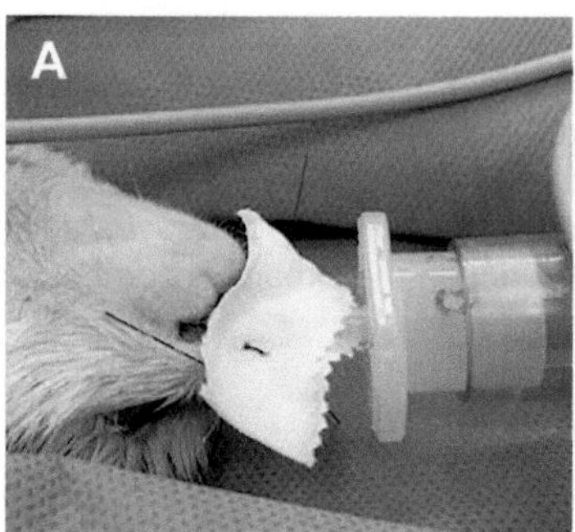

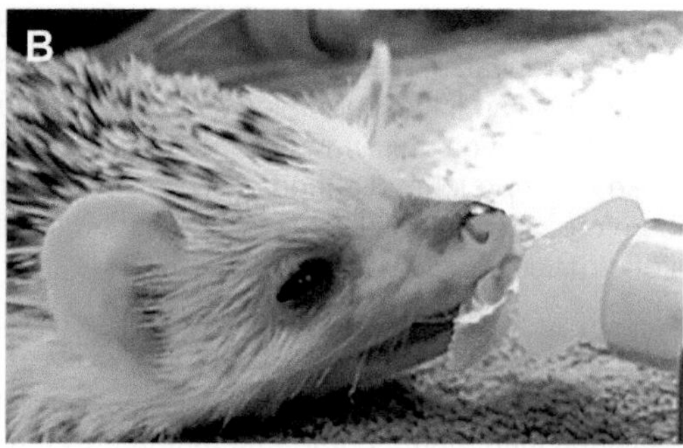

Fig. 4. Sutured endotracheal tube placement in a hedgehog.

recovery.[45] However, less commonly utilized inhalants, such as desflurane, may have an even more rapid recovery and cause less ventilator-induced lung injury in rats.[37,46] Desflurane is also protective against ischemic injury to the myocardium.[47] However, this volatile anesthetic requires a power source to maintain the vaporizer at a constant temperature, making it less commonly utilized[48] Sevoflurane has been associated with less reperfusion injury to the myocardium as compared to propofol total intravenous anesthesia (TIVA).[49] Although this study only looked at perfusion of the myocardium, inferences may be made to maintained perfusion to other tissues in the body. This may become more important for patients that are already hypoperfused prior to the induction of anesthesia. Although TIVA is sometimes preferred in patients that are already cardiovascularly unstable, sole propofol infusions require a very high dose (0.8 mg/kg/min).[50] Ketamine-dexmedetomidine has been utilized for maintenance of a surgical plane of anesthesia in healthy rabbits, and this could be a consideration of rabbits that are cardiovascularly stable but needing invasive airway diagnostics or procedures.[38]

As with all anesthetized patients, minimizing inhalant reduces the risk of negative sequelae. The minimum alveolar concentration (MAC) of volatile anesthetics is well conserved across species and gives a starting point for a vaporizer setting. However, we frequently utilize MAC reducing drugs to reduced inhalant requirements. Utilization constant rate infusions (CRI) may spare the critically ill small mammal from as significant hypoventilation, hypotension, and other complications. Reduction in maintenance amounts of injectable anesthetics for TIVA can be obtained through the addition of ketamine.[50]

SUPPORTIVE CARE

Judicious monitoring is imperative to minimize increased morbidity and mortality in critically ill small mammals. Their clinical status can change rapidly, requiring prompt intervention with hypoventilation, hypoxemia, bradycardia, and hypotension. Fluid resuscitation of hypovolemic patients may be required to restore adequate circulating volume and improve tissue perfusion. Increments of 5 to 10 mL/kg administered as a bolus allow for the assessment of response to fluid therapy while hopefully minimizing the risk of volume overload. Maintenance of circulating volume under general anesthesia is typically 5 to 10 mL/kg/h and may need to be adjusted based on hydration status. In a euhydrated small mammal in hypovolemic shock hypertonic saline (2–4 mL/kg) may facilitate lower volume resuscitation. Dextrose supplementation (1%–5%) is often required to maintain normoglycemia, depending on the species and their normal blood glucose level. Active warming is vitally important in the maintenance of body temperature in small mammals, and typically numerous modalities are necessary.

ANESTHETIC COMPLICATIONS

It is common to encounter complications during an anesthetic episode, which often relate to poor tissue perfusion and/or oxygenation. Small mammals typically have a higher heart rate than dogs and cats, and they rely more on this for their cardiac output. Therefore, bradycardia is often treated with anticholinergics. Although atropine is the most rapid acting and useful in an emergency, glycopyrrolate will have a more prolonged effect and may reduce the need for repeated dosing. Up to 60% of rabbits have endogenous atropinesterases that inactivate atropine, so for heart rate support, glycopyrrolate should be preferentially utilized in rabbits.[51] Hypotension despite the treatment of bradycardia is also a common occurrence in small mammalian anesthesia. Due to drug availability, dopamine is often a first-line vasopressor for the treatment of inhalant induced hypotension. However, rabbits are unique in this regard as well, having no response to dopamine in the face of inhalant-induced hypotension. Norepinephrine is the vasopressor of choice for the treatment of hypotension during anesthesia in rabbits, though high-dose phenylephrine may also work.[52,53]

RECOVERY

Continuation of heat support during the recovery period is important, as patients that become hypothermic will have a prolonged recovery. Hypothermia reduces immune responses within tissues, which can predispose a debilitated patient to post-anesthetic complications. During the recovery period, the reversal of sedative agents may hasten recovery. If the endotracheal tube is secured with suture, ensure that these have been clipped to allow for easy extubation when the patient is ready. If vasopressor support was necessary during the anesthetic episode, continue to tailoring it to optimize blood pressure and heart rate. This may need to be continued in the post-operative period in the intensive care unit. Diligence of monitoring in the first 24 to 48 hours after anesthesia is crucial to continuing the supportive management of critically ill small mammals.

AVIAN SPECIES

Introduction

Birds are a very diverse group of patients that vary greatly in size and anatomical features. Compared to similarly sized mammals, they have a large heart with a Type 2B Purkinje system, meaning that the conduction fibers penetrate the ventricular endocardium and epicardium. Due to this, the S wave can have a bigger deflection and should not be confused with ventricular tachycardia.[54] Birds have several cardiovascular adaptations, including a large stroke volume and cardiac output, dense autonomic fibers within the cardiac muscle, and higher blood pressure (mean arterial pressure up to 150 mm Hg). They have numerous unique respiratory adaptations that must be taken into consideration, especially when injury has occurred. There are numerous pneumatic bones, including the vertebrae, ribs, sternum, humerus, pelvis, and femur. If these become injured, then ventilation and oxygenation could be altered. The utilization of IO catheters allows access to the vascular compartment; however, pneumatic bones should never be utilized for an IO catheter. The air exchange in birds is extremely efficient, in part due to the resistance within the air sacs. They have unidirectional flow that moves through three orders of branching of the airways, and a single respiratory cycle is completed with two breaths.[55,56]

Due to their higher metabolic rate, fasting is often minimized to maintain their blood glucose. However, this makes them more prone to still having material within the crop or proximal gastrointestinal system, increasing the risk of aspiration. In birds that are more critically ill, they may have been inappetent for longer than a few hours or may have become injured shortly after a meal. Due to this, the airway should be protected after anesthetic induction. Additionally, monitoring of blood sugar and maintenance of normoglycemia is imperative for metabolic and anesthetic stability.

Avian species are very prone to negative sequelae that often is potentiated by stress.[57,58] Among arrested birds in a tertiary hospital, sedation and anesthesia comprised 3.4% of deaths, with an additional 4.3% arresting post anesthesia.[59] Smaller birds in particular, such as Budgerigars, are more prone to sedation and peri-anesthetic death (16.33%), while other birds collectively have a lower mortality rate (1.76%).[10] Therefore, every effort should be made to prepare all equipment ahead of time and anticipate potential complications so that intervention may be swift. A summary of the advantages and disadvantages of drugs is found later in discussion (**Table 3**).

Sedation

For the initial sedation of avian species, butorphanol (1–2 mg/kg) and/or midazolam (1–2 mg/kg) are frequently utilized due to the good sedative results with presumed minimal cardiovascular effects. The combination of butorphanol and midazolam in healthy psittacine birds is safe and effective.[60] However, in patients that are critically ill, these benefits may be less apparent, as the author has seen the progression of bradyarrhythmias when one or both drugs are given to birds for pre-anesthetic sedation. Sedation with butorphanol at least 10 minutes prior to the induction of anesthesia is recommended, as it reduces that excitatory phase of inhalant anesthetic induction.[61] As an alternative to IM injections, both butorphanol and midazolam can be given IN.[62] In birds that are injured and painful, more energetic, or more dangerous, ketamine (5–10 mg/kg) may be added to aid in sedation, reduce the stress of birds caused by handling, and reduce the amount of inhalant necessary to induce anesthesia in birds.[63] This may be beneficial in more critically ill or injure birds, where the vasodilatory and respiratory depressant effects of inhalants may be detrimental.

Alfaxalone has also been investigated for administration IM in various species, with lower doses being associated with inadequate sedation and high doses being associated with respiratory arrest.[64] As compared to butorphanol-midazolam, alfaxalone alone has been shown to provide more consistent sedation when given IM.[65] Compared to manual restraint, alfaxalone IM sedation has been associated with lower circulating lactate levels and may be a viable alternative to the administration of inhalants for non-invasive procedures.[66] When premedicated with IN butorphanol-midazolam, low doses of alfaxalone IM have allowed for the intubation of birds as well, but may predispose them to hypothermia.[62,67] Additionally, small birds given higher SC doses alone or combined with other premedication experience prolonged sedation.[68] Perceived hyperexcitation in the form of muscle tremors has also been noted in birds given IM alfaxalone, which is improved when combined with midazolam.[69] However, in the author's experience, these drugs can cause precipitate formation and should therefore be given as two separate injections. Combinations of ketamine and alfaxalone have also been investigated, resulting in consistent sedation with moderate excitation present at induction.[70] The risk of apnea would be greater in debilitated patients, so careful choice of dose is recommended when considering alfaxalone as a sedative in critically ill birds. With the increased risk of apnea with alfaxalone, the author tends to choose to add ketamine as discussed above to allow for immobilization while also maintaining ventilatory drive.

Table 3
Summary of advantages and disadvantages of sedatives and anesthetics in avian species

Drug Class	Routes of Administration	Advantages	Disadvantages	References
Benzodiazepines	IM, IV, IN	Safe and effective Synergistic with opioids Reversible MAC reducing	May not be adequate sedation as a sole agent	Psittacines[60,62]
Opioids (butorphanol)	IM, IV, IN	Safe and effective Synergistic with benzodiazepines Reversible MAC reducing May provide some analgesia	May not be adequate sedation as a sole agent	Psittacines[60–62]
Alpha-2 agonists	IM, IV	Reversible	Induces bradycardia which is not well tolerated in small or critically ill birds	
Neurosteroid (Alfaxalone)	IM, SC, IV	Consistent sedation at moderate doses alone compared Reduced anaerobic circulation compared to manual restraint Can be used as IM induction drug MAC reducing Lower risk of apnea when titrated to effect Quick smooth induction when given IV	Low doses alone inadequate for sedation Higher doses given rapidly associated with apnea and cardiovascular depression More prone to hypothermia Not reversible	Psittacines[62,64–68] Chicken[80]
Cyclohexamines (Ketamine, Telazol)	IM, IV	Reduces stress of handling Wide safety margin Synergistic with other premedication	Not reversible Acidic pH (burns with injection)	Psittacines[63,73–75]
Propofol	IV only	Low cost Can be used for TIVA	Transient apnea Provides no analgesia	Chicken/Turkey[76,78] Swan[77]

Abbreviations: IM, intramuscular; IV, intravenous; IN, intranasal; SC, subcutaneous; TIVA, total intravenous anesthesia.

Anesthetic Induction

Unlike in mammalian species, where inhalant induction is a stressful process associated with increased catecholamine release and patient distress, the efficient respiratory system of avians makes mask volatile inhalant induction more appropriate for birds, even when injured.[71] Administration of premedication improves induction quality and reduces the amount of inhalant necessary to allow for intubation.[60] Although both isoflurane and sevoflurane can be utilized to induce anesthesia in avian species, the quality of induction and time for induction and recovery are more favorable with sevoflurane.[61] Therefore, it is recommended to utilize sevoflurane, if available, for ill or injured birds requiring general anesthesia. Unfortunately, pre-oxygenation does not alter the time between apnea and desaturation, which occurs after approximately 25 seconds.[72] Since birds are not tolerant of apnea, ventilatory support should be initiated as soon as possible following anesthetic induction.

As an alternative to inhalant induction, ketamine may be given as part of an induction protocol.[73] In the author's experience a very protective and/or painful bird that requires initial immobilization with injectable medications, such as ketamine, may have a higher drug requirement, regardless of health status. Much higher doses of ketamine have been evaluated in some species and have been found to be safe administered to healthy birds IO or IM.[74] Due to its high safety index, ketamine is a reasonable option for these remote immobilizations but may be associated with prolonged recoveries. Tiletamine-zolazepam combinations have also been utilized in these scenarios.[75] Propofol has also been evaluated in chickens as an induction agent, requiring much higher doses (5–9 mg/kg) than in mammalian counterparts.[76–78] However, transient apnea is a higher risk with this agent administration.[78] Alfaxalone has also been evaluated in some birds as an IV induction agent. Alfaxalone is associated with smoother and quicker induction than inhalant and is MAC reducing.[79] At lower doses and when titrated to effect, minimal respiratory depression has been noted.[80] However, when given at higher doses more rapidly, its use has been associated with more cardiorespiratory depression in healthy birds.[67,79] Therefore, caution and careful titration to effect is recommended in birds that are debilitated.

Orotracheal Intubation

Intubation of these species is simple, as they do not have an epiglottis. Birds have complete tracheal rings, so an uncuffed or Cole ETT should be utilized, securing it with tape attached circumferentially within the oral cavity and around the beak. If orotracheal intubation is not possible due to the presence of a mass, upper airway obstruction, or trauma that restricts access to the rima glottidis, then an air sac may be surgically cannulated to provide oxygen and ventilation.[81]

Anesthetic Maintenance and Monitoring

Anesthesia is typically maintained with volatile anesthetics delivered in oxygen. Sevoflurane is commonly utilized for the maintenance of anesthesia in birds. Although MAC is presumed to be fairly conserved between species, there has been some variation reported in avian species. The maintenance of anesthesia with inhalants has been shown to have similar effects as in other animals, such as hypotension and hypoventilation despite increased respiratory rate.[82] Isoflurane may also be utilized, though MAC also varies by type of bird.[83] Inhalants may be reduced through the utilization of CRI and other techniques. In some species, TIVA is a viable option for maintaining anesthesia in birds. Propofol (0.5–1.2 mg/kg/h) has been utilized in chickens to maintain a surgical plane of anesthesia when combined with analgesics.[76,77] More investigation into the potential utilization for TIVA in birds is needed before the recommendation of this modality.

Most birds will require assisted ventilation with minimal distension of the respiratory system during an anesthetic event, as the method of airway exchange with the capillary is very efficient.[84] Many anesthetists will utilize a pressure limited ventilator to avoid overdistension of the parabronchi. With lower pressures (~5 cm water), there is less reduction of venous return, though cardiovascular depression can still occur.[85,86] Care should be taken when ventilating any critically ill bird, as their cardiac reserve may be diminished. Additionally, it should be expected that if the integrity of the air sac is compromised that oxygenation and ventilation may be diminished, requiring intermittent manual closure of the air sacs to allow for ventilation and minimize the risk of desaturation.[72,85]

Monitoring should be performed utilizing a combination of Doppler, ECG, capnography, pulse oximetry, and core body temperature. Especially in critically ill patients, close monitoring of these parameters as well as blood glucose levels is recommended to ensure the optimization of care. If the cloaca needs to be evaluated under sedation or anesthesia, this should be done prior to the placement of the temperature probe, as this may cause superficial iatrogenic trauma to the area.

Supportive Care

Avian species have a higher body temperature than mammals, and in order to maintain this, multiple environmental heating devices should be utilized to minimize the risk of complications that can increase mortality.[87] This may include heated tables, forced-air heating units, and overhead convection heat sources. Intravenous fluids should be administered, typically at 5 to 10 mL/kg/h, and dextrose supplementation should be provided to maintain blood glucose within normal ranges for that species of bird (typically 200–400 mg/dL).

Anesthetic Complications

In the author's experience, sick birds are much more prone to bradyarrhythmias than their healthy counterparts. Although anticholinergics, such as atropine, may increase the viscosity of respiratory secretions in birds, administration is often necessary to prevent cardiac arrest.[88] In patients that have a high vagal tone, such as with yolk peritonitis, bradyarrhythmias may occur prior to sedation or anesthesia. Often, these pathological bradyarrhythmias may not be responsive to atropine and likely will progress with sedation or induction of anesthesia. Profound atrioventricular block with escape beats in a bird (**Fig. 5**) should not be confused with ventricular tachycardia. Even if critically ill birds are not bradycardic prior to induction, acute bradyarrhythmias may occur during the procedure due to vagal stimulation, requiring temporary cessation of the stimulus and administration of atropine. If ventricular tachycardia does occur, it can be treated with lidocaine given IV as a bolus and then CRI.

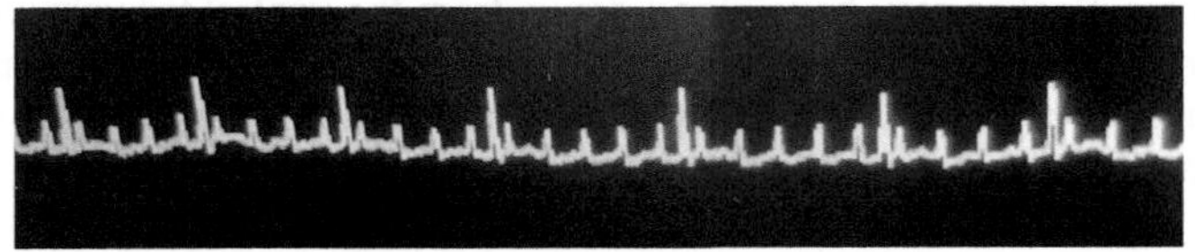

Fig. 5. Third degree atrioventricular block in a 19-year-old Eclectus parrot with severe yolk peritonitis that was not responsive to atropine. The ventricular rate was 80 to 90 bpm while the atrial rate was 350 bpm.

Evidence of hemorrhage should be monitored closely during anesthesia, including blood lost through intravenous catheter placement, phlebotomy, and surgical manipulation. If a patient becomes clinical for blood loss (tachycardic, hypotensive), hypertonic saline (2–4 mL/kg) can be administered over 10 to 20 minutes to aid in volume resuscitation of a euhydrated patient. If excessive hemorrhage occurs, blood can be obtained from a donor (often a chicken) to administer. Discussion of blood transfusions is beyond the scope of this article, however.

Due to the inherent greater risk of avian species to experience peri-anesthetic death, it is important to pre-calculate emergency drug doses.[10] In preparation for catastrophic complications, doses of atropine and epinephrine should be drawn up prior to the initiation of anesthesia to minimize lag time between complication and intervention. Early initiation of cardiopulmonary resuscitation efforts is recommended. Although the return of spontaneous circulation is rare, there is a higher likelihood of success with early intervention during the perianesthetic episode.[89]

Recovery

Following inhalant anesthesia, recovery typically occurs within a few minutes, even when kept at surgical planes.[61,82] Due to the rapid nature of recovery, the ETT should be untaped once inhalant anesthetics are discontinued to facilitate quick and atraumatic extubation. The anesthetist should maintain the bird on oxygen supplementation until extubation, then provide oxygen flow by via face mask until the bird can be safely transferred to ICU for continued monitoring in the post operative period. Reversal of the benzodiazepine may be considered with flumazenil if recovery is delayed. Heat support should be continued throughout the recovery period, as well as fluid therapy ± dextrose supplementation.

REPTILIAN SPECIES

Introduction

As with all exotic companion animals, there are numerous alterations in normal physiology in reptiles as compared to other species. One of the biggest differences is the lower metabolic rate (as low as one-tenth of mammals), and their metabolic rate is tightly linked to their body temperature.[90] The cardiovascular system has many differences. The heart is comprised of three chambers (except for crocodilians), with the ventricles separated by a muscular ridge that changes shape with sympathetic tone.[91] Reptiles also have a renal and hepatic portal systems that take blood from the caudal half of the body through the liver and kidneys prior to entry into systemic circulation, so IM injections should always be given in the cranial half of the body, if feasible.[92,93]

Venous access is much more challenging in reptiles, and sites depend heavily on the animal being worked with. Chelonians can have jugular catheters placed after sedation.[94] If vascular access is critical and a jugular catheter is not feasible, an intraosseous catheter in the bridge of the shell could be a potential location for an intraosseous catheter. Snakes may have blood drawn from the ventral tail vein with manual restraint or palatine vein and heart if anesthetized. Although vascular access is limited in these species, cardiac puncture may result in tamponade and death.[95] In debilitated snakes, cardiac puncture for diagnostic purposes is not recommended, as it may contribute to their demise. An alternative vascular access point in lizards is the placement of an IO catheter. Although this is not recommended for prolonged therapy and carries an elevated risk of limb fracture, an IO catheter allows for temporary vascular access to aid in the resuscitation and treatment of critically ill lizards.

Similar to birds, the respiratory system of reptiles differs significantly from the more "default" mammalian system most practitioners are more familiar with. Air flow in reptiles may also be unidirectional, as in birds, and provide some benefit to these patients that have a low metabolic rate.[96,97] Many have complete tracheal rings and lack an epiglottis. Reptiles also lack a diaphragm, creating a single coelomic cavity instead of a thoracic and abdominal cavity. Reptiles also have different responses to respiratory depression, including less robust responses to hypoxemia, varying degrees of hypoxic pulmonary vasoconstriction, and increased ventilation with hypercapnia.[98,99] Chelonians ventilate through the movement of their limbs, so assisted ventilation is necessary in these species once anesthetized. Snakes have a lower surface area of lung, having only one effective lung.

Due to the anatomical and physiologic challenges noted above with obtaining vascular access to reptiles, sedating reptiles frequently causes anesthetic induction. Sedation and anesthesia carry a higher risk for reptiles (1.49%) than dogs and cats, but they fair better than birds and small mammals.[10] Reptiles are often deemed sedated when they lose the righting reflex, but the level of sedation necessary for a given patient may in part be related to human safety concerns. A chameleon or bearded dragon may require less heavy sedation to safely handle them, while a tegu or water monitor lizard may need stronger immobilization to limit harm to themselves or to personnel. A summary of the advantages and disadvantages of drugs is found later in discussion (**Table 4**).

Sedation and anesthetic induction

Each type of reptile appears to have a different reaction to sedation, including the onset of sedation, length of sedation, side effects, and recovery. This depends on drug choice, route of administration, and dose administered. When working with a debilitated reptile, the anesthetist should consider pros and cons of each drug choice, being thoughtful to choose drugs with limited cardiorespiratory depressant effects and with predictable recovery periods. Reversibility of drugs may also improve outcome. Midazolam has been utilized as a sedative in leopard geckos and ball pythons.[100,101] The reader is cautioned in using midazolam alone in wild caught reptiles, as dysphoria may be noted, making the patients more difficult to handle. Midazolam has been combined with alfaxalone or dexmedetomidine in healthy ball pythons for successful sedation.[101] However, as with other protocols involving alpha-2 agonists that have been discussed, utilization of these sedation protocols has been in healthy individuals, and the effects of the same protocols on debilitated patients may not be tolerated. In red eared sliders, alfaxalone (10–20 mg/kg) given alone IM causes inconsistent sedation that is better at higher doses, with heart rate increasing over time.[102] However, their body temperature also increased during this time, which could increase the metabolism of the drug.

In another study with galliwasps, alfaxalone (15 mg/kg) caused acceptable sedation with a mild decrease in heart rate over time, whereas ketamine (40 mg/kg) was associated with unpredictable and short-lived sedation.[102,103] Ketamine has been utilized at higher doses for the induction of anesthesia in healthy lizards, when combined with other sedatives, including hydromorphone, which produced synergistic sedation.[104–106] When evaluating various drug combinations with ketamine, ketamine-diazepam had the fastest onset time of anesthesia in pond turtles.[107] Any of these effects are going to be made more profound in critically ill reptiles. In the author's experience, a combination of alfaxalone (10–20 mg/kg) and midazolam (1–2 mg/kg) provides good sedation for monitoring the instrumentation of debilitated reptiles, initial non-invasive diagnostics, and intravenous catheter placement, often allowing for

Table 4
Reptilian sedation and anesthesia

Drug Class	Route of Administration	Advantages	Disadvantages	Study Examples
Benzodiazepines	IV, IM, SC, IC	May be used as a sole sedative, especially in young or debilitated patients Reversible Fast onset sedation in turtles when combined with ketamine	Dysphoria/excitability in wild or aggressive animals	Lizards[100] Snakes[101] Chelonians[107,111]
Opioids (hydromorphone)	IV, IM, IC	Synergistic sedation with ketamine		Lizards[106]
Alpha-2 agonists	IV, IM, SC, IC	Synergistic sedation with other agents	Reduced heart rate and cardiac output	Snake[101]
Neurosteroid (Alfaxalone)	IV, IM, SC, IC	Synergistic sedation with other agents With high dose IV bolus, tachycardia Can be used for TIVA	Inconsistent sedation as a sole agent Higher doses associated with prolonged recovery Dose dependent respiratory depression Transient hypertension (2 min)	Snake[101,108,109,113] Lizards[103] Chelonians[102,112]
Cyclohexamines (Ketamine, Telazol)	IV, IM, IC	Synergistic sedation when combined with other agents	Unpredictable short-lived sedation as a sole agent	Lizard[103–106]
Propofol	IV only	No alteration of mean arterial **blood pressure** **Tachycardia**		Snake[113]

Abbreviation: IM, intramuscular; IV, intravenous; SC, subcutaneous; IC, intracoelomic; TIVA, total intravenous anesthesia.

intubation. Alfaxalone has also been evaluated at various doses given IM to corn snakes, with higher doses being associated with a longer sedation period and prolonged recovery.[108] For painful reptiles, hydromorphone (0.1 mg/kg), and ketamine (5–10 mg/kg) may be added and for more fractious patients.

Intracoelomic administration of anesthetics may produce adequate sedation in some snakes.[109,110] Hatchling turtles have been anesthetized with IV administration of midazolam for diagnostic procedures.[111] If IV access has already been obtained, then alfaxalone can be used to induce anesthesia. In loggerhead turtles, there appears to be a dose-dependent respiratory depression, which is similar to other species.[112] Alfaxalone (15 mg/kg) and propofol (15 mg/kg) induce anesthesia in rattlesnakes, both causing an increase in heart rate with sedative effects for about 30 minutes. Alfaxalone was associated with a transient hypertension and apnea in 70% of rattlesnakes given a high IV dose.[109,113] By utilizing injectable anesthetics, the potential for inhalant anesthetic overdose, excitatory phase of induction, and personnel exposure can all be limited.

Inhalant anesthetics can induce anesthesia in reptiles as well.[114] However, this requires much more time for induction than in birds and most reptile patients cannot be handled safely until they are fully anesthetized, which predisposes them to anesthetic overdose.[115] Inhalants cause vasodilation and progressive shunting, leading to ventilation-perfusion derangements that can further prolong recovery from inhalant anesthetics.[116] Both isoflurane and sevoflurane have been evaluated, but when greater than 80% shunting is present, the benefit of utilization of sevoflurane is diminished.[117]

Reptiles should only have non-cuffed ETT utilized. In most reptilian species, intubation is easy due to the unobstructed view of the rima glottidis. However, species variation exists, and some reptiles may have adaptive structures for communication, such as the keeled epiglottis of the pine snake (**Fig. 6**).[118] This may require a smaller than anticipated ETT to be chosen. The ETT can be secured to the head with tape around the jaw, similar to securing an ETT in birds.

Anesthetic Maintenance and Monitoring

Historically, volatile anesthetics have been utilized for the maintenance of general anesthesia in reptiles. However, this method requires hyperventilation to maintain

A

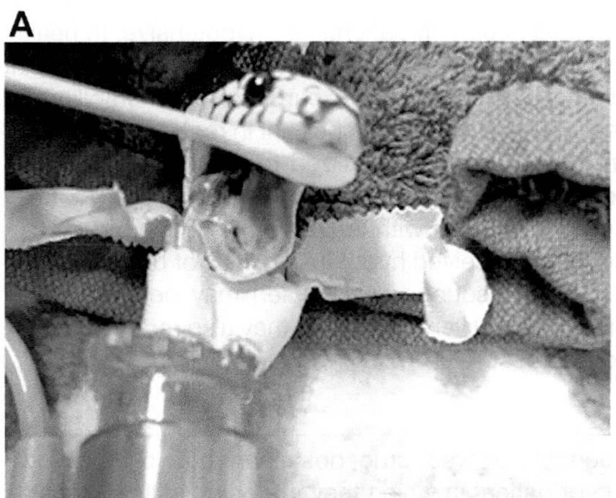

B

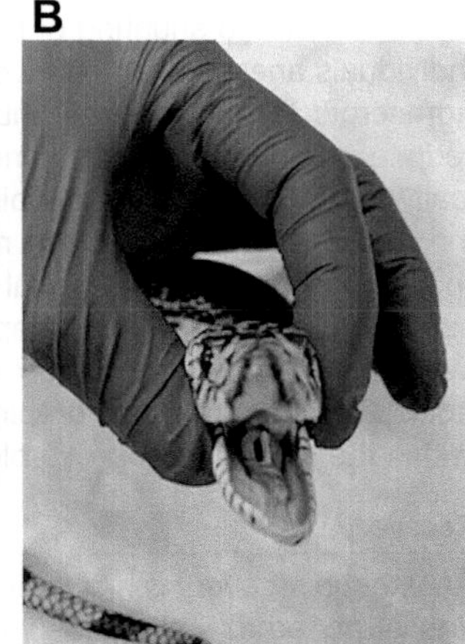

Fig. 6. Comparison of rima glottidis on a typical snake (*A*) and a pine snake that has a keeled epiglottis (*B*).

anesthetic depth in addition to the delivery of inhalant in oxygen as a carrier gas, which reduces the ventilatory drive in reptiles.[66] Recent investigations into total intravenous anesthesia utilizing alfaxalone as an infusion have been evaluated by the author, though to date are not published. Reptiles, including chelonians and lizards, have been anesthetized with alfaxalone TIVA for invasive surgical procedures, requiring less ventilation and therefore allowing for normocapnia.

Monitoring of reptiles is similar to other species. A Doppler probe can be placed over the heart on the ventral aspect of the patient, or it may be placed in the oral cavity with the crystal facing the palate. For chelonians, a special adapter (see **Fig. 1**D) can be directed toward the heart at the level of the pectoral muscles. Although traditional ECG is challenging, esophageal ECG probes (see **Fig. 2**C) can be connected to multiparameter models and allow for heart rate and rhythm monitoring in these patients. Mainstream capnography can be utilized to monitor ventilation. With a low metabolic rate, respiratory rates as low as one breath every 3 minutes may be all that is necessary to maintain normocapnia. When utilizing inhalants, higher respiratory rates are necessary to maintain adequate anesthetic depth. Due to the low surface area of the lung of snake, care should be taken to not over distend these patients, utilizing lower peak inspiratory pressures.

Supportive Care

The route of administration of fluid therapy will depend on if IV access has been obtained and the hydration status of the patient. If there is no IV access, then subcutaneous administration may be considered. Previous recommendations for Reptile Ringers solutions are now being determined as unfounded.[119] In reptiles that are hypovolemic, resuscitation with a balanced crystalloid may be a better option to restore acid-base and electrolyte imbalances.[120]

Hypothermia has been associated with reduced response to ventilatory changes, acid-base status, and oxygen consumption in some reptiles, so maintenance of appropriate body temperature for a given species is recommended.[121] Metabolic and heart rate increase as temperature increases, so maintenance of normal temperature aids in reducing other complications.

Anesthetic Complications

Due to the lack of separation between the ventricles in the three chambered heart, reptiles are prone to shunting of blood, especially if patients are hypotensive. In healthy individuals anesthetized with volatile anesthetics, interventions gauged at increasing adrenergic tone to reduce shunting of blood improve cardiovascular stability and reduce anesthesia recovery times. This is even more important in reptiles that are critically ill. Both atropine and epinephrine have been utilized to hasten recovery from inhalant anesthetics in some reptiles.[122–124] However, this does not appear to be the case with snakes (personal communication with S. Divers). Although blood pressure is difficult to evaluate in reptilians, perceived hypotension (lack of bleeding of tissue when cut, poor cardiac contraction sounds on Doppler) may be treated with epinephrine or atropine. Norepinephrine (delivered as a CRI) may also reduce shunting within the heart and improve blood pressure.[125]

Recovery

Anesthetic recovery is highly dependent on what drug, dose, and route of administration is utilized as well as the type of patient in which they are being utilized. Inhalant anesthetic use is associated with prolonged recoveries, greater than 200 minutes in snapping turtles; the administration of epinephrine or electrical stimulation at GV-26 being associated with quicker recovery times.[122] When volatile anesthetics are used, the administration of IM epinephrine has been shown to hasten recovery times in loggerhead turtles.[124] Similarly, the administration of epinephrine to alligators has been shown to make anesthetic recovery more rapid.[123] Atropine has also been utilized to eliminate shunting in tortoises under inhalant anesthesia, allowing for lower isoflurane administration amounts and potentially improve recovery.[64]

With injectable anesthetics, loggerhead turtles given only intravenous alfaxalone recover in 30 to 90 minutes, depending on the dose utilized.[112] Terrapins can have a prolonged recovery of up to 126 minutes with IM alfaxalone, while IV administration of a single bolus is associated with shorter time to recovery (29–45 minutes).[126] Galliwasps given 5 mg/kg IV may take over 70 minutes to recover. Given IV in the same species, 15 mg/kg causes predictable short recovery.[102,103] Ketamine (40 mg/kg), on the other hand, has been associated with prolonged recovery, when used as a sole agent.[103] Higher doses of ketamine-diazepam in pond turtles have hastened recoveries, though a gender bias appeared to exist with males recovering faster than females.[107] Alfaxalone TIVA has been associated with predictable recovery times, quicker than seen with inhalant anesthetic episodes in reptiles. Long-acting dissociatives, such as tiletamine-zolazepam, are not recommended for use in reptiles due to profoundly prolonged recovery times. In the author's experience, a snapping turtle administered tiletamine-zolazepam prior to referral for an upper gastrointestinal scope took 5 days to recover normal ambulation, requiring heat support and hydration maintenance with intravenous fluids until it was able to voluntarily move and ingest food again. Recovery can be hastened through the utilization of reversal agents, such as flumazenil for benzodiazepines, where available, though resedation has been noted in some instances.[127,128]

Future Directions

As more owners are expecting supportive care of their exotic animals when they become sick or injured, the veterinarian is faced with the realization that a single

Table 5
Example sedation protocols for various exotic companion animals

Species	Drug combination	Dose	Things to watch for
Small mammals	Butorphanol	2 mg/kg IM	
	Midazolam	2 mg/kg IM	
	+/− Ketamine	5 mg/kg IM	May make patient intubatable
	+/− Alfaxalone	1–2 mg/kg IM	May make patient intubatable, myoclonus
Birds	Butorphanol	2 mg/kg IM	
	Midazolam	2 mg/kg IM	
	+/− Ketamine	5–10 mg/kg IM	May make patient intubatable
Reptiles	Midazolam	1–2 mg/kg IM	Dysphoria when given alone in healthy wildlife
	Alfaxalone	10–20 mg/kg IM	May take 60–80 min post injection for reusability, paddling/tremors when given as sole agent
	+/− Hydromorphone	0.1 mg/kg IM	Synergistic sedation
	+/−Ketamine	5–10 mg/kg IM	May make patient intubatable

These are example protocols and may not be safe for all patients; appropriate knowledge of the drug, dose, patient type, and patient health status are necessary when utilizing any anesthetic agents.

Table 6
Example anesthetic protocols for various exotic companion animals

Species	Premedication	Induction	Maintenance	Special Tips
Small rodents	Midazolam 1–2 mg/kg IM	If IVC in place: • Ketamine 5 mg/kg IV • ± Alfaxalone 2 mg/kg IV titrated to effect	Volatile anesthetic (choose one) • Isoflurane • Sevoflurane	Prone to bradycardia and arrest
	Opioid (choose one) • Butorphanol 1–2 mg/kg IM • Hydromorphone 0.2–0.3 mg/kg IM	If no IVC in place: • Tight fitting mask induction with Sevoflurane 5% in oxygen until relaxation • Then can maintain with flow by Inhalant titrating to effect or attempt intubation	MAC reduction • Lidocaine 2 mg/kg then 3–6 mg/kg/h • Local anesthesia as appropriate (2–4 mg/kg lidocaine)	Intubation often extremely challenging • May require scope assistance • Stylet recommended • May laryngospasm – have topical lidocaine available • Have very small ETT available • Consider LMA for rabbits • Prone to upper airway obstruction/mucus plug formation
	+/– Ketamine 5 mg/kg IM			Blood pressure maintenance • Maintenance crystalloids 10 mL/kg/h ± dextrose supplementation • If hemorrhage, consider hypertonic saline 2–4 mL/kg IV bolus • Maintain normal heart rate with anticholinergics +/– norepinephrine 0.1–0.5 mcg/kg/min
	+/– Alfaxalone 3 mg/kg IM			Rabbits have a couple of oddities • do not respond to atropine and therefore need to have bradycardia treated with glycopyrrolate • Norepinephrine is the vasopressor of choice May require reversals to hasten recovery

Birds	Opioid (choose one) • Butorphanol 2 mg/kg IM or IV • Fentanyl 30 mcg/kg IV +/– Midazolam 2 mg/kg IM or IV +/– Ketamine 5 mg/kg IM (if needed to place IVC)	If IVC in place, Ketamine 5 mg/kg IV If no IVC in place, tight fitting mask with sevoflurane 5% in oxygen until relaxation and able to intubate	Volatile anesthetic (choose one) • Isoflurane • Sevoflurane MAC reduction • Lidocaine 2 mg/kg then 3–6 mg/kg/h • ±Fentanyl 50 mcg/kg/h • Local anesthesia as appropriate (2–4 mg/kg lidocaine)	Must use Cole tube for intubation Blood pressure maintenance • Maintenance crystalloids 10 mL/kg/h • Maintain appropriate heart rate with anticholinergics • ± Hypertonic saline 2–4 mL/kg if documented hemorrhage • If persistent hemorrhage/ documented blood loss, consider whole blood transfusion (use chicken as donor) May require the reversal of sedatives

(*continued on next page*)

Table 6
(continued)

Species	Premedication	Induction	Maintenance	Special Tips
Reptiles	Alfaxalone 10–20 mg/kg IM	May be able to intubate on premedication protocol	Alfaxalone TIVA 0.05–0.2 mg/kg/min IV or IO • Discontinue at closure • Extubation ~100 min post cessation	Do NOT need to supplement oxygen
	Midazolam 1–2 mg/kg IM	+/– Ketamine 1 mg/kg IM	Alternative if no IV or IO access • Volatile anesthetics (Sevoflurane or Isoflurane)	Ventilate to normocapnia (may only be a breath every 1–2 min) • If use inhalants, will need to hyperventilate to maintain adequate anesthetic depth • Maintenance crystalloids at 3–5 mL/kg/h • May require norepinephrine blood pressure support (shown in reptiles with limbs)
	Hydromorphone 0.2 mg/kg IM			Reversal of benzodiazepine recommended (0.07–0.14 mg/kg)
	+/– Ketamine 5 mg/kg IM			Maintain normothermia to hasten recovery

These are example protocols and may not be safe for all patients; appropriate knowledge of the drug, dose, patient type, and patient health status are necessary when utilizing any anesthetic agents.

sedation or anesthetic protocol is not best for all patients. When working with wildlife, this is also a consideration, as health status may not be able to be assessed prior to anesthesia. As we expand our knowledge of the pharmacokinetics and pharmacodynamics of drugs in healthy and critically ill exotics, tailored therapy allows for improved quality of care to be provided. Each individual species has its own unique anatomy and physiology that influence the effects of drugs in vivo, opening the door for a plethora of research avenues to investigate in a variety of species both in health and during illness.

SUMMARY

Sedation and anesthesia in veterinary exotic animals are challenging due to the variety of patients that are treated and inherent risks in treating them. To safely perform diagnostics and therapeutics on these patients, sedation and/or anesthesia is often required. Example sedation and anesthetic protocols are provided (**Tables 5** and **6**, respectively). However, attention to detail is a must, as well as knowledge of idiosyncrasies of each species and potential side effects of each drug to improve patient outcomes. By anticipating complications based on the patient characteristics and drug profiles, safety of sedation and anesthesia can be improved in these minor species.

CLINICS CARE POINTS

- To perform diagnostics and therapeutic care for exotic patients that are sick or injured, sedation and/or anesthesia is frequently required.
- It is important for the clinician to consider drug choice, route of administration, and dose based on the unique characteristics of the type of patient as well as potential comorbidities.
- Appropriate preparation of equipment and supplies, including in the event of an emergency, is necessary prior to the administration of anesthetics to exotic ill or injured patients.
- When possible, the utilization of drugs with a wide safety margin and/or those that are reversible may aid in the successful anesthesia of these patients.

DISCLOSURE

Dr H.N. Trenholme has been in contact with Jurox regarding becoming a potential partner for research, but to date, no goods or services have been provided.

REFERENCES

1. McNally EM, Robertson SA, Pablo LS. Comparison of time to desaturation between preoxygenated and nonpreoxygenated dogs following sedation with acepromazine maleate and morphine and induction of anesthesia with propofol. Am J Vet Res 2009;70(11):1333–8.
2. Duke-Novakovski T, Fujiyama M, Beazley SG. Comparison of mainstream (Capnostat 5) and two low-flow sidestream capnometers (VM-2500-S and Capnostream) in spontaneously breathing rabbits anesthetized with a Bain coaxial breathing system. Vet Anaesth Analg 2020;47(4):537–46.
3. Tweed WA. A non-rebreathing coaxial anaesthesia system: dependence of end-tidal gas concentrations on fresh gas flow and tidal volume. Anaesthesia 1997;52(3):237–41.

4. Ekbom K, Assareh H, Anderson RE, et al. The effects of fresh gas flow on the amount of sevoflurane vaporized during 1 minimum alveolar concentration anaesthesia for day surgery: a clinical study. Acta Anaesth Scand 2007;51(3): 290–3. https://doi.org/10.1111/j.1399-6576.2006.01235.x.
5. Crooks CJ, West J, Morling JR, et al. Pulse oximeter measurements vary across ethnic groups: an observational study in patients with COVID-19. Eur Respir J 2022;59(4):2103246.
6. Mosley CA, Dyson D, Smith DA. The cardiovascular dose–response effects of isoflurane alone and combined with butorphanol in the green iguana (Iguana iguana). Vet Anaesth Analg 2004;31(1):64–72.
7. Schuetze S, Manig A, Ribes S, et al. Aged mice show an increased mortality after anesthesia with a standard dose of ketamine/xylazine. Laboratory Animal Res 2019;35(1):8.
8. Smiler KL, Stein S, Hrapkiewicz KL, et al. Tissue response to intramuscular and intraperitoneal injections of ketamine and xylazine in rats. Lab Anim Sci 1990; 40(1):60–4.
9. Das RG, North D. Implications of experimental technique for analysis and interpretation of data from animal experiments: outliers and increased variability resulting from failure of intraperitoneal injection procedures. Lab Anim 2007;41(3): 312–20.
10. Brodbelt DC, Blissitt KJ, Hammond RA, et al. The risk of death: the Confidential Enquiry into Perioperative Small Animal Fatalities. Vet Anaesth Analg 2008; 35(5):365–73.
11. Huynh M, Poumeyrol S, Pignon C, et al. Intramuscular administration of alfaxalone for sedation in rabbits. Vet Rec 2015;176(10):255.
12. Knutson KA, Petritz OA, Thomson AE, et al. Intramuscular Alfaxalone–Butorphanol–Midazolam Compared with Ketamine–Butorphanol– Midazolam in New Zealand White Rabbits. J Am Assoc Lab Anim 2022;61(5):475–81.
13. Bradley MP, Doerning CM, Nowland MH, et al. Intramuscular Administration of Alfaxalone Alone and in Combination for Sedation and Anesthesia of Rabbits (Oryctolagus cuniculus). J Am Assoc Lab Anim 2019;58(2):216–22.
14. Santangelo B, Micieli F, Mozzillo T, et al. Transnasal administration of a combination of dexmedetomidine, midazolam and butorphanol produces deep sedation in New Zealand White rabbits. Vet Anaesth Analg 2016;43(2):209–14.
15. d'Ovidio D, Marino F, Noviello E, et al. Sedative effects of intramuscular alfaxalone in pet guinea pigs (Cavia porcellus). Vet Anaesth Analg 2018;45(2):183–9.
16. Doerning CM, Bradley MP, Lester PA, et al. Effects of subcutaneous alfaxalone alone and in combination with dexmedetomidine and buprenorphine in guinea pigs (Cavia porcellus). Vet Anaesth Analg 2018;45(5):658–66.
17. Álvarez ER, Solé LV, Mateo AG de C. Comparison of subcutaneous sedation with alfaxalone or alfaxalone-midazolam in pet guinea pigs (Cavia porcellus) of three different age groups. J Am Vet Med Assoc 2022;260(9):1–7.
18. Sixtus RP, Pacharinsak C, Gray CL, et al. Differential effects of four intramuscular sedatives on cardiorespiratory stability in juvenile guinea pigs (Cavia porcellus). PLoS One 2021;16(11):e0259559.
19. Ambros B, Knych HK, Sadar MJ. Pharmacokinetics of hydromorphone hydrochloride after intravenous and intramuscular administration in guinea pigs (Cavia porcellus). Am J Vet Res 2020;81(4):361–6.
20. Milloway MC, Posner LP, Balko JA. Sedative and cardiorespiratory effects of intramuscular alfaxalone and butorphanol at two dosages in ferrets (Mustela putorius furo). J Zoo Wildlife Med 2021;51(4):841–7.

21. Mazaheri-Khameneh R, Sarrafzadeh-Rezaei F, Asri-Rezaei S, et al. Evaluation of clinical and paraclinical effects of intraosseous vs intravenous administration of propofol on general anesthesia in rabbits. Vet Res Forum Int Q J 2011;3(2): 103–9.
22. Allweiler S, Leach MC, Flecknell PA. The use of propofol and sevoflurane for surgical anaesthesia in New Zealand White rabbits. Lab Anim 2009;44(2):113–7.
23. Santos M, Viñuela A, Vela AA, et al. Single-syringe ketamine–propofol for induction of anaesthesia in rabbits. Vet Anaesth Analg 2016;43(5):561–5.
24. Ko JC, Thurmon JC, Tranquilli WJ, et al. A comparison of medetomidine-propofol and medetomidine-midazolam-propofol anesthesia in rabbits. Lab Anim Sci 1992;42(5):503–7.
25. Tutunaru AC, Şonea A, Drion P, et al. Anaesthetic induction with alfaxalone may produce hypoxemia in rabbits premedicated with fentanyl/droperidol. Vet Anaesth Analg 2013;40(6):657–9.
26. Navarrete-Calvo R, Gómez-Villamandos RJ, Morgaz J, et al. Cardiorespiratory, anaesthetic and recovery effects of morphine combined with medetomidine and alfaxalone in rabbits. Vet Rec 2014;174(4):95.
27. Grint NJ, Smith HE, Senior JM. Clinical evaluation of alfaxalone in cyclodextrin for the induction of anaesthesia in rabbits. Vet Rec 2008;163(13):395.
28. Marsh MK, McLeod SR, Hansen A, et al. Induction of anaesthesia in wild rabbits using a new alfaxalone formulation. Vet Rec 2009;164(4):122.
29. Grint NJ, Murison PJ. A comparison of ketamine–midazolam and ketamine–medetomidine combinations for induction of anaesthesia in rabbits. Vet Anaesth Analg 2008;35(2):113–21.
30. Gleason NR, Gallos G, Zhang Y, et al. Propofol Preferentially Relaxes Neurokinin Receptor-2-induced Airway Smooth Muscle Contraction in Guinea Pig Trachea. Anesthesiology 2010;112(6):1335–44.
31. Schwenke DO, Cragg PA. Comparison of the depressive effects of four anesthetic regimens on ventilatory and cardiovascular variables in the guinea pig. Comparative Med 2004;54(1):77–85.
32. Schmitz S, Tacke S, Guth B, et al. Comparison of Physiological Parameters and Anaesthesia Specific Observations during Isoflurane, Ketamine-Xylazine or Medetomidine-Midazolam-Fentanyl Anaesthesia in Male Guinea Pigs. PLoS One 2016;11(9):e0161258.
33. Cook DJ, Housmans PR. Mechanism of the Negative Inotropic Effect of Propofol in Isolated Ferret Ventricular Myocardium. Anesthesiology 1994;80(4):859–71.
34. Kongsayreepong S, Cook DJ, Housmans PR. Mechanism of the Direct, Negative Inotropic Effect of Ketamine in Isolated Ferret and Frog Ventricular Myocardium. Anesthesiology 1993;79(2):313–22.
35. Cook DJ, Carton EG, Housmans PR. Mechanism of the Positive Inotropic Effect of Ketamine in Isolated Ferret Ventricular Papillary Muscle. Anesthesiology 1991;74(5):880–8.
36. Bone L, Battles AH, Goldfarb RD, et al. Electrocardiographic values from clinically normal, anesthetized ferrets (Mustela putorius furo). Am J Vet Res 1988; 49(11):1884–7.
37. Hedenqvist P, Roughan JV, Antunes L, et al. Induction of anaesthesia with desflurane and isoflurane in the rabbit. Lab Anim 2001;35(2):172–9.
38. Sayce LJ, Powell ME, Kimball EE, et al. Continuous Rate Infusion of Ketamine Hydrochloride and Dexmedetomidine for Maintenance of Anesthesia during Laryngotracheal Surgery in New Zealand White Rabbits (Oryctolagus cuniculus). J Am Assoc Lab Anim 2020;59(2):176–85.

39. Smith JC, Robertson LD, Auhll A, et al. Endotracheal tubes versus laryngeal mask airways in rabbit inhalation anesthesia: ease of use and waste gas emissions. Contemp Top Lab Anim 2004;43(4):22–5.
40. Fusco A, Douglas H, Barba A, et al. V-Gel® Guided Endotracheal Intubation in Rabbits. Frontiers Vet Sci 2021;8:684624.
41. Engbers S, Larkin A, Rousset N, et al. Comparison of a Supraglottic Airway Device (v-gel®) with Blind Orotracheal Intubation in Rabbits. Frontiers Vet Sci 2017;4:49.
42. Kujime K, Natelson BH. A method of endotracheal intubation of guinea pigs (Cavia porcellus). Lab Anim Sci 1981;31(6):715–6.
43. Longley L. Rodent anaesthesia. Anaesth Exot Pets 2008;59–84.
44. Timm KI, Jahn SE, Sedgwick CJ. The palatal ostium of the guinea pig. Lab Anim Sci 1987;37(6):801–2.
45. Hikasa Y, Yamashita M, Takase K, et al. Prolonged Sevoflurane, Isoflurane and Halothane Anaesthesia in Oxygen Using Rebreathing or Non-rebreathing System in Cats. J Vet Medicine Ser 1998;45(1-10):559–75.
46. Lin X, Ju YN, Gao W, et al. Desflurane Attenuates Ventilator-Induced Lung Injury in Rats with Acute Respiratory Distress Syndrome. BioMed Res Int 2018;2018:7507314.
47. Piriou V, Chiari P, Lhuillier F, et al. Pharmacological preconditioning: comparison of desflurane, sevoflurane, isoflurane and halothane in rabbit myocardium. Bja Br J Anaesth 2002;89(3):486–91.
48. Caldwell JE. Desflurane Clinical Pharmacokinetics and Pharmacodynamics. Clin Pharmacokinet 1994;27(1):6–18.
49. Lotz C, Stumpner J, Smul TM. Sevoflurane as opposed to propofol anesthesia preserves mitochondrial function and alleviates myocardial ischemia/reperfusion injury. Biomed Pharmacother 2020;129:110417.
50. Cruz FS, Carregaro AB, Raiser AG, et al. Total intravenous anesthesia with propofol and S(+)-ketamine in rabbits. Vet Anaesth Analg 2010;37(2):116–22.
51. Liebenberg SP, Linn JM. Seasonal and sexual influences on rabbit atropinesterase. Lab Anim 1980;14(4):297–300.
52. Gosliga JM, Barter LS. Cardiovascular effects of dopamine hydrochloride and phenylephrine hydrochloride in healthy isoflurane-anesthetized New Zealand White rabbits (Oryctolagus cuniculus). Am J Vet Res 2015;76(2):116–21.
53. Uccello O, Sanchez A, Valverde A, et al. Cardiovascular effects of increasing dosages of norepinephrine in healthy isoflurane-anesthetized New Zealand White rabbits. Vet Anaesth Analg 2020;47(6):781–8.
54. Keene BW, Flammer K. ECG of the month. J Am Vet Med Assoc 1991;198(3):408–9.
55. McLelland J., Larynx and trachea, In: King A. and McLelland J., *Form and Function in birds*, 1989, London, Academic Press, 69–103.
56. Harvey EP, Ben-Tal A. Robust Unidirectional Airflow through Avian Lungs: New Insights from a Piecewise Linear Mathematical Model. PLoS Comput Biol 2016;12(2):e1004637.
57. Mans C, Guzman DSM, Lahner LL, et al. Sedation and Physiologic Response to Manual Restraint After Intranasal Administration of Midazolam in Hispaniolan Amazon Parrots (Amazona ventralis). J Avian Med Surg 2012;26(3):130–9.
58. Maho YL, Karmann H, Briot D, et al. Stress in birds due to routine handling and a technique to avoid it. Am J Physiology-regulatory Integr Comp Physiology 1992;263(4):R775–81.

59. Seamon AB, Hofmeister EH, Divers SJ. Outcome following inhalation anesthesia in birds at a veterinary referral hospital: 352 cases (2004–2014). J Am Vet Med Assoc 2017;251(7):814–7.
60. Kubiak M, Roach L, Eatwell K. The Influence of a Combined Butorphanol and Midazolam Premedication on Anesthesia in Psittacid Species. J Avian Med Surg 2016;30(4):317–23.
61. Anjana RR, Parikh PV, Mahla JK, et al. Comparative evaluation of isoflurane and sevoflurane in avian patients. Vet World 2021;14(5):1067–73.
62. Conner CM, Hoppes SM, Stevens BJ, et al. Intranasal butorphanol and midazolam administered prior to intramuscular alfaxalone provides safe and effective sedation in Quaker parrots (Myiopsitta monachus). Am J Vet Res 2022;1–8. https://doi.org/10.2460/ajvr.22.08.0140.
63. Paula VV, Otsuki DA, Auler JOC, et al. The effect of premedication with ketamine, alone or with diazepam, on anaesthesia with sevoflurane in parrots (Amazona aestiva). BMC Vet Res 2013;9(1):142.
64. Greunz EM, Limn D, Bertelsen MF. Alfaxalone Sedation in Black-cheeked Lovebirds (Agapornis nigrigenis) for Non-invasive Procedures. J Avian Med Surg 2021;35(2):161–6.
65. Escalante GC, Balko JA, Chinnadurai SK. Comparison of the Sedative Effects of Alfaxalone and Butorphanol-Midazolam Administered Intramuscularly in Budgerigars (Melopsittacus undulatus). J Avian Med Surg 2018;32(4):279–85.
66. Balko JA, Lindemann DM, Allender MC, et al. Evaluation of the anesthetic and cardiorespiratory effects of intramuscular alfaxalone administration and isoflurane in budgerigars (Melopsittacus undulatus) and comparison with manual restraint. J Am Vet Med Assoc 2019;254(12):1427–35.
67. Romano J, Hasse K, Johnston M. Sedative, cardiorespiratory, and thermoregulatory effects of alfaxalone on Budgerigars (*Melopsittacus undulatus*). J Zoo Wildlife Med 2020;51(1):96–101.
68. Perrin KL, Nielsen JB, Thomsen AF, et al. Alfaxalone anesthesia in the Bengalese finch (Lonchura domestica). J Zoo Wildlife Med 2017;48(4):1146–53.
69. Whitehead MC, Hoppes SM, Musser JMB, et al. The Use of Alfaxalone in Quaker Parrots (Myiopsitta monachus). J Avian Med Surg 2019;33(4):340–8.
70. Chang S, Pierre CBLSt, Ambros B. Comparison of Sedative Effects of Alfaxalone-Ketamine and Alfaxalone-Midazolam Administered Intramuscularly in Chickens. J Avian Med Surg 2022;36(1):21–7.
71. Nishiyama T, Aibiki M, Hanaoka K. Haemodynamic and catecholamine changes during rapid sevoflurane induction with tidal volume breathing. Can J Anaesth J Can D'anesthésie. 1997;44(10):1066–70.
72. Pierre CLSt, Desprez I, Chang S, et al. Effect of preoxygenation before isoflurane induction and rocuronium-induced apnea on time until hemoglobin desaturation in domestic chickens (Gallus gallus domesticus). Vet Anaesth Analg 2021;48(4):524–31.
73. Azizpour A, Hassani Y. Clinical evaluation of general anaesthesia in pigeons using a combination of ketamine and diazepam. J S Afr Vet Assoc 2012;83(1):12.
74. Kamiloglu A, Atalan G, Kamiloglu NN. Comparison of intraosseous and intramuscular drug administration for induction of anaesthesia in domestic pigeons. Res Vet Sci 2008;85(1):171–5.
75. Lin HC, Todhunter PG, Powe TA, et al. Use of xylazine, butorphanol, tiletamine-zolazepam, and isoflurane for induction and maintenance of anesthesia in ratites. J Am Vet Med Assoc 1997;210(2):244–8.

76. Santos EAR, Monteiro ER, Herrera JR, et al. Total intravenous anesthesia in domestic chicken (Gallus gallus domesticus) with propofol alone or in combination with methadone, nalbuphine or fentanyl for ulna osteotomy. Vet Anaesth Analg 2020;47(3):347–55.
77. Müller K, Holzapfel J, Brunnberg L. Total intravenous anaesthesia by boluses or by continuous rate infusion of propofol in mute swans (Cygnus olor). Vet Anaesth Analg 2011;38(4):286–91.
78. Schumacher J, Citino SB, Hernandez K, et al. Cardiopulmonary and anesthetic effects of propofol in wild turkeys. Am J Vet Res 1997;58(9):1014–7.
79. Villaverde-Morcillo S, Benito J, Garca-Snchez R, et al. Comparison of isoflurane and alfaxalone (Alfaxan) for the induction of anesthesia in flamingos (*Phoenicopterus roseus*). J Zoo Wildlife Med 2014;45(2):361–6.
80. Mastakov A, Henning J, Gier R de, et al. Induction of General Anesthesia With Alfaxalone in the Domestic Chicken. J Avian Med Surg 2021;35(3):269–79.
81. Brown C, Pilny AA. Air sac cannula placement in birds. Lab Anim 2006; 35(7):23–4.
82. Botman J, Gabriel F, Dugdale AHA, et al. Anaesthesia with sevoflurane in pigeons: minimal anaesthetic concentration (MAC) determination and investigation of cardiorespiratory variables at 1 MAC. Vet Rec 2016;178(22):560.
83. Mercado JA, Larsen RS, Wack RF, et al. Minimum anesthetic concentration of isoflurane in captive thick-billed parrots (Rhynchopsitta pachyrhyncha). Am J Vet Res 2008;69(2):189–94.
84. Maina JN. Spectacularly robust! Tensegrity principle explains the mechanical strength of the avian lung. Resp Physiol Neurobi 2007;155(1):1–10.
85. Touzot-Jourde G, Hernandez-Divers SJ, Trim CM. Cardiopulmonary effects of controlled versus spontaneous ventilation in pigeons anesthetized for coelioscopy. J Am Vet Med Assoc 2005;227(9):1424–8.
86. Edling TM, Degernes LA, Flammer K, et al. Capnographic monitoring of anesthetized African grey parrots receiving intermittent positive pressure ventilation. J Am Vet Med Assoc 2001;219(12):1714–8.
87. Rembert M, Smith J, Pettifer G, et al. Comparison of traditional thermal support with the forced-air warmer system in Hispaniolan Amazon parrots (Amazona ventralis). Vet Anaesth Analg 2002;29(2):110–1.
88. Gunkel C, Lafortune M. Current techniques in avian anesthesia. Seminars Avian Exot Pet Med 2005;14(4):263–76.
89. Crawford A, Abelson A, Gladden J, et al. Retrospective evaluation of cardiopulmonary arrest and resuscitation in hospitalized birds: 41 cases (2006–2019). J Vet Emerg Crit Car 2022;32(4):491–9.
90. Piercy J, Rogers K, Reichert M, et al. The relationship between body temperature, heart rate, breathing rate, and rate of oxygen consumption, in the tegu lizard (Tupinambis merianae) at various levels of activity. J Comp Physiol B 2015; 185(8):891–903.
91. Jensen B, Moorman AFM, Wang T. Structure and function of the hearts of lizards and snakes. Biol Rev 2014;89(2):302–36.
92. Holz P, Barker IK, Burger JP, et al. The effect of the renal portal system on pharmacokinetic parameters in the red-eared slider (Trachemys scripta elegans). J Zoo Wildl Medicine Official Publ Am Assoc Zoo Vet 1997;28(4):386–93.
93. Yaw TJ, Mans C, Johnson SM, et al. Effect of injection site on alfaxalone-induced sedation in ball pythons (Python regius). J Small Anim Pract 2018;59(12): 747–51.

94. Mans C. Venipuncture techniques in chelonian species. Lab Anim 2008;37(7): 303–4. https://doi.org/10.1038/laban0708-303.
95. Comolli JR, McHale B, Kehoe S, et al. Cardiac Tamponade Following Cardiocentesis in a Ball Python (Python regius). J Herpetological Medicine Surg 2022;32(2):116–8.
96. Farmer CG. Unidirectional flow in lizard lungs: a paradigm shift in our understanding of lung evolution in Diapsida. Zoology 2015;118(5):299–301.
97. Cieri RL, Farmer CG. Computational Fluid Dynamics Reveals a Unique Net Unidirectional Pattern of Pulmonary Airflow in the Savannah Monitor Lizard (Varanus exanthematicus). Anat Rec 2020;303(7):1768–91.
98. Taylor EW, Leite CAC, McKenzie DJ, et al. Control of respiration in fish, amphibians and reptiles. Braz J Med Biol Res 2010;43(5):409–24.
99. Skovgaard N, Abe AS, Andrade DV, et al. Hypoxic pulmonary vasoconstriction in reptiles: a comparative study of four species with different lung structures and pulmonary blood pressures. Am J Physiology-regulatory Integr Comp Physiology. 2005;289(5):R1280–8.
100. Doss GA, Fink DM, Sladky KK, et al. Comparison of subcutaneous dexmedetomidine–midazolam versus alfaxalone–midazolam sedation in leopard geckos (Eublepharis macularius). Vet Anaesth Analg 2017;44(5):1175–83.
101. Yaw TJ, Mans C, Johnson S, et al. Evaluation of subcutaneous administration of alfaxalone-midazolam and dexmedetomidine-midazolam for sedation of ball pythons (Python regius). J Am Vet Med Assoc 2020;256(5):573–9.
102. Shepard MK, Divers S, Braun C, et al. Pharmacodynamics of alfaxalone after single-dose intramuscular administration in red-eared sliders (Trachemys scripta elegans): a comparison of two different doses at two different ambient temperatures. Vet Anaesth Analg 2013;40(6):590–8.
103. Kleinschmidt LM, Hanley CS, Sahrmann JM, et al. Randomized controlled trial comparing the effects of alfaxalone and ketamine hydrochloride in the Haitian giant galliwasp (Celestus warren). J Zoo Wildlife Med 2018;49(2):283–90.
104. Barrillot B, Roux J, Arthaud S, et al. Intramuscular administration of ketamine-detomidine assures stable anaesthesia needed for long-term surgery in the Argentine tegu Salvator merianae. J Zoo Wildlife Med 2018;49(2):291–6.
105. Fink DM, Doss GA, Sladky KK, et al. Effect of injection site on dexmedetomidine-ketamine induced sedation in leopard geckos (Eublepharis macularius). J Am Vet Med Assoc 2018;253(9):1146–50.
106. Rasys AM, Divers SJ, Lauderdale JD, et al. A systematic study of injectable anesthetic agents in the brown anole lizard (Anolis sagrei). Lab Anim 2019; 54(3):281–94.
107. Adel M, Sadegh AB, Arizza V, et al. Anesthetic efficacy of ketamine–diazepam, ketamine–xylazine, and ketamine–acepromazine in Caspian Pond turtles (Mauremys caspica). Indian J Pharmacol 2017;49(1):93–7.
108. Rockwell K, Boykin K, Padlo J, et al. Evaluating the efficacy of alfaxalone in corn snakes (Pantherophis guttatus). Vet Anaesth Analg 2021;48(3):364–71.
109. Webb JK, Keller KA, Chinnadurai SK, et al. Optimizing the pharmacodynamics and evaluating the cardiogenic effects of the injectable anesthetic alfaxalone in prairie rattlesnakes (Crotalus viridis). J Zoo Wildlife Med 2021;52(4):1105–12.
110. Strahl-Heldreth DE, Clark-Price SC, Keating SCJ, et al. Effect of intracoelomic administration of alfaxalone on the righting reflex and tactile stimulus response of common garter snakes (Thamnophis sirtalis). Am J Vet Res 2019;80(2): 144–51.

111. Harms CA, Piniak WED, Eckert SA, et al. Sedation and anesthesia of hatchling leatherback sea turtles (Dermochelys coriacea) for auditory evoked potential measurement in air and in water. J Zoo Wildlife Med 2014;45(1):86–92.
112. Phillips BE, Posner LP, Lewbart GA, et al. Effects of alfaxalone administered intravenously to healthy yearling loggerhead sea turtles (Caretta caretta) at three different doses. J Am Vet Med Assoc 2017;250(8):909–17.
113. Bertelsen MF, Buchanan R, Jensen HM, et al. Pharmacodynamics of propofol and alfaxalone in rattlesnakes (Crotalus durissus). Comp Biochem Physiology Part Mol Integr Physiology 2021;256:110935.
114. Mans C, Sladky K, Schumacher J. General Anesthesia. In: Divers S, Stahl S, editors. Mader's reptile and Amphibian medicine and surgery. Third. St. Louis, Elsevier; 2019. p. 447–74.
115. Hodgson DS. Anesthetic concentrations in enclosed chambers using an innovative delivery device. Vet Anaesth Analg 2007;34(2):99–106.
116. Hicks JW, Wang T. Functional role of cardiac shunts in reptiles. J Exp Zool 1996; 275(2-3):204–16.
117. Williams CJA, Malte CL, Malte H, et al. Ectothermy and cardiac shunts profoundly slow the equilibration of inhaled anaesthetics in a multi-compartment model. Sci Rep-uk 2020;10(1):17157.
118. Young BA, Sheft S, Yost W. Sound production in Pituophis melanoleucus (Serpentes: Colubridae) with the first description of a vocal cord in snakes. J Exp Zool 1995;273(6):472–81.
119. Parkinson LA, Mans C. Evaluation of subcutaneously administered electrolyte solutions in experimentally dehydrated inland bearded dragons (Pogona vitticeps). Am J Vet Res 2020;81(5):437–41.
120. Camacho M, Quintana M del P, Calabuig P, et al. Acid-Base and Plasma Biochemical Changes Using Crystalloid Fluids in Stranded Juvenile Loggerhead Sea Turtles (Caretta caretta). PLoS One 2015;10(7):e0132217.
121. Branco LG, Portner HO, Wood SC. Interaction between temperature and hypoxia in the alligator. Am J Physiology-regulatory Integr Comp Physiology 1993; 265(6):R1339–43.
122. Goe A, Shmalberg J, Gatson B, et al. Epinephrine or GV-26 electrical stimulation reduces inhalant anesthetic recovery time in common snapping turtles (Chelydra serpentina). J Zoo Wildlife Med 2016;47(2):501–7.
123. Gatson BJ, Goe A, Granone TD, et al. Intramuscular epinephrine results in reduced anesthetic recovery time in American alligators (Alligator mississippiensis) undergoing isoflurane anesthesia. J Zoo Wildlife Med 2017;48(1):55–61.
124. Balko JA, Gatson BJ, Cohen EB, et al. Inhalant anesthetic recovery following intramuscular epinephrine in the loggerhead sea turtle (Caretta caretta). J Zoo Wildlife Med 2018;49(3):680–8.
125. Schnellbacher R, Comolli J. Constant Rate Infusions in Exotic Animals. J Exot Pet Med 2020;35:50–7.
126. Kischinovsky M, Duse A, Wang T, et al. Intramuscular administration of alfaxalone in red-eared sliders (Trachemys scripta elegans) – effects of dose and body temperature. Vet Anaesth Analg 2013;40(1):13–20.
127. Sadar MJ, Ambros B. Use of Alfaxalone or MidazolamDexmedetomidineKetamine for Implantation of Radiotransmitters in Bullsnakes (Pituophis catenifer sayi). J Herpetological Medicine Surg 2018;28(3–4):93–8.
128. Larouche CB, Beaufrre H, Mosley C, et al. Evaluation of the effects of midazolam and flumazenil in the ball python (Python regius). J Zoo Wildlife Med 2019;50(3): 579–88.

Fluid Therapy in Exotic Animal Emergency and Critical Care

Lily Parkinson, DVM, Dipl ACZM, Cert Aq V, Dipl ACVECC

KEYWORDS

- Colloid • Crystalloid • Dehydration • Hypovolemia • Maintenance • Replacement
- Resuscitation

KEY POINTS

- Classical Starling's forces are now recognized as inadequate to explain fluid movement in mammalian and non-mammalian patients.
- Mammalian approaches to fluid therapy are likely inappropriate for non-mammalian species.
- Intravascular "shock boluses," hypertonic crystalloid resuscitation, and colloid fluid resuscitation are likely unnecessary in non-mammalian patients.

INTRODUCTION

Despite being a mainstay of treatment for many medical conditions, fluid therapy remains understudied and poorly understood in human and domestic animal medicine, much less in non-domestic care. Fluid administration can be essential for directly treating medical conditions (eg, hypovolemic, distributive, or certain obstructive or metabolic shock states) or providing adjunct support to patients (eg, anorexic patients not taking in any fluids). Fluid therapy encompasses the use of crystalloids (isotonic, hypertonic, and hypotonic), colloids, and blood products (packed red blood cells, plasma, albumin, platelets, cryoprecipitate, fresh whole blood, and so forth) and can be utilized to address hypoperfusion, dehydration, electrolyte abnormalities, acid-base derangements, and blood component loss. This article reviews newer fluid therapy concepts emerging in human and domestic small animal medicine and interweaves contrasting non-domestic species physiology that may affect fluid therapy in these patients, as a useful review for the exotic animal practitioner. While depth of knowledge on exotic animal fluid therapy is severely lacking, this review aims to help the clinician make the most informed decision possible when developing a fluid treatment protocol.

Brookfield Zoo, Chicago Zoological Society, 3300 Golf Road, Brookfield, IL 60513, USA
E-mail address: Lily.Parkinson@czs.org

Vet Clin Exot Anim 26 (2023) 623–645
https://doi.org/10.1016/j.cvex.2023.05.004
vetexotic.theclinics.com
1094-9194/23/

Body Fluid Composition

When assessing fluid needs and constructing a treatment plan, it is essential to consider a patient's normal fluid status. Total body water (TBW) is the term for all water that is found in a patient's body systems. In mammals, TBW comprises 60% to 70% of an animal's mass, with approximately two-thirds of that water found within cells (the intracellular compartment). The remaining third is found extracellularly, which is divided between intravascular fluid (plasma [4%–5% of body weight]), interstitial fluid (15%–18% of body weight), lymph, and transcellular fluids (**Fig. 1**).[1]

Percentage of water within an animal's total body mass is variable: birds, similar to mammals, tend to have 60% to 70% of their body weight made up of water, whereas amphibians have 70% to more than 80% total body water, and fish are in the middle with around 63% to 75%.[2] Extensive research has been performed in numerous reptile species with many reptiles made up of 60% to 75% water.[3] While a lot of research remains to be done on fluid distribution in many different species, some specifics have been elucidated. TBW has been found to be similar between different species of waterfowl, but marine birds have more of their TBW present in the extracellular fluid compartment and they appear (as one would expect) to be more tolerant of taking on high salt loads.[4]In reptiles, marine and terrestrial species had less overall TBW when compared to freshwater species, and more of their TBW was present in the extracellular space.[5]This means that more fluid was present in the plasma, lymph, interstitium, and transcellular fluids with less fluid present within cells in those species that do not have access to freshwater at all times, which may be an important fluid reservoir for these species.[5]Saltwater crocodiles (*Crocodylus porosus*) appear to be an exception and were found to have a very high TBW of 81.1% when living in estuarine environments and a lower, but still high, TBW of 75.7%

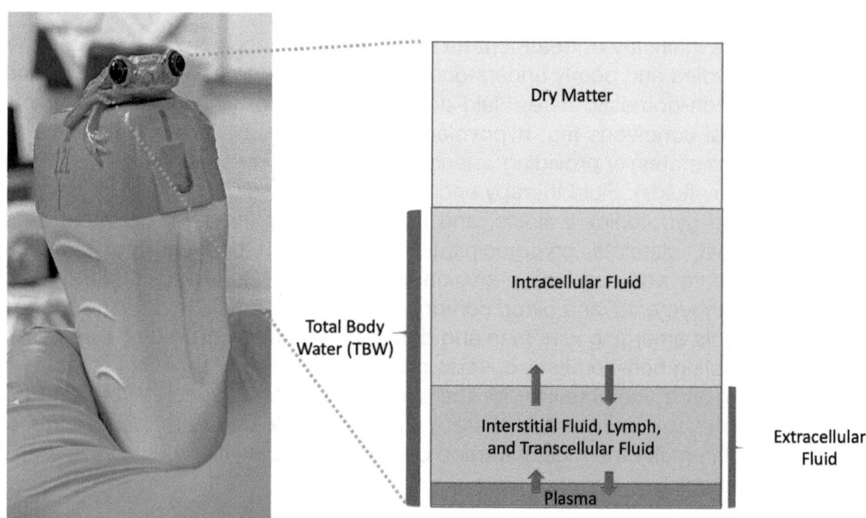

Fig. 1. Infographic representing the different body compartments of this lemur leaf frog (*Hylomantis lemur*). Most body weight in all exotic animal patients is made up of fluid, with total body water broken down into intracellular and extracellular fluid compartments. The extracellular fluid is further divided into the interstitial fluid, lymph, and transcellular fluid and the plasma. Non-mammalian taxa exchange fluid between the plasma and the other extracellular fluid compartments much more readily than mammalian taxa.

when living in a marine environment.[3]On the other end of the spectrum, reptiles living in desert conditions were found to have extremely low TBW during certain seasons, with chuckwallas (*Sauromalus obesus*) having only 40.2% TBW in the autumn.[3]

As a clinician, it is essential to remember that the most commonly sampled portion of TBW, the plasma, represents only a small fraction of the fluid the clinician should be considering within a patient (see **Fig. 1**).[6]New research and paradigm shifts in clinical thinking are beginning to highlight the importance of other fluid compartments that are not so easily sampled or assessed. Traditionally, plasma fluid and its movement to other extracellular fluid compartments was thought to occur due to Starling's forces, with hydrostatic and oncotic forces in blood vessels and the interstitium determining fluid flux. Currently, the *endothelial glycocalyx*, a gel-like layer of molecules that lines the endothelium of blood vessels, is known to be an essential determinant of fluid flux in mammals.[7,8]Starling's forces (differing hydrostatic and oncotic pressures) between the intravascular space/plasma and the subglycocalyx fluid compartment, rather than the interstitium, are now considered the drivers of fluid flux in mammals (**Fig. 2**). As a consequence, the lymphatic system is gaining further prominence; it is now understood to be the most significant route for fluid return to the systemic circulation in mammals.[9,8]

It is not known if non-mammalian species possess an endothelial glycocalyx, but lymph and the lymphatic systems that exist to transport fluid once it is out of the systemic vasculature have been studied and found to vary widely amongst taxa. In mammals, lymph is the fluid filtered out of blood vessels and into lymphatic vessels after traversing an interstitial space. These lymphatic vessels then drain back into the systemic circulation's venous system. The rate of lymph flow returning to the vasculature is very low in mammals, therefore *the lymphatic system plays little to no role in maintaining plasma volume in these species*.[10]This is not the case, however, with other animals. While mammals only turn over 0.03% to 0.1% of their plasma volume per minute with assistance from the lymphatics, snakes will experience a rate of turnover of 0.2% to 0.7% of the plasma volume/minute, fish turn over 0.9% of their plasma

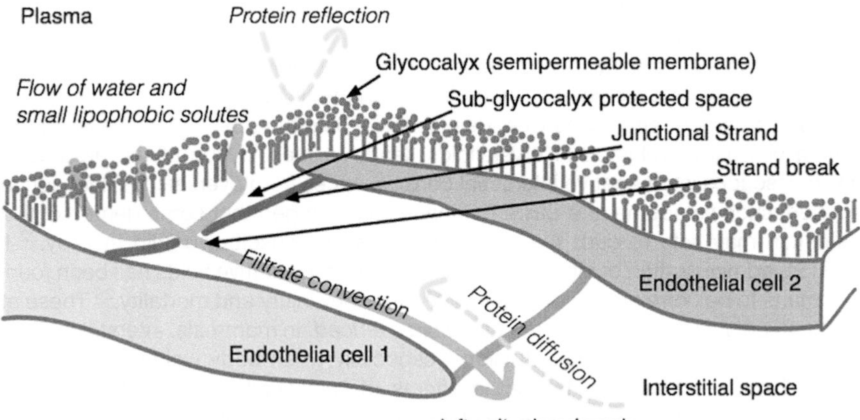

Fig. 2. A drawing illustrating the fluid dynamics and protein movement currently understood to occur between the plasma and the sub-glycocalyx. (TE Woodcock, MBBS MPhil FRCA, Plasma volume, tissue oedema, and the steady-state Starling principle, BJA Education, Volume 17, Issue 2, February 2017, Pages 74–78, https://doi.org/10.1093/bjaed/mkw035.)

volume every minute and some anurans can exchange 3% to 5% of their plasma volume with their lymphatic system every minute.[10,11] Starling's forces cannot explain fluid movement in anurans or fish,[12–14] and lymphatics and fluid movement remain poorly understood in avian species, but also cannot be accounted for via Starling's force equations alone.[15,16]

While lymph may not exchange with the plasma rapidly in mammals, the interstitium has more recently been found to play a major role in mammalian fluid dynamics. The interstitium, a network of glycosaminoglycans, helps give tissues their structure. This structure dictates tissues' relative rigidity, which determines the compliance of different organs.[17] Since the interstitium is difficult to sample and study, it has only recently been discovered that the interstitium can non-osmotically store excess salt, influence blood pressure, start the cascade of systemic inflammatory response syndrome (SIRS) when compromised by digestive enzymes that enter into it during hypovolemic states, and cause inflammatory edema formation when its hydrostatic pressure decreases.[18] In addition to vascular permeability or "leakiness," *interstitial compliance appears to be a major determinant of plasma exchange rates in many animals.*[19]

While discussions of body water distribution and dynamics can appear dry and academic, these physiologic differences likely have important implications for clinicians treating patients with fluids. In mammals, an important distinction needs to be made between *perfusion* and *hydration*. Poor perfusion equates to hypovolemia, or low amounts of fluid in the intravascular space (the plasma). Hydration typically refers to the level of TBW a patient possesses—a dehydrated patient might have adequate intravascular fluid volume, but depleted fluid levels in its other fluid compartments, typically with the extracellular fluid compartment's interstitium losing the most relative fluid volume.[20] With slow exchange from the lymph and interstitium to the plasma, mammals require distinctive treatments when addressing hypovolemia versus dehydration via fluid therapy. *When a mammalian patient is in hypovolemic shock, intravenous or intraosseous fluid support is required to quickly reestablish perfusion: blood and oxygen delivery to tissues (often termed resuscitative fluid therapy). When a mammalian patient is dehydrated, fluid therapy can be administered orally, rectally, intravenously, intraosseously, and/or subcutaneously to correct the dehydration, and the fluids typically need to be administered much more slowly to allow equilibration between the different fluid compartments.*[21]

While fluids have emerged as an essential treatment for many conditions in human and domestic animal medicine, new concerns on the deleterious effects of fluid therapy have emerged recently as well. Resuscitative fluid therapy, especially when performed with large volumes of crystalloids, leads to the thinning of the glycocalyx, which cascades into negative interstitial consequences from overzealous fluid administration, such as edema and SIRS. Evidence has emerged that some degree of fluid restriction may help to curb the negative effects of resuscitative fluid therapy.[22] In addition, administration of high levels of chloride in resuscitative fluids has been found in humans to be correlated with higher rates of kidney injury and mortality.[23] These effects can be summed up under the term *fluid overload*. In mammals, interstitial or pulmonary edema or body cavity effusions, especially when body weight increases by 5% to 10%, are typical of the acute effects of fluid overload. Fluid overload has been linked to an increase in adverse outcomes and mortality in human and mammalian veterinary medicine, and a large push to only utilize the minimum amount of fluids required in treatment has emerged.[24] It is unclear if these concepts of fluid overload are directly applicable to non-mammalian patients, as will be discussed in the next section. It is interesting to note, though, in regards to pulmonary edema, that pulmonary surfactant works to counteract and prevent pulmonary edema in mammals and it appears to do the same in reptiles—and reptiles have 7 to 10 times more per unit area than mammals.[25] It is also interesting to note that 3.5 times more fluid loading (120 mL/kg) in a study in chickens (*Gallus domesticus*) was required to induce pulmonary edema, while 33 to 40 mL/kg induced pulmonary edema in mice.[26,27]

Applying these new principles and knowledge from mammalian fluid therapy to non-mammalian patients without more extensive research into their fluid therapy needs is likely a mistake. Given the higher exchange rates between the lymph and interstitium and the intravascular plasma, *birds, reptiles, and fish appear to compensate for fluid loss more readily than mammals and may require larger fluid volumes (in relation to their TBW) than a comparable mammal case when finally presenting to a veterinarian*, as discussed in the next section. Automatically applying new principles of mammalian fluid restriction cannot be recommended at this time. In addition, the makeup of the ideal fluid for each taxa is far from elucidated and chloride content may not have as large of an effect on the kidneys in non-mammalian patients.

Taxonomic Responses to Hypovolemia

In addition to a higher baseline plasma exchange rate in non-mammalian vertebrates, these taxa appear to have the ability to significantly upregulate the replacement of plasma volume from the lymph and interstitium when challenged with hypovolemia. Hemorrhage is the most immediate and direct cause of hypovolemia and hypoperfusion. Mammals can experience hypovolemic shock from hemorrhaging as little as 15% to 20% of their blood volume (15–20 mL/kg of blood in dogs and 10–15 mL/kg of blood in cats).[28] Mammals do not tolerate blood loss nearly as well as birds, fish, or reptiles.[29,14] In fact, avian species have exhibited extraordinary abilities to survive large amounts of hemorrhage (at least 50% of their blood volume).[30]

In a study directly comparing the response of rats and domestic chickens to hemorrhage, a 4 mL blood loss (approximately 17 mL/kg in the chickens and 13 mL/kg in the rats) showed that cardiac output (CO) decreased by 43% and mean arterial pressure by 25% in the rats as the blood was removed. Chickens, by contrast, had only a 4% decrease in CO and 15% decrease in MAP throughout the relatively higher mL/kg fluid loss. Perhaps even more surprisingly, the typical mammalian response to increase total peripheral resistance (increase the "squeeze" of blood vessels to maintain a better blood pressure and better perfusion when blood is lost) did not occur in the chickens—their total peripheral resistance fell by 13%! The rats, meanwhile, had a 65% increase in their total peripheral resistance.[31] While the exact mechanism for how the chickens withstood this hemorrhage so well was not determined in that study, further research has shown that chickens are extremely efficient at mobilizing interstitial fluid to replace lost plasma volume.[32] Ducks were also shown to use interstitial fluid mobilization when experiencing significant blood loss (25% of blood volume removed).[33] Birds also have an additional advantage in recovering from hemorrhage with their rapid erythropoietic capabilities allowing them to replace lost red blood cells more quickly (chickens have a maximum red blood cell lifespan of 35 days whereas humans have a maximum 90 day red blood cell lifespan).[34–36]

While avian species have exhibited extraordinary abilities to survive large amounts of hemorrhage (50%–60% of blood volume), the hemorrhage is not without consequence for the bird, arguing for the utility of fluid therapy.[37] In one study, when only 10 mL/kg of blood was removed, mitochondrial swelling still occurred in the birds' kidneys, and the degree of swelling increased with increasing hypovolemia.[38] Japanese quail also were able to increase their reticulocytosis and ability to replenish lost red blood cells better when receiving saline to replenish blood lost via hemorrhage than when no fluids were administered.[39] And while quail showed less evidence of heart and liver damage after 30% of their circulating blood volume was removed than mammals, signs of the negative consequences of the hemorrhage could still be seen, such as hypoxemic injury to organs.[40] This suggests that fluid therapy is indicated in birds with hypovolemia.

The ability to mobilize extravascular, extracellular fluid when challenged with hemorrhage plays out in numerous studies throughout multiple non-mammalian species and taxa. When rainbow trout were challenged with hemorrhage, they were able to mobilize fluid from a secondary circulatory system that can replace up to 40% of their blood volume nearly instantaneously.[14] The definitive identity of this piscine secondary circulatory system (lymphatic system, secondary microcirculatory system, or other) is not fully elucidated at this time, but it is clear that its presence provides fish with an excellent ability to handle larger blood loss volumes than mammals.[10] Similarly, snakes have been shown to survive and maintain normal perfusion pressures with up to 122% of their blood volume being lost via hemorrhage over the course of one to 2 hours as long as they were allowed to drink water. While cardiovascular reflexes played a role in the snakes maintaining adequate arterial pressures, absorption of extravascular fluid was the most significant occurrence in snakes withstanding such a severe challenge.[41,11,42] Freshwater turtles with 48% to 80% of their blood volume withdrawn actually increased their blood volumes to 30% higher levels than their pre-hemorrhage state and survived with 80% blood loss without being given access to water.[43] Once again, *the ability to withstand such extraordinary levels of hemorrhage and hypovolemia can be attributed to fluid recruitment into the vasculature from the extracellular fluid compartment.*[43]

Finally, despite amphibians' perceived susceptibility to dehydration and fluid loss, some studies have shown that they have a remarkable ability to withstand blood loss. One study showed that the lymph system and lymph hearts helped to replenish intravascular volume when 78% of a toad's original intravascular volume was removed.[44] Mobilization of lymph through various mechanisms appears to be essential to anuran's ability to survive large volume hemorrhage.[45] Lymph hearts are central to this process, as anurans that underwent lymph heart ablation passed away days later from hemoconcentration without any induced hemorrhage.[10]

In addition to the benefit of lymph heart assistance with acute intravascular fluid loss, these patients may also have additional alternate responses to blood loss that mammals cannot achieve. Fish, amphibians, and reptiles have a trabecular, sponge-like ventricle in their heart, unlike the compact muscular ventricular walls found in birds and mammals. This alternative anatomy appears to have a large impact on the ejection fraction that can be achieved by these hearts. *The typical ventricular ejection fraction of mammals and birds is around 50%; in comparison, the ventricular ejection fraction in these trabecular ventricles is nearly 100%.*[15] And while their contribution and exact physiologic significance to hypovolemia and dehydration is not known, it is also interesting to note that lymph hearts are also present in some avian species (namely ratites) as well as turtles, snakes, lizards, and crocodilians.[10] Some research also suggests that the non-mammalian cardiovascular response to catecholamines (namely epinephrine and norepinephrine) can differ greatly from the expected mammalian response (often mirroring the lack of increased systemic vascular resistance outlined in the hemorrhagic shock studies above), which further suggests alternate responses to hypovolemia and dehydration in these patients.[46–48] All of these physiologic differences should be taken into account when designing future fluid therapy research and considering theoretical fluid therapy approaches.

Taxonomic Responses to Dehydration

As previously discussed, dehydration is a fluid-depleted state in which a patient's intravascular volume has been maintained, but a more chronic fluid loss has occurred, usually from the interstitial compartment of an animal's extracellular fluid.[21] Undoubtedly, large differences in where and how fluid is lost in different species will be found when further research is performed. In small herbivorous mammalian patients, such as rabbits, guinea pigs, chinchilla, and degus, the gastrointestinal tract likely serves as a large body water compartment, just as in horses, and this should be accounted for when assessing hydration and formulating a rehydration plan.[21] Chelonian patients also appear to have a relatively large fluid compartment in their gastrointestinal tract and urinary bladders that might provide a fluid reservoir when needed and should be accounted for when assessing dehydration and formulating a correction plan.[49,50] And, as previously discussed, anurans appear to be remarkably tolerant of dehydration, with some species tolerating up to 45% of their body weight as evaporative water losses[51]and some reptiles live in a clinically dehydrated state during certain seasons with very low TBW.[3]Seasnakes have been reported to survive for 6 to 7 months with clinical dehydration during their natural life history.[52] All of this data argues that *small exotic companion animals may be far more dehydrated than would be assumed by initial evaluation if assessed merely as though they were small domestic animal patients* (eg, *dogs and cats). When these exotic patients are exhibiting clinical dehydration, they may have already utilized additional fluid stores that domestic patients don't have.*

Small exotic companion mammals also have higher fluid requirements than dogs and cats even when not dehydrated, with healthy chinchillas consuming up to 120 mL of water per kg per day, rabbits up to 150 mL/kg/day, and guinea pigs up to 200 mL/kg/day.[53,54] Given how difficult it can be to determine when an animal will respond positively to additional fluid therapy, a focus on emerging fluid responsiveness assessments in mammalian medicine (such as passive leg raises, point of care ultrasound, and so forth), will hopefully be investigated and incorporated into fluid management in exotic animals soon.[55] Overall, *a focus on a fluid-restrictive approach as is emerging in human and small animal domestic medicine cannot be endorsed for exotic animals at this time.* Further trends in mammalian medicine of providing fluid therapy more as an acid-base corrective measure rather than a specific amount or type of fluid may be a useful and recommended approach in exotic species, but research is needed to determine if this is the case. While this approach has only recently been adopted in human medicine, it has already been fully embraced in bovine medicine.[56,57]

Due to the physiologic differences discussed above, exotic animal patients may present with large fluid deficits. Even in common domestic animal patients (dogs and cats), estimating dehydration on physical examination to develop a fluid plan is extremely imprecise,[58] so with the vast number of exotic species with highly variable external features, clinician assessment of dehydration level in exotic species is expected to be inaccurate. At this time, the most important assessment for hydration level and fluid requirements in exotic animal species is utilizing changes in weight of the animal and weights of all fluid outputs.[59] Encouraging owners to obtain weekly weights on their animals and weighing any hospitalized patients at least daily, if not multiple times per day, while also attempting to weigh or otherwise quantify fluid outputs will provide the best information for devising a fluid plan in an exotic animal patient.

Application of Differing Physiologies to Exotic Animal Fluid Therapy

Mammalian *resuscitative fluids* are typically given intravenously and are frequently given as boluses of "shock doses," which are usually a mL/kg dose based upon a percentage of the mammal's blood volume that requires replacement. A clinician may give a dog a 20 mL/kg fluid bolus, which might be termed a "quarter shock bolus," aimed to replenish approximately 25% of that dog's blood volume. Non-mammalian physiology suggests that this approach might not be appropriate for these patients. *Given that any fish, herptile, or bird that is determined to be hypovolemic has likely already also exhausted its interstitial fluid stores (due to their ability to rapidly mobilize this fluid compartment to maintain a normal intravascular volume), planning to replace fluid in increments that are percentages of blood volume may not be the best approach.* Depending on how chronic or acute the development of the hypovolemia is, *it is entirely possible that the patient has lost more than their entire blood volume in fluid before entering a shock state*. An exotic animal practitioner, then, should consider providing that patient more than its blood volume in fluid therapy over the course of its hospitalization. *Providing that fluid subcutaneously, given how rapidly it can be sent to the plasma, may also be a prudent clinical decision*. In many zoologic species, the stress of having an intravenous catheter or prolonged handling to administer fluids intravenously would likely negatively affect a patient. Delivering a single, large, subcutaneous fluid bolus that can be distributed to the vasculature and interstitial space after a quick handling likely provides the least stressful and most impactful treatment for many non-mammalian exotic patients.

While it is not suggested that intravenous catheter placement and fluid administration is never warranted in non-mammalian patients (certainly administration of drugs intravenously, especially during surgical procedures is very advantageous), the tenet in mammalian medicine that a hypovolemic patient must be resuscitated with intravenous fluid boluses may not hold true in non-mammalian patients.

Small mammal fluid therapy

As previously discussed, many new concepts are arising in mammalian fluid therapy; cognizance of fluid overload and microcirculatory resuscitation are coming into greater focus.[60] An exotic animal veterinarian can likely apply their small domestic animal fluid therapy treatment principles to their ferret patients. It is important to remember the higher fluid requirement for the small herbivorous species, though, and it may be useful to watch the literature for further information on intragastric and other enteric fluid therapies that are being investigated, as GI water plays a disproportionate role in these patients.[61,62] Studies show that guinea pigs have approximately 100 mL of water in their gastrointestinal tract per kilogram of body weight and rabbits have approximately 75 mL of GI water/kg of body weight.[63,64] For perspective, dogs have around 5% of their body weight made up of water in their GI tract, which is less than 10% of their TBW; when fasted, GI water drops to around 1% of TBW. Rabbits have approximately 10% of their body weight comprised of GI water, which is 15% of their TBW; when fasted, gut water decreases to less than 10% of TBW.[65] With the frequent administration of pre-formulated herbivore diets to many small exotic companion mammals via syringe feeding or feeding tubes, utilizing the water incorporated into these diets as a portion of the fluid treatment for a patient would be prudent and could be utilized to more directly replenish normal GI fluid levels. As previously discussed, small herbivores have higher maintenance fluid consumption than domestic carnivores, with healthy chinchillas consuming up to 120 mL of water per kg per day, rabbits up to 150 mL/kg/day, and guinea pigs up to 200 mL/kg/day.[53,54] Achieving the administration of these higher fluid requirements can more easily be accomplished by utilizing oral water supplementation in addition to parenteral therapies (**Fig. 3**).

Example Fluid Therapy Plans

3.25 kg rabbit with gastrointestinal ileus

- Weighed 3.50 kg at last wellness exam
- Appears to be dehydrated on exam, but no evidence of hypovolemia/cardiovascular instability
- 3.50 kg -3.25 kg = 0.25 kg= 250 mL of potential fluid loss
- Maintenance fluid needs (patient is currently not eating or drinking): 3.50 kg x 150 mL/kg/day = 525 mL/day
- Total fluid needs over next 48 hours: 525 mL x 2 + 250 mL = 1,300 mL
- Possible fluid plan:
  - 150 mL SQ balanced, isotonic crystalloid (BIC) q8h
  - 65 mL of water mixed into an herbivore critical care diet and fed via syringe or esophageal feeding tube q8h
  - This would result in 1300 mL of fluid being administered over 48 hours, and these treatments could be backed down at later treatment times if the rabbit begins eating and drinking on its own

420-g African Grey parrot presenting with dystocia

- Administered 25 mL BIC given at triage exam
- Bloodwork performed several hours after triage—all fluid absorbed; sodium 157 mEq/L and osmolality 335 mOsm/L; new weight 430 grams—outputs of 5 grams feces/urates and 10-gram egg
- 5 mL BIC given IV during 30-minute egg removal procedure (10 mL/kg/hr estimated based upon bird's higher metabolic rate) and then 20 mL additional BIC given SQ at conclusion of procedure and catheter removed to avoid additional blood loss/stress due to evidence of dehydration after high initial BIC dose
- Next morning, weighs 435 grams with 10 grams feces/urates (presumably high insensible fluid loss in incubator, possibly higher fluid loss that evaporated due to post-obstructive diuresis, fluid all absorbed, patient likely not eating/drinking normally)→administer 15 mL BIC SQ to replace measured outs and account for suspected insensible losses
- Monitor water and food intake closely

150-gram Bearded Dragon with general debilitation

- History indicates patient isn't soaked and has been lethargic for 2 weeks
- Very dull on triage examination
- As a desert species, patient likely was quite dehydrated before passing over into the level of hypovolemia (which caused dull mentation), presume 15% dehydration
- Start with 10% dehydration of current weight (likely much lower than "healthy weight") = 0.150 x 0.10 = 0.015 L = 15 mL BIC → give as two 7.5 mL SQ BIC doses with the 2nd dose administered when the first dose is absorbed
- Place in incubator and monitor, if mentation improves the next day, provide warm water soak, weighing patient prior to and after soaking daily, if no response and fluids are absorbed, check osmolality/electrolytes, and consider 5% dehydration replacement (7.5 mL BIC SQ)

175-gram Emerald Tree Boa with general debilitation

- Boa is lethargic/abnormal for past 2-3 days since shedding
- Very dull on triage examination; weight last week = 200 grams
- Replace lost weight → give 25 mL SQ BIC in various areas along body and mist/"rain" on boa and maintain high humidity during hospitalization
- If patient improves in 2-3 days, reweigh prior to tube feeding; new weight = 190 grams, give 10 mL water with tube feeding formula or injected into force fed prey item to replace weight deficit from "normal," if no improvement, administer 10 mL BIC SQ and repeat replacing deficit from "healthy" weight every 2-3 days until patient able to eat or be tube fed

Fig. 3. Examples on how the author might approach various clinical cases when creating and implementing fluid plans. Since there is no high-quality evidence to support any fluid therapy protocols, these examples are based upon basic physiology research and the author's experience.

Avian fluid therapy

Avian patients are frequently very stressed and are prone to trauma when multiple handling events occur. They may also try to remove intravenous catheters and cause themselves further blood loss and stress from placement of these items. Because birds appear able to recruit interstitial fluid exceptionally well, *administration of subcutaneous (SQ) fluids is likely an appropriate treatment modality, even in patients in a shock state.* It is important to remember that the added stress of prolonged handling of a critically ill bird may also cause death. Supporting their systemic vascular pressure via IV fluids may also not be as essential as in mammalian patients, with chickens not increasing their systemic vascular resistance until a MAP of 25 mm Hg was achieved via hemorrhage.[66] Ducks appear to respond more strongly to catecholamines in their peripheral vasculature than chickens, however, so further research in multiple bird species is surely needed.[67] Further research is undoubtedly needed to directly compare IV and SQ fluid routes in avian patients experiencing hypovolemic shock as well, but avian physiology could support a quick triage exam with SQ fluid administration prior to placing the patient in a warm, dark, oxygenated incubator as the most advantageous initial treatment option.

The amount of fluid that should be administered to a bird will likely be highly variable based upon the species and the chief complaint. Just like in mammals, it appears that physical examination parameters don't provide a reliable indicator of a bird's degree of dehydration,[68] so an approach that does not rely on physical examination parameters is likely best. When a bird presents on emergency and appears unstable, it is prudent to handle that patient as little as possible. In clinics that frequently see avian patients, preparing a chart of frequently treated patients and their typical weights is recommended, so that an appropriate amount of fluid can be drawn up in preparation for patient handling (**Fig. 4**). For an avian patient to appear unstable (often only indicated by a dull mentation, as most birds, if they were experiencing adequate cerebral perfusion, would be alert and/or anxious at the hospital), it is likely experiencing shock. There are many types of shock, but the majority benefit from fluid therapy (**Fig. 5**).[69] Cardiogenic shock appears to be the only type of shock where fluids are strictly contraindicated; if signs of cardiogenic shock are detected on a triage examination (heart murmur, coelomic effusion), then fluid administration can be aborted.

While no well-validated evidence exists on the correct amount of fluid to administer to an unstable, emergency bird patient, having 5% of a bird's body weight in fluid ready for administration during the triage examination appears to be an excellent starting point (see **Fig. 4**)—the clinician can always elect to administer only a portion of the fluids. This speculative starting amount is derived from the hemorrhagic shock studies performed in birds indicating that birds appeared to enter a shock state when around 50% of their blood volume (around 50 mL/kg of fluid, which is 5% of their body weight) was removed. Fifty mL/kg of fluid can usually be administered in the inguinal webbing of a bird comfortably, usually on one side, but it can be split between both inguinal webs if necessary.

The suggested approach to reduce stress for a bird patient presenting on emergency, even if not deemed unstable, would be to turn on a warm, oxygenated incubator and place the bird's travel carrier on a scale. Zero the bird's carrier with the bird in it while drawing up the fluids listed on the pre-prepared emergency chart (see **Fig. 4**) as well as any other emergency treatments or interventions. The patient can then be quickly removed from the carrier and an incoming weight can be obtained and recorded from the weight difference. A quick triage examination can be

Example Emergency Avian Fluid Chart

Species	Typical Weight	Emergency Fluid Dose to Draw Up
African Grey Parrot	500 grams	25 mL
Cockatiel	100 grams	5 mL
American Budgerigar	30 grams	1.5 mL
Macaw Species	1.0 kg	50 mL

Fig. 4. An example avian fluid therapy chart that a clinic could create for emergencies. The chart can be adapted to the species most frequently seen at a practice and the weights most frequently seen at that practice.

Types of Shock	Possible Causes
Hypovolemic	Hemorrhage, severe dehydration (GI losses, polyuria, third spacing), burns
Cardiogenic	Congestive heart failure, cardiac arrhythmias, drug overdose (β-blockers, Ca^{2+} channel blockers, anesthetics)
Obstructive	Gastric, intestinal, or mesenteric volvulus, intravascular parasites, large vessel thrombus, cardiac tamponade (pericardial effusion, etc) or a mass effect impeding on large vessel
Distributive	Sepsis, anaphylaxis, catecholamine excess (fear, pheochromocytoma), heatstroke, Addisonian crisis, traumatic brain injury, seizures
Metabolic	Cytopathic hypoxia (sepsis), hypoglycemia, mitochondrial dysfunction, toxic exposures (cyanide, bromethalin)
Hypoxemic	Severe anemia or dyshemoglobinemia (methemoglobinemia, carbon monoxide), pulmonary dysfunction (5 causes of hypoxemia: V/Q mismatch, hypoventilation, low inspired O2, shunt, diffusion impairment)

Fig. 5. Types of shock and disease processes that can cause that type of shock. Overall, fluids can be utilized to address immediate perfusion problems occurring in most types of shock during the initial stabilization phase of treatment, other than cardiogenic shock.

performed, and the fluids can be administered. The actual amount administered can be adjusted based upon the patient's actual weight and clinician's triage examination findings. The bird can then be placed in the warm incubator and kept as stress-free as possible while a history is taken and other treatment plans are configured.

Once a bird has been hospitalized, the long-term fluid plan needs to be devised based upon numerous factors. As previously discussed, administering fluids based upon body weight and weight of fecal and urine outputs is an excellent approach, but blood work can also give clues to the degree of fluid loss that should be replaced. Baseline body weights and blood work parameters are ideal information to obtain at avian wellness examinations, and the value of these diagnostics in future emergencies can be discussed with owners. Blood osmolality, packed cell volume (PCV), total solids (TS), and sodium elevations have all been shown to correlate with the degree of dehydration in birds in several studies.[68,70–72] Urea and creatinine have also been found to increase with dehydration in pigeons.[70] These changes are often not easy to detect on bloodwork without having that individual patient's baseline values, but if these values are clearly elevated, then the clinician can assume their patient is still in a fluid deficit. Without further research to definitively determine the correct approach, intermittent SQ fluid therapy is likely the best approach. An example fluid therapy plan is outlined in **Fig. 3**.

Herptile fluid therapy

Besides the stress of handling involved with intravenous fluid therapy, additional care needs to be taken with IV/IO fluid therapy in reptiles, as the pressure in the systemic and pulmonary vasculature can have strong effects on the degree of right-to-left shunting present in that reptile. In a sick herptile, maximizing oxygen delivery to the systemic circulation may be essential; altering the pressure in the systemic and pulmonary vasculature will determine the degree of right-to-left and left-to-right shunting occurring.[73,74] Given the low systemic blood pressures present in herptiles,[75] altering the pressure in the systemic vasculature by administering large volumes of intravenous fluids could alter cardiac flow in unexpected ways. And, as previously discussed, herptiles appear capable of maintaining their low systemic blood pressures exceptionally well when faced with large volume hemorrhage without intravenous fluid replenishment.[41] Allowing the herptile to absorb fluid and determine its own systemic vasculature pressure may be preferable, but research should investigate this process further. Like avian species, plasma sodium, PCV, TS, and osmolality appears to increase when a herptile is in a fluid deficit.[3,76] Unlike in avian species, a veterinarian typically has a bit more time to consider the fluid therapy plan for a herptile patient, due to their slightly lower stress levels when compared to birds, so weighing the patient and calculating a fluid plan based upon previous weights or subjective impressions on level of dehydration can be more easily accomplished in these patients. Practitioners often try to be conservative in fluids administered to herptile patients due to thoughts on lower metabolic rates and fluid requirements in these patients. Studies show many reptiles and amphibians taking in very large volumes of fluids all at once after a period of experimentally induced dehydration, and with ill patients they may have an even greater fluid deficit that will need to be corrected prior to recovery.[77]

Lizard fluid therapy. Much like avian patients, lizards may become stressed from handling and immobilization/sedation for IV catheter placement. Intravenous access in lizards can also be technically difficult. Lizards frequently have an adequate subcutaneous space to accommodate fluid administration, and if a lizard is kept warm and given SQ fluids, even in a hypovolemic state, *their physiology would suggest that intravascular and interstitial fluid volumes could be restored*. Depending on the mental status of the lizard patient (any chance of drowning or aspiration should be avoided), a combination of SQ fluids and a bowl of water for drinking or soaking could be provided (see **Fig. 3**).

Snake fluid therapy. Snakes have been found to have an extraordinary ability to withstand vascular fluid loss and they have difficult-to-catheterize veins and arteries. Given that they also often have limited SQ space *a combination of SQ fluids, prey items injected with additional fluids, orally gavaged fluids, and/or a water bowl for soaking/drinking might be the best approach in a hypovolemic snake* (see **Fig. 3**). Remember that snakes have been shown to lose greater than their entire blood volume in hemorrhagic shock models, so administering larger than expected fluid volumes may be required when treating these patients.[41,78,11]

Amphibian fluid therapy. Amphibians are already almost exclusively treated with topical immersion baths of fluid, which appears appropriate given their natural history, ability to absorb fluids through their skin, and their astounding ability to mobilize their lymph back into their systemic vasculature. There is some evidence that amphibians can reduce their skin's permeability to fluids when very dehydrated in an effort to prevent further water loss,[51] so SQ fluid administration (which will result in an intralymph injection in any SQ space in an anuran) could also be an option for direct intravascular fluid administration that would quickly be returned to the systemic vasculature (**Fig. 6**).[79] Amphibians appear to develop a very high sodium level when dehydrated, so measuring this level in the blood or lymph could be important clinical information for a veterinarian.[80]

Fish fluid therapy

Fish have very low whole body interstitial compliance and appear to mobilize fluid into their main circulatory system from a secondary circulatory system. With fluid not being

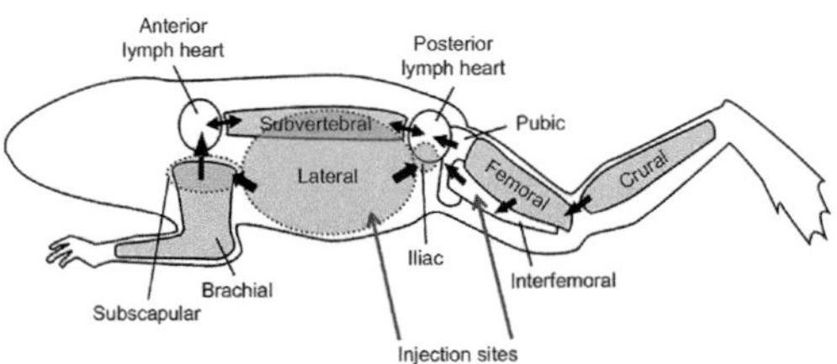

Fig. 6. A diagram of the many different lymph structures present in a typical anuran. The injection sites being shown were for contrast administration in the study from which the figure is referenced. (Reproduced/adapted with permission from Michael S. Hedrick, Kasper Hansen, Tobias Wang, Henrik Lauridsen, Jesper Thygesen, Michael Pedersen, Visualising lymph movement in anuran amphibians with computed tomography, J Exp Biol, 2014, **Fig. 1**.)

supplied by the interstitium and fish possessing very little SQ space, SQ fluids are not really feasible in these patients. The best solution for fluid administration, likely involves the manipulation of the water in which the fish is living. There will be vast differences in the recommendations based upon if the fish is a freshwater, brackish water, or saltwater species. It is also important to note that some fish drink water from their surrounding environment and some do not; there does not appear to be an easily generalizable pattern.[2]Elasmobranchs maintain hyperosmolarity in their plasma to seawater with the help of urea and trimethylamine N-oxide (TMAO) and many other aquatic species have unique approaches to their osmoregulation, which is beyond the scope of this article.[81]Since many fish drink water and regulate intake and uptake of water and ions through their gastrointestinal tract, fluids via gavage or enema during an examination may be an approach to providing fluid support to these species as well.[81,82]As always, more research is warranted.

Invertebrate fluid therapy

Invertebrates encompass a dizzying array of life histories and anatomic and physiologic differences. In general, invertebrates have a relatively open circulatory system and hemolymph, so intravascular fluid resuscitation is not possible. Oral fluid therapy and fluids injected directly into areas of hemolymph are two valid approaches for fluid resuscitation in invertebrates (**Fig. 7**).[83,84]

Fluid Selection

Crystalloids

Fluids can generally be considered crystalloids or colloids. Crystalloids are aqueous solutions containing solutes, such as electrolytes or glucose.[85] Many different types of crystalloid fluids are available commercially that can be considered for exotic patients. Other additional specially-prepared fluid solutions have been suggested for these unique patients, including amphibian, reptile, and elasmobranch Ringer's solutions.[86–88] A crystalloid's tonicity (ie, hypotonic, isotonic, or hypertonic) and osmolality are generally considered when selecting what would be most appropriate for a certain patient. A crystalloid's tonicity generally helps determine if a fluid is a *maintenance* or a *replacement fluid. Maintenance fluids are intended to help replace water losses that occur with normal bodily functions (often termed sensible and insensible losses).* These losses are often pure water or low electrolyte water losses, and therefore *maintenance fluids are hypotonic solutions.*[89] Dextrose is frequently added to these fluids to make them iso-osmolar to the patient, so that hemolysis and other cellular damage

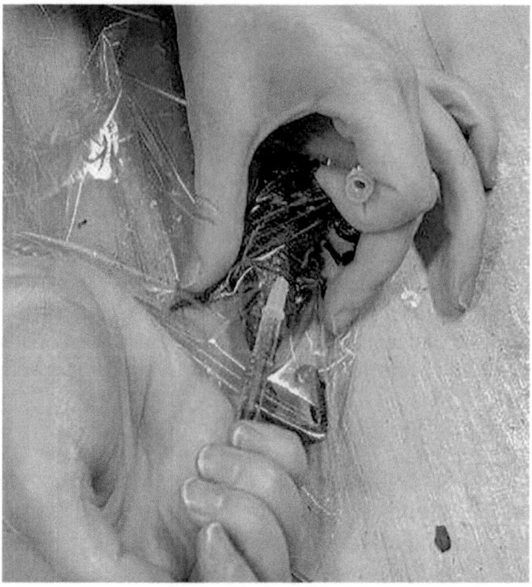

Fig. 7. Administration of specialized fluids created to be a scorpion hemolymph replacement fluid directly into the hemolymph. Restraint within a plastic bag and injection through the plastic bag and into the body of the patient can be an ideal technique for many terrestrial invertebrates.

does not occur as a result of its administration. Once the dextrose is administered in a mammal, the dextrose is quickly metabolized and the resultant hypotonic fluid is overwhelmingly expected to shift into the intracellular fluid compartment.[85] Recent studies with the administration of dextrose (the D-isomer of glucose) to bearded dragons and sea turtles indicate that *reptiles don't appear to quickly metabolize or process the dextrose administered*, with hyperglycemia persisting up to 48 hours after administration.[90,91] Without rapid metabolic processing of the glucose, these fluids would not effectively become hypotonic and function as intended. Studies in rehabilitating sea turtles found fluids with dextrose to be the least effective at returning critically ill sea turtles to a normal acid-base status.[90,92] Subcutaneously administered dextrose also created an additional fluid compartment and removed fluid from already dehydrated pigeons.[71] In addition, the hyperglycemia induced by the dextrose may be harmful in itself. Hyperglycemia is tied to negative outcomes in hospitalized humans[93,94] and chelonians with hyperglycemia examined at a large Taiwanese veterinary hospital had an increased chance of dying while in the hospital.[95] So despite initial theorizing that reptile Ringer's solution (a 1:1 solution of a balanced crystalloid and 5% dextrose) would be the best fluid composition for reptile patients,[87,96] *this does not appear to be the case.* Dextrose administered orally may be considered for hospitalized avian patients. Hospitalized birds will require gavage feeding if they are not eating while hospitalized, due to their rapid metabolism. While additional nutrients via a feeding formula are recommended to feed enterocytes and support the bird beyond its fluid needs, a study in pigeons did reveal that oral 5% dextrose was able to effectively rehydrate dehydrated pigeons.[71]

Crystalloids that are more frequently utilized in human and small animal medicine are isotonic crystalloids. These fluids are meant to match the osmolality of the patient's plasma and a *balanced isotonic crystalloid (BIC) aims to mimic the electrolyte makeup of a patient's plasma as well*. With this composition, *these fluids aim to replenish extracellular fluid losses and are typically referred to as a replacement fluid.*[85] Replacement fluids cannot mimic or be balanced for every mammalian species, so they certainly cannot be expected to match or mimic the plasma of every exotic species. Fortunately, *mammalian and non-mammalian taxa don't appear to require exact iso-osmolarity in the fluids they receive. In general, commercial BICs appear to be safe and effective in exotic patients.*

A concern with utilizing replacement fluids extensively in mammalian patients is their relatively higher sodium and chloride load, particularly with use of 0.9% saline. High chloride loads can be damaging to mammalian kidneys.[85] Significant sodium loads present in mammalian replacement fluids can cause natriuresis, which leads to diuresis, with some studies in horses suggesting that horses were unable to achieve euhydration and experienced rebound dehydration from IV replacement fluid therapy. In addition to diuresis, the high sodium load can lend itself to fluid retention and edema formation.[21] While a great deal of further research is required to fully understand the effects of high sodium and chloride loads in non-mammalian patients, the current evidence appears to show that potassium may be the only electrolyte that truly limits their hydration level as the salt glands and kidneys may be limited on the amount of potassium that can be excreted.[50] Most BICs do have potassium, but, in the author's experience, this level of potassium does not exceed non-mammalian patients' ability to excrete it, likely via the kidneys. Many debilitated patients also benefit from potassium supplementation. *For this reason, no definitive contraindications can be found to utilizing balanced, isotonic, replacement fluids in exotic (both mammalian and non-mammalian) patients at this time.* These replacement fluids are still used nearly exclusively in domestic small animal medicine and should be considered the standard of care for SQ fluids that have been frequently recommended throughout this article.

There is little doubt that response to sodium and chloride changes are vastly different in non-mammalian species. This likely relates to these uricotelic species (species that excrete uric acid as their nitrogen waste product in the urine as "urates") having a relative inability to concentrate their urine to rid themselves of excess electrolytes, but an increased ability to move electrolytes between the plasma and other body water. For example, iguanas became anuric when injected with a heavy salt load and prevented from drinking, in contrast to rats that excreted nearly the entire salt load in urine.[77] Chickens lost fluid almost exclusively from their interstitial fluid compartment when fed a sodium-restricted diet or when administered furosemide. Interestingly, their plasma volume remained unchanged and only their extracellular and interstitial fluid volumes were decreased, which was vastly different than fluid loss seen in domestic cats. The amount of sodium depletion would have led to hypovolemia in a mammal.[97] Additionally, some anurans can withstand a near doubling of their plasma sodium concentration, a change that no mammal could ever survive.[80] It is likely that these differences in non-mammalian species are due to their osmoregulatory organs, namely their gastrointestinal tract (post-renal urine modification) and salt glands. The mammalian kidney is responsible for nearly all mammalian osmoregulation but with no loops of Henle in reptiles and reduced levels in birds, the intestines and salt glands (if present) help with osmoregulation when the bird or reptile cannot excrete the salt load via their kidneys.[98] Marine birds can handle much higher salt loads than other birds, due to their highly functioning salt glands.[4,2] Even newly hatched leatherback sea turtles are able to tolerate large internal electrolyte changes and utilize their salt glands to return to a normal acid-base and electrolyte status that would not be tolerated by mammals.[99]

When considering blood and fluid osmolality in exotic animal medicine, non-mammalian taxa were once assumed to have lower osmolalities than mammalian patients, but recent studies have illustrated that bearded dragons had osmolarities similar to those in dogs and cats (around 295 mOsm/kg)[100] and studies into other lizards species have indicated that they have a variety of different osmolalities, with variability found even between chameleon species.[101] A study on the osmolality of corn snakes indicated that they had a higher average osmolality than dogs and cats of around 344 mOsm/kg.[102] Many of these values are higher than the osmolality of the easily commercially available lactated Ringer's solution (272 mOsm/L), Plasma-Lyte A (294 mOsm/L), and Normosol R (295 mOsm/L). Clinically, these differences are unlikely to have a negative impact when these fluids are administered to non-mammalian exotic patients. If administered SQ, these fluids will likely equilibrate the electrolytes appropriately. If given IV, non-mammalian erythrocytes are much less osmotically fragile than mammalian erythrocytes[103] and these fluids may just provide a slightly hypotonic fluid straddling a maintenance and replacement fluid in those species with typically very high osmolarities.

A final type of crystalloid to consider is a *hypertonic crystalloid*, most commonly hypertonic saline, a 7.2% solution, which generally possesses a tonicity nine times that of normal mammalian plasma. Administration of this fluid in mammals, appears to encourage the mobilization of fluids from the interstitium (or perhaps glycocalyx or sub-glycocalyx space) into the intravascular space (something that non-mammals are already more adept at doing than mammals), which makes this *an ideal fluid for hypovolemic mammals*. After this initial administration, further isotonic crystalloids must be administered to replace fluid pulled from the interstitium.[21] Again, further research is required to make a definitive judgment on the *utility of hypertonic saline in non-mammalian patients, but it appears unlikely to be of great benefit in birds, reptiles, fish, and invertebrates*, as birds, reptiles, and fish already readily pull fluid from the interstitium to maintain intravascular volume and the open circulatory system of invertebrates negates the need for fluid pull into vascular structures.

Colloids

Colloids are crystalloid solutions with large molecular weight structures within them, such as hydroxyethyl starches (*synthetic colloids*) or proteins (*natural colloids*). These starches and proteins tend to not cross the endothelial glycocalyx and therefore exert a force, called the colloid oncotic pressure (COP) between the sub-glycocalyx fluid space and the plasma.[85] Synthetic colloids are falling out of favor and human albumin is gaining favor as a safer colloid option in human medicine, mainly due to acute kidney injury risks from synthetic colloids.[104] Unfortunately, xenotransfusions with human albumin are known to produce transfusion reactions and delayed side effects in other mammalian species, and albumin from exotic animal species is not currently available.[104] Colloids used to be considered essential to treat edema and pull fluid from the interstitium into the intravascular space via the Starling's force of oncotic pressure. This is known to no longer be true, but albumin administration is still considered beneficial in many instances in mammalian medicine as it supports the glycocalyx, which is essential to health and proper fluid balance.[105] Some studies go as far as to claim that albumin directly controls the permeability of the glycocalyx in mammals.[106]

As with all concepts discussed this far, it is unclear if the approach to fluid therapy in mammals and the new paradigms in colloid administration are relevant for non-mammalian patients. *Colloids are mainly utilized in mammalian medicine to provide rapid intravascular volume expansion and to combat interstitial edema*. As previously discussed, *birds, reptiles, and fish are quite capable of intravascular volume expansion without colloid administration* and appear to achieve this without the typical Starling's forces that were originally utilized to justify colloid administration. In addition, interstitial edema appears to occur rarely in non-mammalian patients. In one study, pigeons did not develop edema even when their albumin was decreased to less than 1.0 g/dL with significant hemorrhage. They also clinically rebounded and withstood 39 mL/kg of blood removal.[107] Low colloid osmotic pressure is also frequently present in chronically debilitated loggerhead sea turtles and even in health their albumin and COP were much lower than seen in mammals, but edema does not appear to be a clinical sign exhibited with these changes.[108]

Another important difference between plasma protein in mammals versus birds and reptiles when considering colloids is that *plasma proteins are essential for helping solubilize and excrete uric acid, the nitrogenous end-product of most birds and reptiles*. Since uric acid is normally insoluble in water, protein emulsification is an essential part of these species' physiology, and *synthetic colloids and mammalian proteins will likely not accomplish this essential physiologic role correctly*.[109]

Blood products

A full review of blood transfusions in exotic animal medicine is outside of the scope of this article, but very little is known or published on this topic overall. All transfusions performed thus far appear to be whole blood, packed red blood cell, or plasma transfusions. Non-mammalian exotic patients have very little transfusion literature available. Future research is sorely needed in this area, but, as discussed previously, *non-mammalian exotic patients are surprisingly tolerant of hemorrhage and blood loss as well as low colloid osmotic pressures,* so these patients are often able to survive disease processes leading to severe anemia and/or hypoproteinemia without the aid of a blood transfusion. As discussed above in the fluid therapy section, surviving an insult does not mean that a patient wouldn't benefit from additional supportive care, so future research in mammalian and non-mammalian exotic animal transfusions is highly encouraged.

SUMMARY

Overall, while veterinarians must stay current on the newest fluid therapy research that is emerging in the human medical literature as it often translates into small animal domestic medicine, they are cautioned to not automatically apply these same principles to their non-mammalian exotic patients. Altered physiology in these patients indicates that different fluid volumes, different fluid types, and alternate fluid administration routes may need to be considered. While the state of the literature in exotic animal fluid therapy is sadly lacking, understanding the basic physiology research on the cardiovascular system of these patients can help practitioners conceptualize the response to fluid loss and supplementation, which may help when formulating treatment plans.

CLINICS CARE POINTS

- Subcutaneous fluids are a valid treatment option for hypovolemic avian and herptile patients.
- Commercially-available balanced isotonic crystalloids appear to be a valid treatment option for the majority of exotic animal fluid treatment needs.
- Exotic animal patients may require greater fluid replacement than might be utilized in comparable domestic animal patients.

DISCLOSURE

The author has no conflicts of interest to declare.

REFERENCES

1. Muir WW, Hughes D, Silverstein DC. Editorial: Fluid Therapy in Animals: Physiologic Principles and Contemporary Fluid Resuscitation Considerations. Front Vet Sci 2021;8:744080.
2. Rash R, Lillywhite HB. Drinking behaviors and water balance in marine vertebrates. Marine Biology 2019;166(10).
3. Bradshaw S. Osmoregulation in Lizards. In: Cloudsley-Thompson J, editor. Homeostasis in desert reptiles. Berlin: Springer Link; 1997. p. 39–42.
4. Bennett D, Gray D, Sharp P, et al. Redistribution of extracellular water and sodium may contribute to saline tolerance in wild ducks. Physiol Biochem Zool 2005;78(3):447–55.
5. Thorson T. Body fluid partitioning in reptilia. Copeia 1968;3:592–601.
6. Wellman ML, DiBartola SP, Kohn CW. Applied Physiology of Body Fluids in Dogs and Cats. Fluid, Electrolyte, and Acid-Base Disorders in Small Animal Practice 2012;2–25.
7. Lawrence-Mills SJ, Hughes D, Hezzell MJ, et al. The microvascular endothelial glycocalyx: An additional piece of the puzzle in veterinary medicine. Vet J 2022; 285:105843.
8. Woodcock TE, Woodcock TM. Revised Starling equation and the glycocalyx model of transvascular fluid exchange: an improved paradigm for prescribing intravenous fluid therapy. Br J Anaesth 2012;108(3):384–94.
9. Woodcock TE, Michel CC. Advances in the Starling Principle and Microvascular Fluid Exchange; Consequences and Implications for Fluid Therapy. Front Vet Sci 2021;8:623671.
10. Hedrick MS, Hillman SS, Drewes RC, et al. Lymphatic regulation in nonmammalian vertebrates. J Appl Physiol 2013;115(3):297–308.
11. Lillywhite H, Smits A. Lability of blood volume in snakes and its relation to activity and hypertension. J Exp Biol 1984;110:267–74.
12. Hillman S, Zygmunt A, Baustian M. Transcapillary fluid forces during dehydration in two amphibians. Physiol Zool 1987;60(3):339–45.
13. Hillman SS, Drewes RC, Hedrick MS. Control of blood volume following hypovolemic challenge in vertebrates: Transcapillary versus lymphatic mechanisms. Comp Biochem Physiol Mol Integr Physiol 2021;254:110878.
14. Olson KR, Kinney DW, Dombkowski RA, et al. Transvascular and intravascular fluid transport in the rainbow trout: revisiting Starling's forces, the secondary circulation and interstitial compliance. J Exp Biol 2003;206(Pt 3):457–67.
15. Burggren WW, Christoffels VM, Crossley DA 2nd, et al. Comparative cardiovascular physiology: future trends, opportunities and challenges. Acta Physiol 2014;210(2):257–76.
16. Peltonen LM, Sankari S. Ott's protein osmotic pressure of serum and interstitial fluid in chickens (Gallus gallus): effect of age and gender. J Exp Biol 2011; 214(Pt 4):599–606.
17. Oyama MA, Adin D. Toward quantification of loop diuretic responsiveness for congestive heart failure. J Vet Intern Med 2022;37(1):12–21.
18. Stewart RH. A Modern View of the Interstitial Space in Health and Disease. Front Vet Sci 2020;7:609583.

19. Hancock T, Hoagland T, Hillman SS. Whole-body systemic transcapillary filtration rates, coefficients, and isogravimetric capillary pressures in *Bufo marinus* and *Rana catesbeiana*. Physiol Biochem Zool 2000;73(2):161–8.
20. Mazzaferro E, Powell LL. Fluid Therapy for the Emergent Small Animal Patient: Crystalloids, Colloids, and Albumin Products. Vet Clin North Am Small Anim Pract 2022;52(3):781–96.
21. Crabtree NE, Epstein KL. Current Concepts in Fluid Therapy in Horses. Front Vet Sci 2021;8:648774.
22. Smart L, Hughes D. The Effects of Resuscitative Fluid Therapy on the Endothelial Surface Layer. Front Vet Sci 2021;8:661660.
23. Sen A, Keener CM, Sileanu FE, et al. Chloride Content of Fluids Used for Large-Volume Resuscitation Is Associated With Reduced Survival. Crit Care Med 2017;45(2):e146–53.
24. Hansen B. Fluid Overload. Front Vet Sci 2021;8:668688.
25. Orgeig S, Smits A, Daniels C, et al. Surfactant regulates pulmonary fluid balance in reptiles. Am J Physiol Regul Integr Comp Physiol 1997;273(6):R2013–21.
26. Weidner WJ, Kinnison JR. Effect of hydrostatic pulmonary edema on the inter-parabronchial septum of the chicken lung. Poult Sci 2002;81(10):1563–6.
27. Yoneda K. Fluid-overload pulmonary oedema in mice: The intercellular junctions of bronchiolar epithelium and arterial endothelium. Br J Exp Path 1983;64: 215–24.
28. Linklater A. Management of Hemorrhagic Shock. In: Drobatz KJ, Hopper K, Rozanski E, et al, editors. Textbook of small animal emergency medicine. Hoboken, NJ: John Wiley and Sons, Inc.; 2019. p. 1115–25.
29. Hall K, Drobatz K. Volume Resuscitation in the Acutely Hemorrhaging Patient: Historic Use to Current Applications. Front Vet Sci 2021;8:638104.
30. Wernick MB, Steinmetz HW, Martin-Jurado O, et al. Comparison of fluid types for resuscitation in acute hemorrhagic shock and evaluation fo gastric luminal and transcutaneous PCO2 in leghorn chickens. J Avian Med Surg 2013;27(2): 109–19.
31. Ploucha J, Fink G. Hemodynamics of hemorrhage in the conscious rat and chicken. Am J Physiol Regul Integr Comp Physiol 1986;251(5):R846–50.
32. Ploucha J, Scott J, Ringer R. Vascular and hematologic effects of hemorrhage in the chicken. Am J Physiol Heart Circ Physiol 1981;240(1):H1–17.
33. Djojosugito AM, Folkow B, Kovách AGB. The Mechanisms behind the Rapid Blood Volume Restoration after Hemorrhage in Birds. Acta Physiol Scand 1968;74(1–2):114–22.
34. Rodnan G, Ebaugh JFG, et al. The life span of the red blood cell and the red blood cell volume in the chicken, pigeon, and duck as estimated by the use of Na2Cr51O4 with observations on the red cell turnover rate in the mammal, bird, and reptile. Blood 1957;12(4):355–66.
35. Schindler S, Gildersleeve R. Comparison of recovery from hemorrhage in birds and mammals. Comp Biochem Physiol 1987;87A(3):533–42.
36. Yap KN, Zhang Y. Revisiting the question of nucleated versus enucleated erythrocytes in birds and mammals. Am J Physiol Regul Integr Comp Physiol 2021; 321(4):R547–57.
37. Wernick MB, Steinmetz HW, Martin-Jurado O, et al. Comparison of Fluid Types for Resuscitation in Acute Hemorrhagic Shock and Evaluation of Gastric Luminal and Transcutaneous Pco2in Leghorn Chickens. J Avian Med Surg 2013;27(2): 109–19.

38. Brown T. Effects of bleeding on mitochondrial ultrastructure in the avian kidney. Avian Dis 1985;29(4):1260–5.
39. Schindler S, Gildersleeve R, Thaxton J, et al. Hematological response of hemorrhaged Japanese quail after blood volume replacement with saline. Comp Biochem Physiol 1987;87A(4):933–45.
40. Gildersleeve R, Galvin M, Thaxton J, et al. Hematological response of Japanese quail to acute hemorrhagic stress. Comp Biochem Physiol 1985;81A(2):403–9.
41. Lillywhite H, Ackerman R, Palacios L. Cardiorespiratory responses of snakes to experimental hemorrhage. J Comp Physiol 1983;152:59–65.
42. Smits A, Lillywhite H. Maintenance of blood volume in snakes: transcapillary shifts of extravascular fluids during acute hemorrhage. J Comp Physiol B 1985;155:305–10.
43. Smits A, Kozubowski M. Partitioning of body fluids and cardiovascular responses to circulatory hypovolaemia in the turtle, *Pseudemys scripta elegans*. J Exp Biol 1985;116:237–50.
44. Baustian M. The contribution of the lymphatic pathways during recovery from hemorrhage in the toad *Bufo marinus*. Physiol Zool 1988;61(6):555–63.
45. Hedrick MS, McNew KA, Crossley DA 2nd. Baroreflex function in anurans from different environments. Comp Biochem Physiol Mol Integr Physiol 2015;179: 144–8.
46. Akers T, Peiss C. Comparative study of effect of epinephrine and norepinephrine on cardiovascular system of turtle, alligator, chicken, and opossum. PSEBM (Proc Soc Exp Biol Med) 1963;117:396–9.
47. Baysal F, Vural H. Effects of some catecholamines on the arterial blood pressure of turtle, *Testudo graeca*. Gen Pharmac 1975;6:75–6.
48. Rubanyi G, Huszar L, Kovach A. Comparative physiology of hemorrhage. A study of adrenergic receptor stimulation and blockade in pigeon and mammal. Adv Exp Med Biol 1972;33(0):593–601.
49. Jones TT, Hastings MD, Bostrom BL, et al. Validation of the use of doubly labeled water for estimating metabolic rate in the green turtle (Chelonia mydas L.): a word of caution. J Exp Biol 2009;212(Pt 16):2635–44.
50. Perran Ross J. Water loss in the turtle *Gopherus pollyphemus*. Comp Biochem Physiol 1977;56A:477–80.
51. Hillman SS. Anuran amphibians as comparative models for understanding extreme dehydration tolerance: a unique negative feedback lymphatic mechanism for blood volume regulation. Am J Physiol Regul Integr Comp Physiol 2018;315(4):R790–8.
52. Lillywhite HB, Sheehy CM 3rd, Brischoux F, et al. Pelagic sea snakes dehydrate at sea. Proc Biol Sci 2014;281(1782):20140119.
53. Potter M, Borkowski G. Apparent psychogenic polydipsia and secondary polyuria in laboratory-housed New Zealand white rabbits. Contemp Topics 1998; 37(6):87–9.
54. Wolf P, Cappai MG, Kamphues J. Water consumption in small mammals (dwarf rabbits, Guinea pigs and chinchillas): New data about possible influencing factors. Res Vet Sci 2020;133:146–9.
55. Boysen SR, Gommeren K. Assessment of Volume Status and Fluid Responsiveness in Small Animals. Front Vet Sci 2021;8:630643.
56. Constable PD, Trefz FM, Sen I, et al. Intravenous and Oral Fluid Therapy in Neonatal Calves With Diarrhea or Sepsis and in Adult Cattle. Front Vet Sci 2020;7:603358.

57. Klein-Richers U, Heitland A, Hartmann K, et al. Influence of acetate- vs. lactate-containing fluid bolus therapy on acid-base status, electrolytes, and plasma lactate in dogs. Front Vet Sci 2022;9:903091.
58. Hansen B, DeFrancesco T. Relationship between hydration estimate and body weight change after fluid therapy in critically ill dogs and cats. J Vet Emerg Crit Care 2002;12(4):235–43.
59. Langston C, Gordon D. Effects of IV Fluids in Dogs and Cats With Kidney Failure. Front Vet Sci 2021;8:659960.
60. Cooper ES, Silverstein DC. Fluid Therapy and the Microcirculation in Health and Critical Illness. Front Vet Sci 2021;8:625708.
61. Dias DCR, Ribeiro Filho JD, Viana RB, et al. Comparative Trial of Continuous Flow Enteral and Intravenous Fluid Therapy in Horses. Front Vet Sci 2021;8: 686425.
62. Girisgin AS, Acar F, Cander B, et al. Fluid replacement via the rectum for treatment of hypovolaemic shock in an animal model. Emerg Med J 2006;23(11): 862–4.
63. Hatton GB, Yadav V, Basit AW, et al. Animal Farm: Considerations in Animal Gastrointestinal Physiology and Relevance to Drug Delivery in Humans. J Pharm Sci 2015;104(9):2747–76.
64. Merchant HA, McConnell EL, Liu F, et al. Assessment of gastrointestinal pH, fluid and lymphoid tissue in the guinea pig, rabbit and pig, and implications for their use in drug development. Eur J Pharm Sci 2011;42(1–2):3–10.
65. Cizek L. Total water content of laboratory animals with special reference to volume of fluid within the lumen of the gastrointestinal tract. Am J Physiol Legacy Content 1954;179(1):104–10.
66. Ploucha J, Bursian S, Ringer R, et al. Effects of severe hemorrhagic hypotension on the vasculature of the chicken. Proc Soc Exp Biol Med 1982;170:160–4.
67. Wilson J, West N. Cardiovascular responses to neurohormones in conscious chickens and ducks. Gen Comp Endocrinol 1986;62:268–80.
68. Vanderhasselt RF, Buijs S, Sprenger M, et al. Dehydration indicators for broiler chickens at slaughter. Poult Sci 2013;92(3):612–9.
69. de Laforcade A, Silverstein DC. Shock. In: Silverstein DC, Hopper K, editors. Small Animal Critical Care Medicine. Second Edition. Saint Louis: Elsevier; 2015. p. 26–30.
70. Lumeij JT. Plasma urea, creatinine and uric acid concentrations in response to dehydration in racing pigeons (Columba livia domestica). Avian Pathol 1987; 16(3):377–82.
71. Martin H, Kollias GV. Evaluation of water deprivation and fluid therapy in pigeons. J Zoo Wildl Med 1989;20(2):173–7.
72. Roberts J, Dantzler WH. Glomerular filtration rate in conscious unrestrained starlings under dehydration. J Exp Biol 1989;4(2):R836–9.
73. Hicks J, Ishimatsu A, Molloi S, et al. The mechanism of cardiac shunting in reptiles: A new synthesis. J Exp Biol 1996;199:1435–46.
74. Jensen B, Moorman AF, Wang T. Structure and function of the hearts of lizards and snakes. Biol Rev Camb Philos Soc 2014;89(2):302–36.
75. Schulte K, Kunter U, Moeller MJ. The evolution of blood pressure and the rise of mankind. Nephrol Dial Transplant 2015;30(5):713–23.
76. Parkinson L, Mans C. Effects of furosemide administration to water-deprived inland bearded dragons (Pogona vitticeps). American Journal of Veterinary Research 2018;79(11):1204–8.

77. Kaufman S, Fitzsimons J. Cellular dehydration as a stimulus to drinking in the common iguana, Iguana iguana. In: Peters G, Fitzsimons J, Peters-Haefeli L, editors. Control mechanisms of drinking. Berlin: Springer-Verlag; 1975. p. 47–52.
78. Lillywhite H, Smith L. Haemodynamic responses to haemorrhage in the snake, *Elaphe obsoleta obsoleta*. J Exp Biol 1981;94:275–83.
79. Hillman SS, Hedrick MS, Withers PC, et al. Lymph pools in the basement, sump pumps in the attic: The anuran dilemma for lymph movement. Physiol Biochem Zool 2004;77(2):161–73.
80. Hillman S. Physiologic correlates of differential dehydration tolerance in anuran amphibians. Copeia 1980;1980(1):125–9.
81. Larsen EH, Deaton LE, Onken H, et al. Osmoregulation and excretion. Compr Physiol 2014;4(2):405–573.
82. Parkinson L, Gaines B, Nollens H. Effect of a Nutrient Enema on Serum Nutrient Concentrations in White-Spotted Bamboo Sharks (Chiloscyllium Plagiosum). J Zoo Wildl Med 2019;50(1):55–61.
83. Dombrowski D, De Voe R. Emergency care of invertebrates. Vet Clin North Am Exot Anim Pract 2007;10(2):621–45.
84. Pellett S, Bushell M. Emergency care and first aid of invertebrates. Companion Animal 2015;20(3):182–6.
85. Rudloff E, Hopper K. Crystalloid and Colloid Compositions and Their Impact. Front Vet Sci 2021;8:639848.
86. Hadfield CA, Whitaker BR. Amphibian Emergency Medicine and Care. Seminars Avian Exot Pet Med 2005;14(2):79–89.
87. Prezant RM, Jarchow JL. Indications and applications of clinical techniques in the Green Iguana. Seminars Avian Exot Pet Med 1997;6(2):63–74.
88. Vergneau-Grosset C, Cruz Benedetti IC. Fish Sedation and Anesthesia. Vet Clin North Am Exot Anim Pract 2022;25(1):13–29.
89. DiBartola SP, Bateman S. Introduction to Fluid Therapy. Fluid, Electrolyte, and Acid-Base Disorders in Small Animal Practice 2012;331–50.
90. Camacho M, Quintana Mdel P, Calabuig P, et al. Acid-Base and Plasma Biochemical Changes Using Crystalloid Fluids in Stranded Juvenile Loggerhead Sea Turtles (Caretta caretta). PLoS One 2015;10(7):e0132217.
91. Parkinson L, Mans C. Evaluation of subcutaneously administered electrolyte solutions in experimentally dehydrated inland bearded dragons (*Pogona vitticepsl).* Am J Vet Res 2020;81(5):437–41.
92. Inurria A, Santana A, Casal AB, et al. Comparison Between Effects of Four Crystalloid Solutions on Acid-Base and Electrolyte Abnormalities in Stranded Juvenile Loggerhead Sea Turtles (Caretta caretta). Front Vet Sci 2022;9:855744.
93. Lleva RR, Inzucchi SE. Hospital management of hyperglycemia. Curr Opin Endocrinol Diabetes Obes 2011;18(2):110–8.
94. Plummer MP, Bellomo R, Cousins CE, et al. Dysglycaemia in the critically ill and the interaction of chronic and acute glycaemia with mortality. Intensive Care Med 2014;40(7):973–80.
95. Colon V, Di Girolamo N. Prognostic value of packed cell volume and blood glucose concentration in 954 client-owned chelonians. J Amer Vet Med Assoc 2020;257(12):1265–72.
96. Schumacher JP. Fluid Therapy in Reptiles. In: Fowler M, Miller R, editors. Zoo and wild animal medicine, current therapy6. St Louis, MO: Elsevier; 2008. p. 160–4.

97. Harris K, Koike T. The effects of dietary sodium restriction on fluid and electrolyte metabolism in the chicken (*Gallus domesticus*). Comp Biochem Physiol 1977; 58A:311–7.
98. McWhorter TJ, Caviedes-Vidal E, Karasov WH. The integration of digestion and osmoregulation in the avian gut. Biol Rev Camb Philos Soc 2009;84(4):533–65.
99. Reina R, Jones T, Spotila J. Salt and water regulation by the leatherback sea turtle *Dermochelys coriacea*. J Exp Biol 2002;205:1853–60.
100. Dallwig R, Mitchell MA, Acierno MJ. Determination of Plasma Osmolality and Agreement Between Measured and Calculated Values in Healthy Adult Bearded Dragons (Pogona vitticeps). J Herpetol Med Surg 2010;20(2–3):69–73.
101. Perry SM, Acierno MJ, Mitchell MA. Measuring the Level of Agreement between Osmometer and Calculated Plasma Osmolalities in Two Species of Chameleons, Furcifer pardalis and Chamaeleo calyptratus. J Herpetol Med Surg 2021;31(1).
102. Sanchez-Migallon Guzman D, Mitchell M, Acierno M. Determination of plasma osmolality and agreement between measured and calculated values in captive male corn snakes (*Pantherophis [Elaphe] guttatus guttatus*). J Herp Med Surg 2011;21(1):16–9.
103. Aldrich K, Saunders D, Sievert L, et al. Comparison of erythrocyte osmotic fragility among amphibians, reptiles, birds, and mammals. Trans Kans Acad Sci 2006;109(3/4):149–58.
104. Adamik KN, Yozova ID. Colloids Yes or No? - a "Gretchen Question" Answered. Front Vet Sci 2021;8:624049.
105. Montealegre F, Lyons BM. Fluid Therapy in Dogs and Cats With Sepsis. Front Vet Sci 2021;8:622127.
106. Dull RO, Hahn RG. The glycocalyx as a permeability barrier: basic science and clinical evidence. Crit Care 2022;26(1):273.
107. Cornelius S, Klugman K, Hattingh J. Effects of haemorrhage on colloid osmotic pressure in the pigeon. Comp Biochem Physiol 1982;71A:337–9.
108. Hoffmann HR, Perrault JR, Bandt C, et al. Plasma Colloid Osmotic Pressure in Chronically Debilitated Loggerhead Sea Turtles (Caretta Caretta). J Zoo Wildl Med 2019;50(2):362–8.
109. Braun EJ. Integration of organ systems in avian osmoregulation. J Exp Zool 1999;283(7):702–7.

Urine Output Monitoring and Acute Kidney Injury in Mammalian Exotic Animal Critical Care

Stacey Leonatti Wilkinson, DVM, DABVP, (Reptile and Amphibian)

KEYWORDS

• Acute • Diuretic • Exotic companion mammal • Fluid therapy • Kidney

KEY POINTS

- Acute Kidney Injury (AKI) is a sudden, severe decrease in kidney function, leading to the retention of uremic waste and subsequent fluid, electrolyte, and acid-base abnormalities.
- Numerous causes of AKI exist, and successful treatment depends on identifying and properly treating the underlying cause, along with proper fluid support, correction of electrolyte and acid-base disturbances, supportive care, and urine output monitoring.
- Exotic species present numerous challenges when managing AKI. Their small size can make IV/IO and urinary catheterization difficult, especially without sedation or anesthesia.
- Exotic animals tend to hide clinical signs of illness until disease is advanced, so distinguishing acute from chronic kidney disease can be difficult, and can make cases more difficult to manage.
- Prognosis for AKI overall is guarded to poor, though with proper identification and aggressive treatment, patients can recover. In some cases, permanent renal damage occurs that needs chronic management.

INTRODUCTION

Acute kidney injury (AKI) is defined as a sudden, severe decrease in kidney function. This leads to the retention of uremic wastes, abnormalities in circulating fluids and electrolytes, and acid-base imbalances.[1,2] Much of the knowledge of pathophysiology, causes, diagnosis, and treatment of AKI stems from small animal medicine (dogs and cats) and is then extrapolated to exotic species. Most exotic companion mammal species with AKI will follow a similar progression and can be managed similarly, with some individual species variation. An overview of AKI will be presented here, with further information pertaining to exotic companion mammals.

Avian and Exotic Animal Hospital of Georgia, 118 Pipemakers Circle Suite 110, Pooler, GA 31322, USA
E-mail address: drw@avianexotichospital.com

Vet Clin Exot Anim 26 (2023) 647–672
https://doi.org/10.1016/j.cvex.2023.05.005
1094-9194/23/

PATHOPHYSIOLOGY

Categories of AKI include prerenal, renal (intrinsic), and postrenal. Prerenal AKI arises when the hydrostatic pressure within the glomerular tuft is too low to cause the movement of plasma ultrafiltrate into Bowman's capsule, leading to the retention of nitrogenous wastes in the bloodstream.[3,4] Prerenal AKI occurs secondary to decreases in renal blood flow or abnormal perfusion, typically a complication of conditions that cause hemodynamic abnormalities such as severe dehydration, hypotension, hypovolemia, shock, and so forth.[3,4] It does not initially cause morphologic abnormalities in the kidneys and can be reversible with the correction of hemodynamic changes, but it can lead to primary renal AKI due to renal ischemia if not corrected.[3,4]

Postrenal AKI typically develops when a blockage in urine outflow causes intranephron hydrostatic pressure to increase and prevent ultrafiltration at the glomerular tuft, thus preventing the creation of new urine.[4] This leads to the retention of nitrogenous wastes in the blood, although only if both kidneys are affected by the blockage. If one kidney remains unaffected and has normal function, it can compensate for the drastic drop in GFR.[3,4] Postrenal AKI can rapidly be corrected by treating the underlying cause, but if the distal urine outflow obstruction is not relieved, intrarenal pressure can increase, leading to tubular epithelial damage and interstitial inflammation and edema, causing primary renal AKI.[1,4] Postrenal AKI can also develop with leakage of urine into the retroperitoneal or peritoneal cavities. In these circumstances, GFR remains normal; however, azotemia develops as nitrogenous wastes are reabsorbed into circulation from the peritoneal or retroperitoneal spaces.[4]

The clinical course of renal AKI can be divided into four phases. Phase one, initiation, occurs during and immediately after the insult to the kidneys when pathologic damage to the kidney occurs.[2,3] GFR is reduced and direct tubular damage occurs, which leads to hypoxia, ATP depletion, formation of free radicals, cellular damage, and Na^+/K^+-ATPase pump dysfunction. Cellular basement membranes are damaged which results in tubular casts, increased backpressure from these casts, and further reduction in GFR.[3] Renal ischemia is increased by inflammation and afferent arteriolar vasoconstriction.[3] During phase two, extension, the processes of ischemia, hypoxia, inflammation, and cellular injury continue and lasts 1 to 2 days.[2,3] Clinical signs and laboratory abnormalities may or may not be evident during the first two phases, though this is the ideal time to intervene and attempt treatment. Phase three, maintenance, is characterized by the stabilization of GFR at its nadir and may last days to weeks.[2,3] Azotemia and uremia are present, and oliguria or anuria may occur during this stage, though urine production is highly variable. Apoptosis continues but renal blood flow increases, leading to tubular repair.[3] In phase four, recovery, renal tubular repair occurs and GFR improves.[2,3] Marked polyuria may develop secondary to the partial restoration of renal tubular function and diuresis of accumulated solutes. This typically marks the beginning of this phase, and may last for weeks to months.[3] Renal function may improve, return to normal, or the animal may be left with residual renal dysfunction.

Because the kidneys receive approximately 20% to 25% of circulating cardiac output, they are extremely susceptible to ischemic damage. Ischemia results in renal hypoperfusion, decreased nephrotoxin distribution volume, decreased tubular flow, and increased vasoconstriction.[1,2] This vasoconstriction in turn decreases GFR.[1,2] Necrosis resulting in tubular cell death incites inflammation, and the inflammatory response is now recognized in playing a major role in AKI. Many of these inflammatory mechanisms are being investigated as potential targets for the prevention or treatment of AKI.[2,5,6]

AKI can also cause distant organ injury which can contribute to or be the cause of death. AKI is associated with increased levels of proinflammatory cytokines consistent with systemic inflammatory response syndrome (SIRS).[2] The end result of cytokine release is inflammation, neutrophil accumulation, endothelial injury, increased lung capillary permeability, and noncardiogenic pulmonary edema.[2,7] Cardiac changes such as cellular apoptosis, cardiac hypertrophy, increased cardiac macrophages, and mitochondrial damage have been found in experimental models of AKI.[2,8] Acute uremia can be associated with encephalopathy though the exact mechanism is unknown.[2,6]

CAUSES

There are many potential causes of AKI in animals with some variations among species groups. **Box 1** lists common causes for most domestic species while **Box 2** contains additional causes found in various exotic companion mammal species. Many of the causes of AKI in domestic species apply to exotics as well, while some conditions are species specific (eg, lily ingestion in cats, *Encephalitozoon cuniculi* infection in rabbits, and so forth). While the exact cause of AKI remains undetermined in many cases, it is important to make every effort to identify the etiology due to its potential influence on treatment and prognosis. Grading schemes for AKI have been developed for humans and for dogs and cats through the International Renal Interest Society (IRIS) (**Table 1**). This has not been applied to exotic animals.

DIAGNOSIS

History and Physical Examination

Many clinical signs of AKI are nonspecific, and most patients will have a history of illness of only hours to days. Obtain a thorough history including any previous medications or toxin exposure. Clinical signs may include lethargy, anorexia, nausea/vomiting (in species which are able to), diarrhea, melena, polydipsia, polyuria, stranguria, hematuria, or oliguria/anuria.[2,9] Physical exam findings can include weakness, lethargy, signs of dehydration, hypothermia or fever, tachycardia or bradycardia, malodorous breath, oral ulcerations, hypersalivation, palpable renomegaly or abdominal pain, enlarged urinary bladder, and peripheral edema.[1,2,9] History of chronic kidney disease may be present. Remember many exotic patients are extremely adept at hiding their clinical signs of illness until disease is advanced. Some patients may be extremely critical at presentation, and even minimal restraint can be too much for them to handle. Some patients may also have progressed to a more chronic form of disease by the time they show signs.

Clinical Pathology

Initial laboratory evaluation should include a complete blood count, biochemistry profile, assessment of acid-base status, urinalysis, and urine culture in mammals. Leukocytosis may be present with pyelonephritis or other infectious agents, but a stress leukogram, leukopenia, hemoconcentration, or anemia may be present as well.[1,2,9] In mammals, BUN and creatinine may be elevated, but a lack of azotemia does not rule out AKI.[1,2] Other biochemical changes may include hyperphosphatemia, hypo- or hypercalcemia, hypo- or hypernatremia, hypo- or hyperkalemia, and metabolic acidosis.[1,2,9] Hyperkalemia is common with obstructive AKI or animals that are in the oliguric/anuric phase.[2]

Urinalysis can be performed in exotic companion mammals just as in dogs and cats. Isosthenuria will typically be present with AKI, whereas prerenal causes of azotemia

Box 1
Common causes of acute kidney injury in the dog and cat[2,3]

- Nephrotoxins
  - Organic Compounds
    - Ethylene glycol
    - Solvents
    - Pesticides
    - Heavy metals
      - Lead
      - Mercury
      - Arsenic
      - Bismuth
      - Zinc
  - Drugs
    - Antibiotics
      - Aminoglycosides
      - Cephalosporins
      - Tetracyclines
      - Sulfonamides
      - Penicillins
      - Vancomycin
      - Fluoroquinolones
    - Amphotericin B
    - Chemotherapeutics
      - Cisplatin and carboplatin
      - Doxorubicin
      - Methotrexate
    - Cyclosporine
    - Azathioprine
    - ACE-inhibitors
    - Mannitol, other diuretics
    - Allopurinol
    - Cimetidine
    - Methoxyflurane
    - Lipid-lowering drugs
    - Non-steroidal anti-inflammatory drugs
    - Penicillamine
    - Vitamin D analogs
    - Thiacetarsamide
  - Plants
    - Grapes and raisins
    - Lilies (cats)
  - Other Toxins
    - Envenomation (snake, bee, and so forth)
    - Hemoglobin/myoglobin
    - Melamine/cyanuric acid
    - Radiographic contrast agents (possible)
    - Superphosphate fertilizer
    - Vitamin D containing rodenticides
- Infectious
  - Bacterial pyelonephritis
  - Leptospirosis
  - Babesiosis
  - Leishmaniasis
  - Lyme Disease
  - Rocky Mountain Spotted Fever
  - Feline Infectious Peritonitis (FIP)

- Ischemia
  - Hypovolemia/dehydration
  - Hypotension – including anesthesia
  - Hyperviscosity
    - Hyperglobulinemia
    - Polycythemia
  - Disseminated intravascular coagulation
  - Renal vessel thrombosis
  - Shock
    - Hemorrhagic
    - Septic
    - Traumatic
    - Burns
  - Decreased cardiac output
  - Heat stroke
- Obstructive
  - Calculi
  - Mucous plugs/dried blood
  - Neoplasia
  - Blood clots
  - Urethral or ureteral strictures
- Other
  - Systemic inflammatory response syndrome
  - Hypercalcemia
  - Pancreatitis
  - Cardiac failure
  - Hepatic failure
  - Sepsis
  - Amyloidosis
  - Immune-mediated glomerulonephritis
  - Urine leakage into the abdomen
  - Neoplasia
    - Lymphoma
    - Adenocarcinoma
    - Sarcoma/hemangiosarcoma
    - Nephroblastoma

would be suspected with an elevated urine-specific gravity.[2] Glucosuria may be seen with tubular damage.[1,2] Urine pH varies based on species. Urine sediment should be examined for red and white blood cells, bacteria, casts, and crystals. Calcium carbonate crystals are normal in rabbits and guinea pigs. The presence of casts suggests ongoing renal damage.[1] Proteinuria is often present, and a urine protein:creatinine ratio can help quantify this.

There are numerous novel biomarkers of kidney injury currently under investigation in human medicine. Only in recent years have these biomarkers started to be investigated in veterinary patients. Currently, none have been evaluated in exotic species other than in laboratory settings from which findings may be extrapolated to domestic species. The advantage of these novel biomarkers is improved sensitivity and specificity for the diagnosis of AKI as compared with serum creatinine and blood urea nitrogen (BUN).[9–12] Of these, symmetric dimethylarginine (SDMA) has become the most widely used in cats and dogs as it has been shown to correlate well with reduced GFR and is a more specific, sensitive, and accurate marker of renal function compared to serum creatinine.[10] It has not been verified in exotic species, though there has been one preliminary study that shows promise in ferrets.[13]

Box 2

Additional common causes of AKI more specific to exotic species[33,34,44,56,59,60,63,75,94,99,113,114]

Ferrets
- Aleutians disease (parvovirus)
- Systemic coronavirus (ferret FIP-like disease)
- Bacterial nephritis and pyelonephritis
- Renal cysts (common in ferrets, rarely a cause of disease)
- Lymphoma, rarely other neoplasia
- Grape/raisin toxicity (anecdotal)
- Zinc or copper toxicity
- Obstructive
  - Urolithiasis – cysteine, struvite
  - Prostatomegaly/periprostatic cysts secondary to adrenocortical disease
  - Preputial neoplasia

Rabbits
- Encephalitozoon cuniculi
- Urolithiasis and urinary sludge – calcium carbonate or other calcium salts
- Bacterial nephritis and pyelonephritis
- Nephrocalcinosis and Vitamin D toxicity
- Neoplasia (nephroblastoma)
- Herniation of urinary bladder through the inguinal ring
- Renal adipose deposition – secondary to anorexia, hepatic lipidosis, pregnancy toxemia

Guinea Pigs
- Urolithiasis – calcium carbonate
- Bacterial nephritis and pyelonephritis
- Excessive Vitamin D consumption

Chinchillas
- Urolithiasis – calcium carbonate
- Obstruction secondary to paraphimosis (fur ring), balanoposthitis

Mice
- Pyelonephritis
- Obstruction due to infection of the preputial glands or bulbourethral glands
- Klossiella muris
- Hydronephrosis
  - Occurs more commonly in certain genetic strains
  - Obstruction secondary to retrograde movement of seminal plugs in the urethra

Rats
- Hydronephrosis as with mice
- Nephrocalcinosis – dietary factors, strain related
- Pyelonephritis
- Trichosomoides crassicauda
- Neoplasia

Hedgehogs
- Pyelonephritis
- Neoplasia

Sugar Gliders
- Renal Klossiellosis – *Klossiella dulcis n.* sp
- Obstruction secondary to enlarged cloacal and paracloacal glands
  - Neoplasia
  - Hyperplasia/cysts
  - Impaction/infection
- Obstruction secondary to self-mutilation of the penis
- Copper toxicity

Avian
- Neoplasia – primary and metastatic
- Nutritional
  - Excessive dietary calcium or Vitamin D3
  - Hypovitaminosis A
  - Iron storage disease
  - Renal lipidosis
- Infectious
  - Bacterial nephritis – ascending infection from cloaca, hematogenous spread
  - Fungal nephritis
    - Aspergillosis – local invasion from air sac, hematogenous spread
    - Cryptococcosis
    - Microsporidiosis
  - Parasitic
    - Coccidia (*Eimeria* spp.)
    - Cryptosporidiosis
    - Trematodes/cestodes
    - hemoparasites
  - Viral
    - Polyomavirus
    - Adenovirus
    - Pigeon Paramyxovirus 1
    - Bornavirus
    - West Nile Virus
- Toxin
  - Capture myopathy and subsequent myoglobinuric nephrosis
  - Vitamin D containing rodenticides – both primary and secondary (eating rodents that have been affected by toxicosis)
  - Heavy Metal
    - Lead
    - Zinc
    - Mercury – especially mercury containing fish
    - Arsenic
  - Crude oil
  - NSAIDs
    - Diclofenac
    - Ketoprofen
  - Allopurinol – experimentally
  - Aminoglycosides
  - Garlic and onion
  - Plant or fungal toxins on feed
- Obstructive – cloacolith, ureterolith (urate concretions), egg retention
- Trauma

Reptiles
- Infectious
  - Bacterial nephritis
  - Fungal nephritis
  - Microsporidia (particularly *E pogonae*)
  - Viral
    - Inclusion body disease (Arenavirus)
    - Ranavirus (chelonians)
    - Picornavirus (tortoises)
    - Adenoviruses (lizards)
    - Herpesviruses (chelonians)
  - Parasitic
    - *Spironucleus* (*Hexamita*) protozoa
    - Entamoeba invadens
    - Intranuclear coccidia (tortoises)
    - *Cryptosporidium* sp. (rare)
    - *Klossiella* coccidia (boas)

Myxosporidia protozoa (chelonians)
Styphlodora renalis and *S. horrida* trematodes (boas and pythons)
Spirorchid flukes (aquatic chelonians)
Urolithiasis - cloacal uroliths or ureteroliths causing obstruction
Cold stunning (sea turtles)
Hypovitaminosis A
Hypervitaminosis D
Neoplasia (renal adenocarcinoma)
Aminoglycosides
Excessive protein ingestion
Severe dehydration – secondary to inappropriate husbandry

Amphibians
Infectious
Bacterial nephritis – ascending infection or septicemia
Fungal nephritis
Viral
Ranavirus
Lucke's renal adenocarcinoma (herpesvirus)
Parasitic
Trematode flukes
Oligochaete worms
Myxozoa
Coccidia (various species)
E ranarum, other protozoa
Hypovitaminosis A
Dehydration
Urolithiasis/cystic calculi
Toxin
Oxalate nephropathy (plant ingestion)
Heavy metals
Copper
Cadmium
Lead
Zinc
Volatile compounds in glue used for PVC piping
Water quality abnormalities
Numerous possibilities in free ranging amphibians

Tests to identify specific causes of AKI should be performed based on the clinical history and species. In domestic animals these can include ethylene glycol or other toxin levels, testing for Leptospirosis or other infectious agents, serum cholecalciferol levels, and so forth.[2,9] Blood pressure measurements should also be obtained to monitor both for hypotension, which can exacerbate AKI, and hypertension which can occur secondary to kidney disease.[9] In exotic species, tests chosen will be based on the species, both as a matter of what may be most common in those animals and the ability to obtain a test result safely and effectively. Some exotics may be too small to obtain enough blood or urine for certain tests, some may be too weak to handle lab sampling on presentation, or it may be impractical to obtain certain tests from certain animals based on size or temperament. Blood pressure measurements are routinely obtained in rabbits (doppler or oscillometric) and can also be obtained in ferrets and guinea pigs, but as patient size decreases, measurements become difficult to impossible to measure. Blood pressure cuffs are not made for small species and often even in patients where measurement is feasible, it may require sedation or anesthesia which is not ideal in patients with AKI. Additional testing will be discussed with each species group.

Table 1
International Renal Interest Society classification system for acute kidney injury[2]

Grade	Blood Creatinine (mg/dL	Clinical Description
I	<1.6	Nonazotemic AKI: a. documented AKI: historical, clinical, laboratory, or imaging evidence of AKI, clinical oliguria/anuria, volume responsiveness[a] b. progressive nonazotemic increase in blood creatinine; ≥0.3 mg/dL within 48h c. measured oliguria (<1 mL/kg/h) or anuria over 6h
II	1.7–2.5	Mild AKI: a. Documented AKI and static or progressive azotemia b. Progressive azotemic increase in blood creatinine; >0.3 mg/dL within 48h, or volume responsiveness c. Measured oliguria (<1 mL/kg/h) or anuria over 6h
III	2.6–5.0	Moderate to severe AKI:
IV	5.1–10.0	a. Documented AKI and increasing severities of azotemia
V	>10.0	and functional renal failure

[a] Volume responsiveness is an increase in urine production to greater than 1 mL/kg/h over 6h and/or decrease in serum creatinine to baseline over 48h.

Diagnostic Imaging

Various imaging techniques can be useful in determining the underlying cause of AKI. Radiographs can aid in determining the size and shape of the kidneys and presence of urolithiasis.[2,9] Ultrasonography is more helpful for precise measurement of renal size, echogenicity of the parenchyma, identification of cysts or masses, or pyelectasia with pyelonephritis.[2,9] Intravenous urography is not typically beneficial in AKI because animals with an elevated serum creatinine lack sufficient renal function to excrete and concentrate the contrast medium and iodinated contrast media are potentially nephrotoxic.[2]

CT and MRI may be used as well. In domestic species, advanced imaging does not usually provide more information than ultrasound and has the disadvantage of often requiring sedation or general anesthesia.[2] However, given the limitations of ultrasound in many exotic species and the ease of obtaining a CT scan with sedation only, in these patients, CT may prove more useful than in domestic animals.

Cytology and Histopathology

A renal aspirate may be performed in cases where amyloidosis, lymphoma or other neoplasia is suspected.[2,9] Histopathologic examination of the renal tissue will yield the most information about the chronicity of the disease process and may identify a certain cause, but in many cases, it may not identify the cause, but only the result of the damage to the renal tissue.[2,9] Renal biopsy is indicated when the results would change the therapy or prognosis and benefits must outweigh the risks (anesthesia, bleeding, and so forth). This is considered on a case-by-case basis and will be easier to obtain in some species than others.

TREATMENT

Treatment of AKI should be initiated as soon as possible and requires intensive patient monitoring. The goals of therapy are to preserve and restore renal hemodynamics, increase solute excretion, decrease toxicity of nephrotoxic agents, maintain urine output, and correct fluid, acid-base, and electrolyte abnormalities.[1,2,9] Treatment is most successful during the initiation and extension phases of AKI, and the underlying cause must be identified and treated if possible.[1,2,9] Administration of nephrotoxic drugs should be discontinued. Vomiting should be induced (in species where this is appropriate) in animals with recent toxin ingestion, and animals that have been exposed to certain toxins should receive the antidote, if available. Activated charcoal should be administered toxin ingestion cases where vomiting cannot be induced (as in most exotic species). If pyelonephritis is suspected, or in endemic areas of certain infectious diseases, empiric therapy with antibiotics should be started. More specific therapies will be discussed with each species group.

Fluid Therapy

Intravenous (IV) fluid therapy is the mainstay of treatment for all animals with AKI. IV fluid therapy helps to correct dehydration, reverse azotemia, and correct electrolyte and acid-base abnormalities.[1,2,9] In many exotic species, IV catheterization is extremely difficult due to patient size, inability to visualize a vein, difficulty maintaining peripheral vein catheterization, or a tendency of patients to chew or become tangled in fluid lines (**Fig. 1**). If these small patients are extremely dehydrated or hypovolemic, a peripheral vein may not be visible. An alternative option in these animals is intraosseous (IO) catheterization; any therapies given IV can also be administered IO (**Fig. 2**). The preferred sites for IO catheterization are the proximal tibia, femur, and humerus in mammals. Typically, in these debilitated patients, an IO catheter can be placed using local analgesia and either a spinal needle or hypodermic needle based on the size of the bone. Placement can be confirmed with two view radiographs, and the needle is covered with an IV

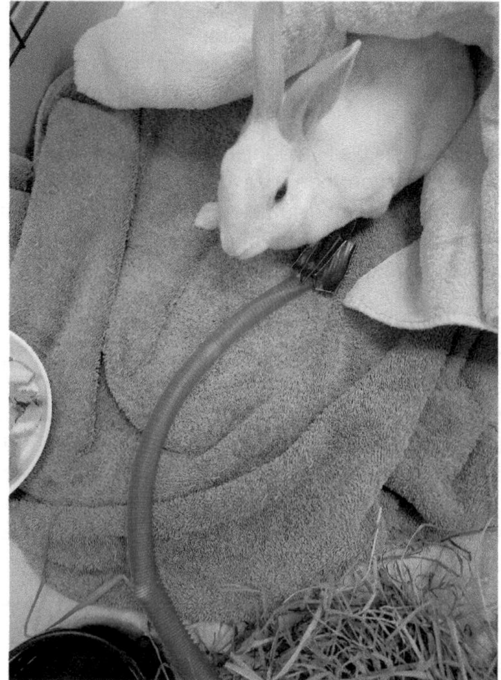

Fig. 1. Domestic rabbit (*Oryctolagus cuniculus*) receiving IV fluid therapy through a cephalic vein IV catheter. Note the plastic tubing covering the IV fluid line to protect it from chewing by the patient. (Photo courtesy Daniel Johnson).

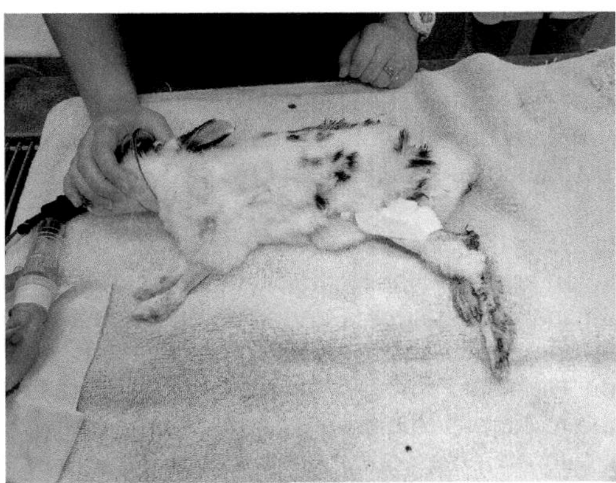

Fig. 2. IO catheter placement in the proximal tibia of a domestic rabbit (*Oryctolagus cuniculus*). The rabbit's extremely debilitated condition (visible in the photo) necessitated the placement of an IO instead of IV catheter under brief gas anesthesia.

port and secured to the limb with tape and either sutures or other bandage material. In certain situations, subcutaneous (SC) fluids may be necessary if IV or IO fluids cannot be administered; while this is commonplace in exotic species due to patient size, it is less ideal in cases of AKI. However, in some situations, risks of catheter placement outweighs the benefits. Sometimes a large bolus of SC fluids can be given to the patient while client discussions about therapy are taking place. This can help improve perfusion and blood pressure making IV catheterization easier.

Frequent monitoring is necessary to make adjustments in therapy and watch for volume overload. Monitoring parameters include: hydration status, body weight, urine output, mucous membrane color, capillary refill time, heart and respiratory rate, peripheral blood pressure, central venous pressure, packed cell volume and total protein, and serum chemistry parameters including renal values and electrolytes.[1,2,9] Again, in some exotic species, frequent monitoring of bloodwork parameters may be challenging due to the ability to obtain a blood sample on a repeated basis (small vein, instability of the patient, or size of patient limiting the maximum safe blood volume taken). Parameters excluding labwork should be monitored at least every 4 hours.

The initial volume of fluid to be administered can be calculated the same way regardless of the species involved. The formula used is based on the animal's body weight and degree of hydration:

Body weight (kg) x estimated % dehydration x 1000 = fluid deficit in milliliters.

For example, a 2500 g (2.5 kg) rabbit with 8% dehydration would require 200 mL of fluid to replace deficits. Keep in mind for some tiny exotic patients, this may be a very small volume of fluids (example: 100g cockatiel or sugar glider with 8% dehydration would receive 8 mL). This should be replaced over 4 to 12 hours, but can be given more slowly in certain cases (such as cardiac disease) to reduce the risk of volume overload. In addition to the deficit, the animal's normal maintenance fluids should also be given, and estimated ongoing fluid losses (such as from diarrhea, vomiting, and so forth) should be accounted for as well. Maintenance fluid requirements vary by species (44–66 mL/kg/d for canine/feline).[2] Isotonic fluids such as Lactated Ringers (LRS), Plasma-Lyte A, or Normosol-R can typically be administered initially, but the type of fluid should be adjusted based on the patient's fluid and electrolyte status.[1,2] If the patient is hypokalemic, then potassium supplementation is needed. 0.9% saline has historically been recommended for hyperkalemia, however, there is recent evidence to suggest that even though some balanced crystalloid solutions contain potassium, they do not contain enough potassium to worsen hyperkalemia and the benefits of a balanced solution outweighs the risks of using 0.9% NaCl only. The high sodium and chloride levels in 0.9% saline may create negative effects as well.[14] If hypernatremia occurs, then fluids with less sodium such as half strength LRS or 0.45% NaCl with 2.5% dextrose may be used.[1,2]

It is important to note that increasing fluid rates do not necessarily equate to improved renal function and survival. High volumes and rates of fluid have the potential to worsen AKI by increasing edema and venous congestion within the encapsulated kidney, which compresses tubules and intrarenal vessels, further hampering the kidney's function. High fluid amounts can also have adverse effects on cardiopulmonary function, due to increased capillary permeability seen with AKI.[2,9] Fluid overload is associated with adverse consequences and decreased survival, especially because dialysis to remove excess fluid is often not available, and even less so when dealing with exotic pets.[9,15–17] Patients should be carefully monitored for signs of fluid overload such as subcutaneous edema or increased respiratory rate or effort due to pulmonary edema. Urine output should be closely monitored (discussed later in discussion), and other parameters such as body weight, PCV/TS, and central venous pressure (CVP) can be used as well.[2,9] Fluid therapy should be continued until azotemia has resolved or stabilized, then fluid therapy can be tapered by approximately 25% per day.[2,9] Renal values have reached a plateau when there is no change over 24 hrs in a well-hydrated patient.[9] Abrupt discontinuation of fluids can lead to rapid dehydration, especially from post-obstructive or therapeutic diuresis. Some animals may become polyuric with recovery from AKI, and fluid therapy must be adjusted to account for this as well.

Urine Output Monitoring

Measuring urine output is one of the most important, but often most neglected, aspect of monitoring animals with AKI. Urine output monitoring is extremely important when tapering fluids as output should diminish by a corresponding degree to which fluids are tapered; if not, the kidneys are unable to regulate fluid balance adequately.[1] Placement of an indwelling urinary catheter is the most accurate method for monitoring urine volume. However, the benefits of an indwelling catheter must be weighed against risks of ascending infection and the need for sedation/anesthesia to place the catheter.[2] The risk of infection can be reduced by scrupulous attention to sterile placement of the catheter, maintenance of a closed collection system, daily cleaning of the visible portions of the catheter, and changing the catheter every 2 to 3 days as the risk of infection increases after 3 days.[2,18] In exotic companion mammals, catheterization is most commonly used in ferrets and can be performed in guinea pigs and rabbits, but as the size of the patient decreases, the ability to place a catheter becomes increasingly difficult. Maintenance of a urinary catheter in these species is also extremely difficult as many (especially rodents) will attempt to chew at anything unusual. Maintaining a closed collection system can also be quite difficult as again most of these patients will attempt to remove them, or become tangled in the lines with normal movement unless the patient is obtunded or kept sedated. For animals in which catheterization is not practical, absorbent pads can be placed under the patient to estimate urine volume. The pads are weighed before and after use and the urine volume is calculated from the difference. One gram equals approximately 1 mL of urine produced.[2] In species that use a litter box, a nonabsorbent litter can be used so that voided urine samples can be collected and measured. Alternatively, patients can be housed on a grate off the cage floor so urine can be collected. Body weight monitoring can also be helpful.

Management of Oliguria or Anuria

Once the patient has been rehydrated, urine output should rapidly increase. Oliguria in small animal patients is defined as urine output <1 mL/kg/h in a well-hydrated, normotensive patient, with anuria meaning no urine production (<0.08 mL/kg/h).[2] Relative oliguria describes a patient producing 1-2 mL/kg/h of urine despite higher infusion volumes of IV fluids.[2] If urine production is not sufficient, first the patient's hydration status should be reassessed, being sure to account for insensible losses, ongoing losses, volume of urine produced, and so forth and recalculate fluids for the next 4 hours.[2,16,19] If the patient is well hydrated, specific therapy to increase urine flow is the next step in the treatment of oliguria/anuria. There is currently no evidence that these medications (described later in discussion) improve the outcome in human or veterinary AKI patients, but it is thought that if a patient is able to respond to these medical interventions, their kidney injury is likely less severe and, as such, they tend to have a better prognosis.[9] Animals that remain oliguric/anuric for 6 to 12 hrs after medical intervention should be considered as failing to respond.[9] At that point renal replacement therapy (dialysis) is the only option.[9]

The loop diuretic furosemide is the initial drug of choice. While this drug may increase urine output, reduce tubular obstruction, and improve renal blood flow, it does not increase GFR or improve outcome or survival rates in patients with AKI.[2] An initial dose of 2 mg/kg IV is suggested, and if effective, urine output typically increases within 20 to 40 minutes. If the initial dose fails to increase urine production, escalating doses up to 4-6 mg/kg can be administered at hourly intervals and the effective doses continued every 6 to 8 hours.[1,2] Alternatively, a loading dose of 0.66 mg/kg IV followed by a constant rate infusion (CRI) of 0.5 to 1.0 mg/kg/h can be used, and has been shown to be more effective at producing diuresis in normal dogs.[1,19,20] Dosing of furosemide for exotic species is typically extrapolated from small animal medicine, and no studies exist documenting which protocol is preferred. In exotics where IV administration is not possible, intramuscular (IM) administration is useful and effective, but there are species considerations (discussed later in discussion).

Mannitol is an osmotic diuretic that increases renal blood flow, GFR, and tubular fluid flow and acts as a free radial scavenger.[9] In the past it has been recommended as well, but use has fallen out of favor as studies have not shown mannitol to be any more effective than volume expansion alone, and it can contribute to circulatory overload.[1,9,19]

Fenoldopam is a specific dopamine D_1 receptor agonist used to treat emergency hypertension in humans and has gained popularity for use in oliguric or anuric AKI because of its effect on systemic vasodilation and the promotion of diuresis. It has an extremely high affinity for the feline D_1 receptor compared to dopamine.[21] A study in healthy cats using a 2h infusion of fenoldopam at 0.5 μg/kg/min documented an increase in urine output, sodium excretion, fractional excretion of sodium and creatinine clearance within 6h that lasted for at least 24h.[21] However, one study of critically ill cats and dogs with AKI that received fenoldopam showed no improvement in survival to discharge, length of hospital stay, or improvement in renal biochemical parameters when compared with patients with AKI not receiving fenoldopam.[22] The recommended dosage range is 0.1 to 1 μg/kg/min as a constant rate infusion.[9] No literature exists on the use of fenoldopam in exotics other than in lab animal medicine describing use in rats, mice, or rabbits for extrapolation to human use.

Dopamine as a low-dose CRI was used in the past to increase urine output, but numerous studies in humans along with those in small animal patients, have shown no benefit in patients with AKI. Its use can also result in serious adverse effects such as tachyarrhythmias, vasoconstriction, and hypertension; as such it is no longer recommended for therapy in AKI.[2,9] Dopamine usage in exotic animal patients has mainly been restricted to use in managing hypotension during anesthesia. In rabbits, dopamine and phenylephrine at dog and cat doses have not been found to be effective.[23]

Correction of Acid-base and Electrolyte Abnormalities

Metabolic acidosis is common in animals with AKI. Mild metabolic acidosis typically corrects with IV fluid therapy alone. Sodium bicarbonate IV therapy (isotonic solutions only) is typically reserved only for severe cases (pH < 7.1) as this therapy itself has significant risks, including volume overload, pulmonary edema, hypertension, hypernatremia, and cerebrospinal fluid acidosis.[1,2,19] Bicarbonate therapy is rarely used in exotics other than in species large enough to obtain repeated blood samples so that monitoring can be performed. Dosing is extrapolated from domestic species. Blood lactate levels can be measured to assess perfusion status, but clinicians should remember that there are no published reference ranges for exotics and there are many potential causes of hyperlactatemia. There has been some preliminary work done in rabbits and ferrets, showing normal lactate values are significantly higher than dogs and cats.[24] Monitoring trends may still be useful.

Moderate to severe hyperkalemia may occur if the animal is oliguric or anuric, which can lead to life-threatening cardiac arrhythmias. Urine production must be ensured, and mild to moderate hyperkalemia may resolve with IV fluid therapy alone. Severe hyperkalemia may need additional therapy such as calcium gluconate to protect the heart, dextrose, regular insulin, terbutaline, or sodium bicarbonate.[2,19] Hypokalemia may occur from excessive urinary loss, inadequate intake, or GI loss. Potassium may be added to IV fluids and continued orally if needed.

Hyperphosphatemia is a result of decreased renal excretion and is usually addressed by IV fluid therapy.[9] Oral phosphate binders may be added for persistent elevations. Calcium gluconate may be given IV for hypocalcemia, but care must be taken to evaluate both calcium and phosphorus levels to avoid the risk of dystrophic mineralization.

Treatment of Other Uremic Complications

Vomiting is extremely common with AKI in domestic species. The cause is multifactorial, but the ulceration of the GI tract can occur as a result of uremia. Antiemetics such as maropitant, metoclopramide, or ondansetron may be useful. Histamine receptor antagonists such as famotidine and cimetidine or proton-pump inhibitors such as omeprazole, pantoprazole, or esomeprazole may be beneficial as well. Sucralfate is a mucosal protectant for esophageal or gastric ulcers. Dosing is empirical for most exotic species and listed in **Box 3**.

Hypertension is common with AKI and may be exacerbated by IV fluid therapy. Volume overload must be addressed if that is the case. In cases of hypertension secondary to AKI, the calcium channel blocker amlodipine may be used, but caution must be used not to induce hypotension and decrease renal perfusion.[2,9] ACE inhibitors such as enalapril or benazepril should be avoided due to their negative effect on GFR.[2,9]

Animals with AKI are typically anorexic. In domestic species, the placement of a feeding tube allows enteral nutrition, or parenteral nutrition can be given if enteral nutrition is not an option.[2,9] For exotic patients, lack of food intake can lead to its own life-threatening complications (gastrointestinal stasis in herbivores, hypoglycemia in small patients, and so forth). Syringe feeding or gavage feeding via tube is typically easily

Box 3
Dosages of medications useful in patients with AKI.[2]

Dosages provided are for canine/feline patients and may be extrapolated to exotics in cases where pharmacokinetic studies for the species are not available.

Metoclopramide 0.1 to 0.5 mg/kg IV, IM, SQ q8h or 0.01 to 0.02 mg/kg/h IV CRI

Maropitant 1 mg/kg IV or SQ q24 h up to 5 days

Ondansetron 0.1 to 0.2 mg/kg SQ q8h or 0.5 mg/kg loading dose IV then 0.5 mg/kg/h IV CRI

Famotidine 0.5-1 mg/kg IV, SQ, PO q12 to 24h

Ranitidine 1-2 mg/kg IV, SQ, IV q8-12h**no longer available

Cimetidine 5 to 10 mg/kg IV, PO q6-8h

Omeprazole 0.5-1 mg/kg PO q12 h

Pantoprazole 1 mg/kg IV q12 to 24h

Esomeprazole 1 mg/kg IV, SQ q12 h

Sucralfate 250 to 500 mg PO q8-12h

Amlodipine 0.2 to 0.4 mg/kg PO q24 h

accomplished in most exotic patients making the use of feeding tubes less necessary, unless a patient is unable to swallow.

Renal Replacement Therapy

RRT can be considered for patients that remain oliguric or anuric despite appropriate medical therapy, those with refractory hyperkalemia or acid-base disturbances, removal of certain toxins, or for volume overload.[9] These therapies include peritoneal dialysis (PD), hemodialysis (IHD), and continuous renal replacement therapy (CRRT), or even kidney transplantation in cats. While PD can be performed at many 24 hr referral centers, it requires specialized equipment, is labor-intensive, and necessitates experience and understanding of the technique. IHD and CRRT are only available at certain facilities, and data is limited on these therapies in veterinary medicine. There are no reports of RRT in exotic patients other than as lab animal models, other than one report in rabbits.[25–28]

PROGNOSIS

The prognosis for AKI in all species is guarded to poor overall. Reported mortality rates for all causes in canine/feline patients is 45% to 75%, though prognosis can vary based on the cause.[1,2,9] Degree of azotemia is not predictive of outcome, but factors that confer a poorer prognosis include lack of urine production, hypocalcemia, hyperphosphatemia, anemia, and other organ involvement such as sepsis, pancreatitis, and so forth.[1,2,9] Survival with RRT can be 44% to 60%, which sounds favorable, but without this therapy these animals would not have survived.[9,29–31] Despite appropriate therapy, residual kidney disease or incomplete recovery is common and affects about 50% of patients that survive an acute event.[9,32]

Unfortunately, no statistics exist on reported outcomes for exotic species with AKI, however, it can be assumed that survival rates would be similar to lower than domestic species. There are limitations in exotic animal medicine that affect treatment, such as patient size affecting the ability to treat with IV/IO fluids or obtain repeated blood samples for monitoring, and RRT is not an option for exotics at this time. Exotic patients are also extremely adept at hiding their clinical signs of illness until disease is advanced, so these patients are often in critical condition before presenting to the veterinarian, making them more difficult to treat.

EXOTIC COMPANION MAMMALS

Ferrets

Ferrets (*Mustela putorius furo*) with AKI are the closest in anatomy, clinical presentation, and treatment options to domestic species. Clinical signs are similar, though skin turgor for hydration assessment can be difficult as rapid weight loss can occur in ferrets even with acute disease. Similar elevations in parameters on bloodwork are used, though in ferrets creatinine levels are lower than dogs and cats (0.2–0.8 mg/dL) and do not rise as rapidly as other parameters.[33] Therefore, ferret patients with an elevated BUN but normal creatinine may still have AKI, and other parameters and test results need to be evaluated. Treatment protocols and monitoring can be adapted from dogs and cats including fluid therapy, management of electrolyte disturbances, antibiotics, treatment of toxin ingestion, and supportive care.[33,34] Gastrointestinal ulcers are common in ferrets with any illness and can be managed routinely.[35] *Helicobacter* gastritis is commonly associated with ulcers in ferrets, so specific therapy for this disease process may be needed as well. Anorexic ferrets can be syringe fed with a commercial carnivore feeding formula (Oxbow Carnivore Care, Oxbow, Omaha, NE, or Emeraid Carnivore, Lafebers, Cornell, IL). Typically a 24g IV catheter can be placed in the cephalic vein for fluid and medication administration, though care must be taken to keep the ferret from becoming entangled in the IV lines or trying to remove it (**Fig. 3**). Alternatively, the lateral saphenous vein can be used, but IO catheterization may be necessary in extremely debilitated patients.

One of the most common presentations of AKI in ferrets occurs in males due to urethral obstruction. Ferrets with urethral obstruction are often described by clients as straining to defecate when they are actually straining to urinate, or they may exhibit signs such as urine dribbling, hematuria, vocalizing, or acting restless progressing to lethargy and worsening symptoms as their condition deteriorates. Typically, a large, distended, painful bladder is palpable on presentation. The most common causes of this condition include urolithiasis or prostatomegaly secondary to adrenocortical disease, but preputial gland neoplasia (typically adenocarcinoma) is possible as well. Treatment is specific to the underlying disease process, but typically a urinary catheter will need to be placed in order to relieve the obstruction and allow urine flow while comorbidities are managed. A Slippery Sam tomcat urethral catheter (SurgiVet, Smith Medical, Dublin, OH) works well for ferrets as the material is stiff enough to pass around the pelvic flexure of the urethra, the length is appropriate, and the port can be sutured to the skin of the ventral abdomen (**Fig. 4**). Keeping a ferret from removing its own urinary catheter is one of the more difficult points of management. This type of catheter can be attached to a closed collection system for urine output monitoring (1-2 mL/kg/h), but keeping the ferret from becoming entangled in the lines is difficult unless the patient is extremely weak and ill or kept sedated. Often monitoring the weight of urine collected in puppy pads as it drips from the end of the catheter is necessary, and close attention must be paid to the cleanliness of the patient and catheter port to prevent ascending infection. In patients where a urinary catheter cannot be placed, decompressive cystocentesis can be performed (preferably with ultrasound guidance) to relieve a critically full bladder. Temporary or long-term cystotomy tube placement can also be considered.[33]

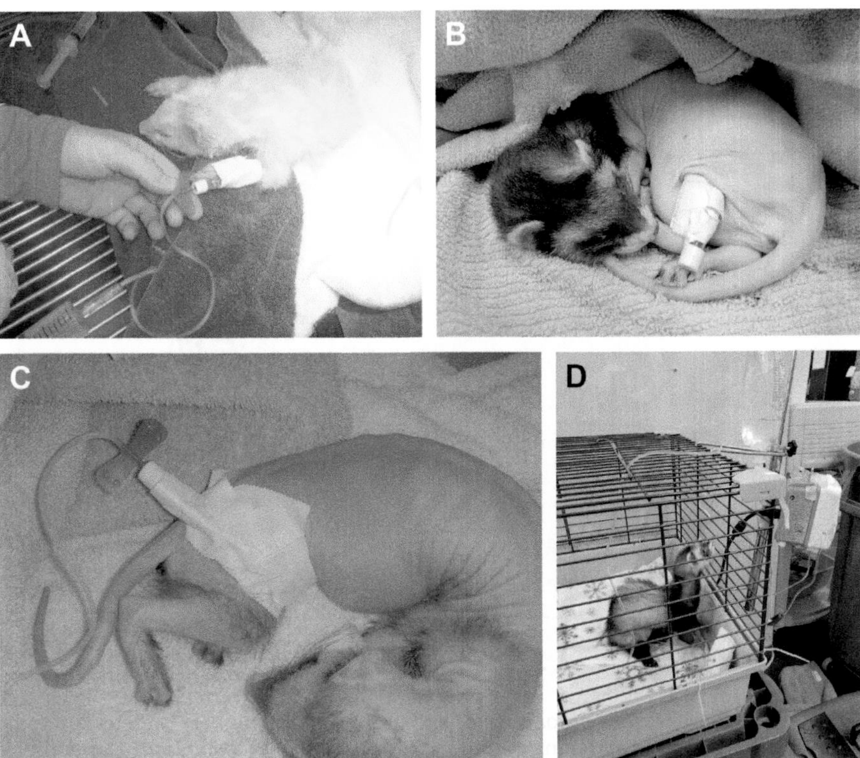

Fig. 3. Domestic ferret (*Mustela putorius furo*) IV and IO catheter placement: (*A*) cephalic vein (*B*) lateral saphenous vein (*C*) proximal femur (*D*) demonstrating the challenges of IV catheter maintenance in an active ferret patient (Photo courtesy Dr. Daniel Johnson.).

Urinary obstruction commonly occurs secondary to urolithiasis, especially in younger patients (**Fig. 5**). Historically the most common urolith type in ferrets was struvite, but in recent years cysteine has become increasingly prevalent, now making up over 90% of submissions to centers of urolith analysis.[36–40] A genetic component to this condition, as found in dogs and humans, has been proposed but there also seems to be a high correlation with feeding grain-free diets containing legumes (peas, lentils, beans).[36] Surgical removal of stones is the only treatment option as medical dissolution is not feasible with cysteine uroliths. Ideally urethroliths will be flushed back into the bladder for removal through cystotomy, though this can be challenging, and risks of urethral tearing, necrosis, and stricture are all possible.

Other causes of urinary obstruction in the male ferret are abnormalities of the prostate caused by adrenocortical disease and preputial neoplasia. Males can develop prostatic hyperplasia, cysts, and abscesses. The description and treatment of adrenocortical disease is well described in any current literature about ferret endocrine diseases. Acute obstruction can be managed by the placement of a urinary catheter and administration of leuprolide acetate to allow the prostate to shrink. Leuprolide will shrink the prostate more quickly than a Deslorelin acetate implant which is used for long-term control.[33] Large associated prostatic cysts have been managed with surgical marsupialization or omentalization of the cyst.[41] Preputial tumors are typically aggressive neoplasms that can require the amputation of the penis and a scrotal

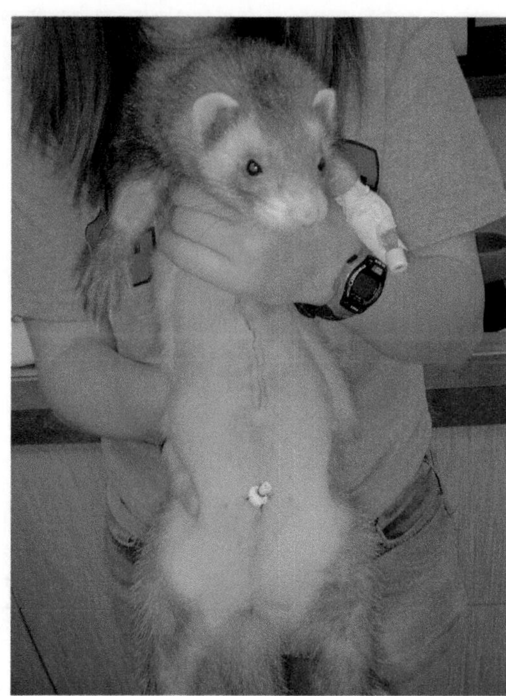

Fig. 4. Male ferret (*Mustela putorius furo*) with a Slippery Sam urinary catheter sutured in place to allow urination and urine output monitoring along with an IV catheter in the cephalic vein for fluid administration. (Photo courtesy Dr. Daniel Johnson.).

urethrostomy in order for the patient to urinate. This is typically a palliative measure as these tumors can be aggressive and metastasize and seem poorly responsive to adjunctive treatment.[35,42]

Rabbits

Rabbits (*Oryctolagus cuniculus*) with AKI often present with similar signs to other species including lethargy, weakness, anorexia, and so forth. Because rabbits cannot vomit, obvious signs of nausea are not present, but anorexia leads to the lack of fecal production in this species (gastrointestinal syndrome, or GI stasis) with subsequent effects well described in the literature. Body temperature at presentation is extremely important in rabbits, as any rabbit with a body temperature below 38.0°C (100.4°F)

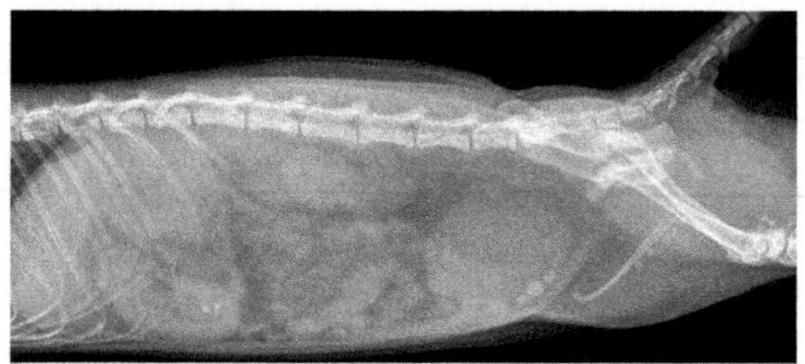

Fig. 5. Right lateral radiographs of a 1 year old neutered male domestic ferret (*Mustela putorius furo*) with cysteine cystoliths and urethroliths causing a urinary obstruction and AKI.

carries a more guarded prognosis, and active rewarming measures should be implemented.[43] Repeated blood sampling can often be obtained readily, and lactate and acid-base status has been evaluated in rabbits.[23] The central ear artery can be used for arterial sampling, though the risk of thrombosis and necrosis of the ear is possible. IV catheterization is typically readily achieved in the rabbit using the cephalic or peripheral ear veins. While the lateral saphenous vein is the largest peripheral vein and easy to catheterize, when a rabbit sits in a normal posture, the legs are fully flexed underneath the body, and maintaining flow through a catheter in this location is difficult. IV lines often need to be protected with thicker plastic tubing to prevent chewing through the line. Urinary catheters are typically easy to place in this species, but maintaining them in place with a closed collection system for urine output monitoring is difficult, again because of this species' propensity to chew though lines or become entangled in them with any movement. While an E-collar can be placed, this does tend to inhibit a rabbit's ability to eat and drink on its own and prevents it from eating cecotrophs. Urine output can be measured with absorbent pads or collection in litter boxes or other grates as previously described.

Rabbits have a higher fluid maintenance rate than most other mammalian species (100–120 mL/kg/d, or 3-4 mL/kg/h) because of the higher water demand of the GI tract.[23,35] Urine specific gravity is more dilute in rabbits compared to other mammals (1.003–1.036) and urine pH is typically alkaline at 8 to 9.23. Normal urine output is also higher than a similar sized carnivore at 1-4 mL/kg/h and can be as high as 5 to 10 mL/kg/h in the diuresis phase of AKI.[23,44] Influence of the diet on the urine is high because an increased proportion of fresh vegetables enhances urine output.[45,46] For this reason, and because a major portion of total body water is present in the GI tract, oral fluid administration can be highly useful in rabbits needing fluid resuscitation. Rabbits prefer to drink from a water bowl rather than a dripper, and so a bowl is recommended to maximize water intake in AKI patients.[45] Anorexic rabbits need to have supplemental nutrition provided to prevent gastrointestinal stasis. Commercial herbivore hand feeding formulas are available (Oxbow Critical Care Herbivore, Emeraid Herbivore) that can be syringe fed multiple times daily and are readily accepted. These feeding formulas are made with water and oral rehydration with these feeding formulas can be incorporated into a holistic treatment approach. In debilitated patients, a nasogastric feeding tube can be considered.

Intraperitoneal fluid administration has been used extensively in rabbits as a model of peritoneal dialysis.[25–27] The principle is to use the peritoneal membrane as a surface of exchange for fluid and solutes but use in pet rabbits is anecdotal.[28] Peritoneal dialysis is very time consuming and labor intensive. This technique is mainly used in case of oliguric or anuric renal failure but is considered as a last option strategy and carries a poor prognosis.

E cuniculi is one of the most common causes of renal disease reported in the rabbit. Many rabbits carry the organism, which is harbored in the kidneys and transmitted through urine. Signs can vary from completely asymptomatic to decreased appetite and weight loss, dehydration, lethargy, and polyuria/polydipsia to fulminant renal failure. This organism can also cause neurologic signs (vestibular disease) and phacoclastic uveitis. Diagnosis is challenging because of the number of animals with positive antibody titers without active infection and the observation that many animals recover spontaneously without treatment.[47] Measurement of IgG, IgM, and C-reactive protein (CRP) are the current preferred diagnostic tests. In patients with renal disease secondary to E. cuniculi, treatment is primarily focused on kidney support.[47] No treatment has been shown to eliminate the organism, and treatment with benzimidazoles is often used successfully but is also controversial as the duration of treatment has not been established and severe bone marrow suppression can result.[47,48]

Urolithiasis and urinary sludge are also common in rabbit patients and are a potential cause of AKI. Stones can form anywhere in the urinary tract and are composed of calcium salts, especially calcium carbonate (**Fig. 6**). Rabbits possess unique calcium metabolism that predisposes to urolith formation.[35,49] Unlike other mammals, rabbits passively absorb calcium from the GI tract independent of Vitamin D_3 and rely on renal excretion to maintain calcium homeostasis; most mammals eliminate excess calcium through the GI tract.[35,49] Higher urinary calcium concentration predisposes rabbits to supersaturation and sludge and urolith formation.[35,49] Clinical signs are similar to other species. Patients with sludge may appear to have urinary incontinence and remain soiled around the rear end. Calcium stones or sludge can easily be seen on radiographs for diagnosis, and because calcium is eliminated in the urine, crystals are always present on urinalysis. Obstructions of the renal pelvis, ureters, and urethra can result in acute kidney injury. Calcium stones cannot be dissolved medically and must be removed via surgery. Cystotomy is straightforward in this species, and techniques for more advanced techniques such as ureteral stenting, nephrotomy, and nephrectomy have been described in the rabbit, though prognosis varies with severity of disease.[50–52] Bladder sludge does not typically result in obstruction or AKI, but can be managed with analgesia, increased fluid intake, exercise, dietary modification, and bladder expression.

Other Exotic Companion Mammals

Management of AKI becomes more challenging in other exotic companion mammals. The smaller the patient, the more difficult it becomes to place an IV catheter, often necessitating IO catheterization, which is challenging as well. In small rodents, preventing chewing and removal of fluid lines is a constant struggle. While a urinary catheter may be placed under anesthesia to relieve obstruction, maintaining one in patient smaller than a guinea pig (*Cavia porcellus*) is difficult, not only due to size but the propensity of the patients (especially rodents and sugar gliders) to chew. In guinea pigs, one must be careful to avoid the intromittent sac during catheterization. IV catheters can be used as a urinary catheter as there are no commercial urinary catheters small enough for patients the size of a rat (*Rattus norvegicus domestica*) or smaller (**Fig. 7**) Often SC fluids are used because of these challenges, so close monitoring is needed

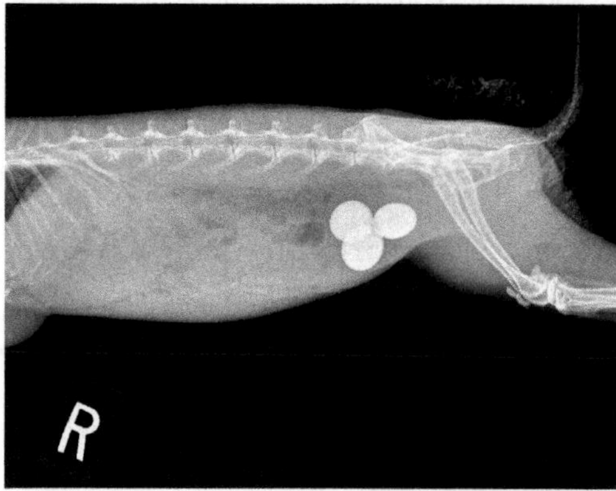

Fig. 6. Right lateral radiograph of a spayed female domestic rabbit (*Oryctolagus cuniculus*) with three calcium carbonate uroliths.

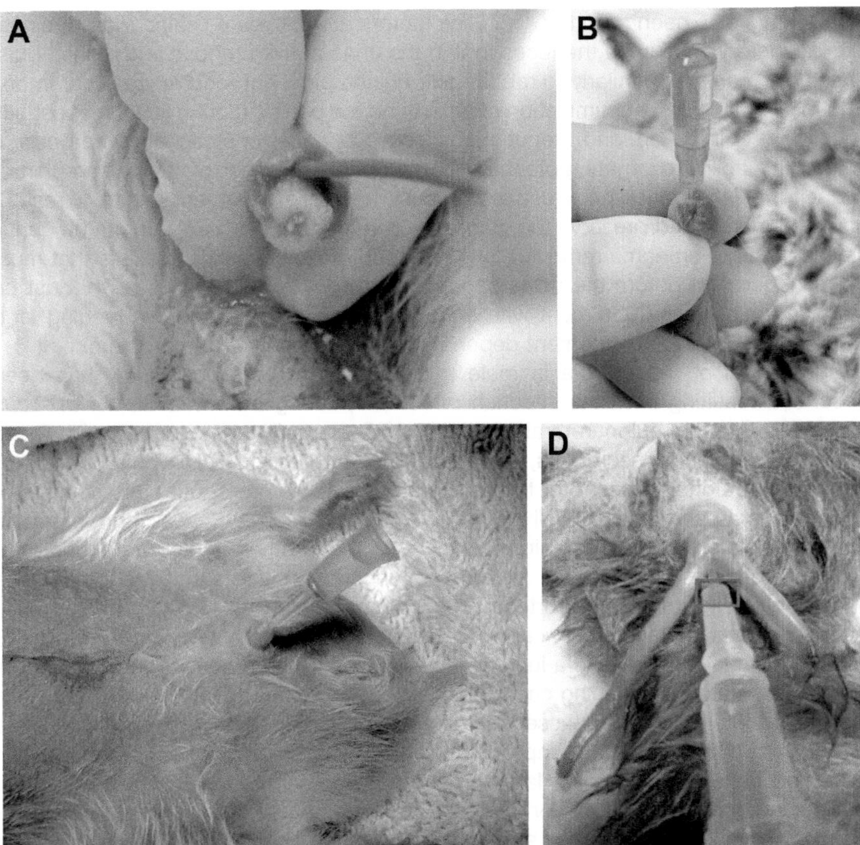

Fig. 7. Urinary catheter placement in a (*A*) male guinea pig (note avoidance of the intromittent sac) (*B*) male chinchilla (*C*) male rat (*D*) male sugar glider ([C] Photo courtesy of Lauren V Powers, DVM, Dipl ABVP; [D] Photo courtesy of Dr. Miwa Yasutsugu.).

to make sure fluids are absorbed and urine is being produced. Small mammals can be maintained on white towels or paper towels to monitor urine output (not particulate bedding) and towels can be weighed to estimate urine output as previously described. Puppy pads with plastic backing are often chewed. Repeated blood analysis to monitor progress is also challenging as obtaining a blood sample may require anesthesia each time, and the smaller the patient, the less blood can be taken safely, especially on a repeated basis. For these reasons, the management of AKI in mammals smaller than a guinea pig often carries a poor prognosis.

Guinea pigs are predisposed to calcium urolithiasis as they possess the same calcium excretion methods as rabbits.[35] They can be managed in a similar manner but recurrence is common. Urolith removal via endoscopy has been described.[53,54] Uroliths often form in the urethra in female guinea pigs and can be removed manually under anesthesia or with the use of a retractor.[55] *Corynebacterium renale* and other bacteria, have been reported in concurrence with uroliths, or as causes of bacterial cystitis and pyelonephritis in guinea pigs.[56]

Chinchillas (*Chinchilla lanigera*) are also predisposed to urolith formation, particularly in males. Most uroliths are composed of calcium carbonate, but semen-matrix calculi have also been reported.[57,58] Risk factors are unclear as chinchillas eliminate excess dietary calcium in the feces, not in the urine as with rabbits and guinea pigs. These are managed similarly to rabbits and guinea pigs, but recurrence is common.

In male chinchillas, accumulation of fur around the penis ("fur ring"), balanoposthitis secondary to infection, and preputial abscesses or adhesions can all compromise a chinchilla's ability to urinate, potentially leading to AKI. In cases of severe paraphimosis, self-mutilation of the penis can also occur. The goal of treatment is to try to restore normal urination and preserve the glans penis. If the tissue is viable, it can be gently cleaned, hair or smegma removed, and replaced. If severe swelling exists that must be managed first before the penis can be replaced. The underlying cause must be managed, along with treatment with antibiotics, analgesia, supportive feeding, and fluid therapy or AKI management depending on the severity of the problem.

Obstruction of the urethra in male mice (*Mus musculus domestica*) has been described resulting from the infection of the preputial glands with *Staphylococcus aureus* and/or the bulbourethral glands with *Pasteurella pneumotropica*.[59] These accessory sex gland secretions, and more rarely urolithiasis, can obstruct the urethra.[35,59] Mice often present for the self-mutilation of the penis, but other sources of penile trauma can occur as well (aggressive breeding activity, cage trauma, and so forth.).[59] Isolate the affected animal, clean and debride the affected area, and treat with antibiotics and analgesia.[59] Uroliths are uncommon in rats, mice, and hamsters and are typically struvite if reported.[59]

Sugar gliders (*Petaurus breviceps*) possess a unique anatomy compared to other small mammals. Males have a long, forked penis, and the urethral opening is at the base of the fork. The opening can be catheterized if needed with a 26g IV catheter, but the catheter cannot be passed all the way to the bladder.[60] They also possess a cloaca with common urinary, reproductive, and gastrointestinal tract openings with paracloacal glands that are similar to anal glands in other mammals. The paracloacal glands can become impacted or infected, and paracloacal cysts have also been reported, all of which can cause stranguria. The glands can be expressed, infection treated with antibiotics, and in the case of recurrent issues or cysts, surgical removal carries a good prognosis.

Cystitis, crystalluria, and urolithiasis have all been reported in sugar gliders. Crystalluria often develops as a result of dietary issues and lack of fluid intake, though lack of proper environment and social structure can contribute as well, as they lead to decrease in normal urination and marking behaviors.[60] Crystals and stones are typically struvite and can be managed with traditional therapies.[60] Urolithiasis can cause urethral obstruction, and surgery is typically required. Underlying causes must be corrected to help prevent recurrence.

Self-trauma and mutilation of the penis can result in difficulty urinating or a urinary obstruction if the trauma extends past the urethral opening. Self-trauma can often occur in gliders who are housed alone as they are highly social animals.[60] It can also occur if there is any abnormality of the penis, excessive breeding, and so forth. as gliders are also known to self-mutilate any area of pain or abnormality.[60] Patients will present for signs of urinary obstruction, and typically an enlarged, firm urinary bladder is palpable. If the trauma is just to the forked portion of the penis, then this can be amputated and the ability to urinate is preserved. However, if the urethra is damaged, surgery to create a new opening to allow urine to pass is possible, though not without potential complications in a patient this size with a tendency to self-mutilate.

Hedgehogs (*Atelerix albiventris*) and other rodents such as degus (*Octodon degus*), prairie dogs (*Cynomys ludovicianus*), hamsters (various species), gerbils (*Meriones unguiculatus*), and so forth all can present with AKI as well for various reasons. The challenges of managing these patients is described above. Prairie dogs and hedgehogs can present difficulties in maintaining IV catheters because of their short limbs, and if a hedgehog curls into a ball, the catheter will obstruct. In some species (rats, hamsters, prairie dogs, degus, hedgehogs), chronic kidney disease in older animals is far more common than AKI, and thus is outside the scope of this review.

SUMMARY

Acute kidney injury can occur in any species, and there are many clinical signs, causes, diagnostics, and treatment options that are conserved across species groups. However, there are many differences in anatomy and physiology along with management challenges that are present with exotic species that are not dealt with in dogs and cats. Patient size often limits the amount of diagnostic testing and certain treatment options. Exotic patients tend to hide their clinical signs of illness – as such, they are often presented when disease is more advanced and any handling or stress can often be fatal, limiting the amount of testing and treatment that can be done initially. Prognosis for AKI is guarded in exotic species as in domestic animals, but if the disease is identified and treated swiftly, patients can often recover, though sometimes permanent kidney damage remains. More advanced therapies and testing options being used for humans, dogs, and cats need further research in exotic animals.

DISCLOSURE

The author declares no conflicts of interest.

CLINICS CARE POINTS

- Monitor similar blood and urine parameters as for dogs and cats (BUN, Crea, electrolytes, and so forth).
- Be conscious of the amount of blood that can be taken at once or over time in small patients.
- Numerous causes of AKI exist – attempt to determine the cause so specific treatment can be initiated.
- IV fluid therapy can be challenging in small or active patients – monitor lines closely for chewing, becoming tangled or occluded, and so forth.
- Monitor for signs of fluid overload similar to domestic species - body weight, PCV/TS, hydration status, urine output, mucous membrane color, capillary refill time, heart and respiratory rate, peripheral blood pressure.
- Monitor urine output – if an indwelling urinary catheter and collection system can be placed in the species being treated, this needs to be monitored closely for tangling or chewing of lines. If not, monitor by collecting urine from cage or weighing bedding.
- Watch for post-obstructive diuresis and correct if needed.
- Furosemide can be used to stimulate urine output.
- Syringe feeding and other supportive care will likely be needed.

REFERENCES

1. Langston C. Acute Kidney Injury. In: Ettinger SJ, Feldman EC, Cote, editors. Textbook of veterinary internal medicine: diseases of the dog and cat. 8th ed. St. Louis: Elsevier; 2017. p. 4650–85.

2. Ross L. Acute kidney injury in dogs and cats. Vet Clin North Am Small Anim 2022; 22:659–72.
3. Monaghan K, Nolan B, Labato M. Feline acute kidney injury: 1. Pathophysiology, etiology, and etiology-specific management considerations. J Feline Med Surg 2012;25:775–84.
4. Claus MA. Pathophysiology of AKI. Proc International veterinary emergency and critical care Symposium. 2017.
5. Han SJ, Lee HT. Mechanisms and therapeutic targets of ischemic acute kidney injury. Kidney Res Clin Pract 2019;38:427–40.
6. Okusa MD, Portilla D. Pathophysiology of acute kidney injury. In: Chertow GM, Marsden PA, Skorecki K, et al, editors. Brenner and Rector's the kidney. 11th edition. St. Louis: Elsevier; 2019. p. 906–39.
7. Faubel S, Edelstein CL. Mechanisms and mediators of lung injury after acute kidney injury. Nat Rev Nephrol 2016;12:48–60.
8. Doi K, Rabb H. Impact of acute kidney injury on distant organ function: recent findings and potential therapeutic targets. Kidney Int 2016;89:555–64.
9. Monaghan K, Nolan B, Labato M. Feline acute kidney injury: 2. Approach to diagnosis, treatment, and prognosis. J Feline Med Surg 2012;25:785–93.
10. Yerramilli M, Farace G, Quinn J, et al. Kidney disease and the nexus of chronic kidney disease and acute kidney injury: the role of novel biomarkers as early and accurate diagnostics. Vet Clin N Am Small Anim 2016;46:961–93.
11. Cobrin AR, Blois SL, Kruth SA, et al. Biomarkers in the assessment of acute and chronic kidney diseases in the dog and cat. J Sm Anim Pract 2013;54:647–55.
12. Paes-Leme FO, Souza EM, Paes PR, et al. Advances in the evaluation of kidney function in the critically ill dog. Front Vet Sci 2021;8:1–5.
13. Montesinos A, Ardiaca M, Bonvehi C, et al. Plasma levels of symmetric dimethylarginine in domestic ferrets *(Mustela putorious furo)* with and without renal disease. Proc Intern Conf Avian Herp Exot Mammal Med 2017;444.
14. Toporek AH, Semler MW, Self WH, et al. Balanced Crystalloids versus Saline in Critically Ill Adults with Hyperkalemia or Acute Kidney Injury: Secondary Analysis of a Clinical Trial. Am J Respir Crit Care Med 2021;203:1322–5.
15. Hansen B. Fluid overload. Front Vet Sci 2021;8:668–88.
16. Langston CA. Effects of IV fluids in dogs and cats with kidney failure. Front Vet Sci 2021;8:659–60.
17. Yerram P, Karuparthi P, Misra M. Fluid overload and acute kidney injury. Hemodial Int 2010;14:348–54.
18. Barsant JA. Urinary tract catheterization and nosocomial infections in dogs and cats. In: Proceedings of the ACVIM Forum. 2010. p.445-447.
19. Langston C. Managing fluid and electrolyte disorders in kidney disease. Vet Clin North Am 2017;47:471–90.
20. Adin DB, Taylor AW, Hill RC, et al. Intermittent bolus injection versus continuous infusion of furosemide in normal adult greyhound dogs. J Vet Intern Med 2003;17: 632–6.
21. Simmons JP, Wohl JS, Schwartz DD, et al. Diuretic effects of fenoldopam in healthy cats. J Vet Emerg Crit Care 2006;16:96–103.
22. Nielsen LK, Bracker K, Price LL. Administration of fenoldopam in critically ill small animal patients with acute kidney injury: 28 dogs and 34 cats (2008–2012). J Vet Emerg Crit Care 2015;25:396–404.
23. Huynh M, Pignon C. Assessment and care of the critically ill rabbit. Vet Clin North Am Exot Anim Pract 2016;19:379–409.

24. Gladden JN, Lennox AM. Emergency and critical care of small mammals. In: Quesenberry KE, Orcutt CJ, Mans C, et al, editors. Ferrets, rabbits, and rodents: clinical medicine and surgery. 4th edition. St. Louis: Elsevier; 2021. p. 595–608.
25. Dziuk E, Siekierzynski M. Experimental model of peritoneal dialysis. Acta Physiol Pol 1973;24:465–72.
26. Gotloib L, Crassweller P, Rodella H, et al. Experimental model for studies of continuous peritoneal dialysis in uremic rabbits. Nephron 1982;31:254–9.
27. Zunic-Bozinovski S, Lausevic Z, Krstic S, et al. An experimental, non-uremic rabbit model of peritoneal dialysis. Physiol Res 2008;57:253–60.
28. Wojick K, Berube D, Barr J III. Clinical technique: peritoneal dialysis and percutaneous peritoneal dialysis catheter placement in small mammals. J Exot Pet Med 2008;17:181–8.
29. Cooper RL, Labato MA. Peritoneal dialysis in cats with acute kidney injury: 22 cases (2001–2006). J Vet Intern Med 2011;25:14–9.
30. Diehl SH, Seshadri R. Use of continuous renal replacement therapy for treatment of dogs and cats with acute or acute-on-chronic renal failure: 33 cases (2002–2006). J Vet Emerg Crit Care 2008;18:370–82.
31. Langston CE, Cowgill LD, Spano JA. Applications and outcome of hemodialysis in cats: a review of 29 cases. J Vet Intern Med 1997;11:348–55.
32. Worwag S, Langston CE. Acute intrinsic renal failure in cats: 32 cases (1997–2004). J Am Vet Med Assoc 2008;232:728–32.
33. Di Girolamo N, Huynh M. Disorders of the urinary and reproductive systems in ferrets. In: Quesenberry KE, Orcutt CJ, Mans C, et al, editors. Ferrets, rabbits, and rodents: clinical medicine and surgery. 4th edition. St. Louis: Elsevier; 2021. p. 39–54.
34. Garbin M, Pablo LS, Alexander AB. Management of hyperkalemia and associated complications in a ferret (*Mustela putortius furo*) with urinary obstruction requiring surgery. J Exot Pet Med 2021;39:4–7.
35. Reavill DR, Lennox AM. Disease overview of the urinary tract in exotic companion mammals and tips on clinical management. Vet Clin N Am Exot Anim Pract 2020;23:169–93.
36. Pacheco RE. Cysteine urolithiasis in ferrets. Vet Clin N Am Exot Anim Pract 2020;23:309–19.
37. Hanak EH, Di Girolamo N, DeSilva U, et al. Composition of ferret uroliths in North America and Europe: 1055 cases (2010-2018). Abstract, presented at: Exotics Conference with AAZV, Saint Louis, MO. 2019.
38. Minnesota Urolith Center. Cystine rising: Ferreting out the cause. In: Minnesota Urolith Center image of the month. 2018. Available at: https://vetmed.umn.edu/urolith-center/image-of-month/cystine-rising-ferreting-out-cause. Accessed November 29, 2022.
39. Nwaokorie EE, Osborne CA, Lulich JP, et al. Epidemiology of struvite uroliths in ferrets: 272 cases (1981-2007). J Am Vet Med Assoc 2011;239:1319–24.
40. Nwaokorie EE, Osborne CA, Lulich JP, et al. Epidemiological evaluation of cystine urolithiasis in domestic ferrets (*Mustela putorius furo*): 70 cases (1992–2009). J Am Vet Med Assoc 2013;242:1099–103.
41. Powers LV, Winkler K, Garner MM, et al. Omentalization of prostatic abscesses and large cysts in ferrets (*Mustela putorius furo*). J Exot Pet Med 2007;16:186–94.
42. van Zeeland YRA, Lennox A, Quinton JF, et al. Prepuce and partial penile amputation for treatment of preputial gland neoplasia in two ferrets. J Small Anim Pract 2014;55:593–6.

43. Di Girolamo N, Toth G, Selleri P. Prognostic value of rectal temperature at hospital admission in client-owned rabbits. J Am Vet Med Assoc 2016;248:288–97.
44. Di Girolamo N, Selleri P. Disorders of the urinary and reproductive systems (rabbit). In: Quesenberry KE, Orcutt CJ, Mans C, et al, editors. Ferrets, rabbits, and rodents: clinical medicine and surgery. 4th edition. St. Louis: Elsevier; 2021. p. 201–19.
45. Tschudin A, Clauss M, Codron D, et al. Water intake in domestic rabbits (*Oryctolagus cuniculus*) from open dishes and nipple drinkers under different water and feeding regimes. J Anim Physiol Anim Nutr 2011;95:499–511.
46. Clauss M, Burger B, Liesegang A, et al. Influence of diet on calcium metabolism, tissue calcification and urinary sludge in rabbits (*Oryctolagus cuniculus*). J Anim Physiol Anim Nutr 2012;96:798–807.
47. Kunzel F, Fisher P. Clinical signs, diagnosis, and treatment of *Encephalitozoon cuniculi* infection in rabbits. Vet Clin North Am Exot Anim Pract 2018;21:69–82.
48. Graham JE, Garner MM, Reavill DR. Benzimidazole toxicosis in rabbits: 13 cases (2003 to 2011). J Exot Pet Med 2014;23:188–95.
49. Wong AD, Gardhouse S, Rooney T, et al. Associations between biochemical parameters and referral centre in pet rabbits with urolithiasis. J Small Anim Prac 2021;62:554–61.
50. Martorell J, Bailon D, Majo N, et al. Lateral approach to nephrotomy in the management of unilateral renal calculi in a rabbit (*Oryctolagus cuniculus*). J Am Vet Med Assoc 2012;240:863–8.
51. Rhody JL. Unilateral nephrectomy for hydronephrosis in a pet rabbit. Vet Clin North Am Exot Anim Pract 2006;9:633–41.
52. Rembeaux H, Langlois I, Burdick S, et al. Placement of ureteral stents in three rabbits for the treatment of obstructive ureterolithiasis. J Small Anim Pract 2021;62:489–95.
53. Pizzi R. Cystoscopic removal of a urolith from a pet guinea pig. Vet Rec 2009;165:148–9.
54. Wenger S, Hatt JM. Transurethral cystoscopy and endoscopic urolith removal in female guinea pigs (*Cavia porcellus*). Vet Clin North Am Exot Anim Pract 2015;18:437–46.
55. Lewis TT, Lennox AM. Nonsurgical removal of urethral uroliths using a self-retaining retractor with elastic stays in female guinea pigs (*Cavia porcellus*): 16 Cases (2006-2019). J Exot Pet Med 2021;36:11–5.
56. Pignon R, Mayer J. Guinea pigs. In: Quesenberry KE, Orcutt CJ, Mans C, et al, editors. Ferrets, rabbits, and rodents: clinical medicine and surgery. 4th edition. St. Louis: Elsevier; 2021. p. 270–97.
57. Higbie CT, DiGeronimo PM, Bennet RA, et al. Semen-matrix calculi in a juvenile chinchilla (*Chinchilla lanigera*). J Exot Pet Med 2019;28:69–75.
58. Martel-Arquette A, Mans C. Urolithiasis in chinchillas: 15 cases (2007-2011). J Small Anim Pract 2016;57:260–4.
59. Frohlich J. Rats and Mice. In: Quesenberry KE, Orcutt CJ, Mans C, et al, editors. Ferrets, rabbits, and rodents: clinical medicine and surgery. 4th edition. St. Louis: Elsevier; 2021. p. 345–67.
60. Johnson-Delaney C. Sugar gliders. In: Quesenberry KE, Orcutt CJ, Mans C, et al, editors. Ferrets, rabbits, and rodents: clinical medicine and surgery. 4th edition. St. Louis: Elsevier; 2021. p. 385–400.

Urine Output Monitoring and Acute Kidney Injury in Non-mammalian Exotic Animal Critical Care

Stacey Leonatti Wilkinson, DVM, DABVP (Reptile and Amphibian)

KEYWORDS

• Acute • Avian • Diuretic • Fluid therapy • Gout • Kidney • Reptile • Urine output

KEY POINTS

- Acute Kidney Injury (AKI) is a sudden, severe decrease in kidney function, leading to the retention of uremic waste and subsequent fluid, electrolyte, and acid-base abnormalities.
- Numerous causes of AKI exist, and successful treatment depends on identifying and properly treating the underlying cause, along with proper fluid support, correction of electrolyte and acid-base disturbances, supportive care, and urine output monitoring.
- Exotic species present numerous challenges when managing AKI. Their small size can make IV/IO and urinary catheterization difficult, especially without sedation or anesthesia. Birds and reptiles are very different anatomically which create different challenges, especially with urine output monitoring.
- Exotic animals tend to hide clinical signs of illness until disease is advanced, so especially in birds and reptiles, distinguishing acute from chronic kidney disease can be difficult, and can make cases more difficult to manage.
- Prognosis for AKI overall is guarded to poor, though with proper identification and aggressive treatment, patients can recover. In some cases, permanent renal damage occurs that needs chronic management.

INTRODUCTION

Acute kidney injury (AKI) is defined as a sudden, severe decrease in kidney function. This leads to the retention of uremic wastes, abnormalities in circulating fluids and electrolytes, and acid-base imbalances.[1,2] Much of the knowledge of pathophysiology, causes, diagnosis, and treatment of AKI stems from small animal medicine (dogs and cats) and is then extrapolated to exotic species. As discussed in the previous article, most exotic companion mammal species with AKI will follow a similar

Avian and Exotic Animal Hospital of Georgia, 118 Pipemakers Circle Suite 110, Pooler, GA 31322, USA
E-mail address: drw@avianexotichospital.com

Vet Clin Exot Anim 26 (2023) 673–710
https://doi.org/10.1016/j.cvex.2023.05.008

progression and can be managed similarly, with some individual species variation. However, the assessment of kidney function and urine output monitoring in avian, reptile, and amphibian species requires different knowledge and techniques compared to the more well-known mammalian paradigms. A brief overview of AKI will be presented here, with further information pertaining to each species group.

PATHOPHYSIOLOGY

As previously discussed in the mammalian article, categories of AKI include prerenal, renal (intrinsic), and postrenal causes of renal insult. Similar categories have not been well described for avian and reptile patients, due to variations in physiology, but similar phenomena can be appreciated. Prerenal AKI arises when the hydrostatic pressure within the glomerular tuft is too low to cause movement of plasma ultrafiltrate into Bowman's capsule, leading to the retention of nitrogenous wastes in the bloodstream.[3–8] Prerenal AKI occurs secondary to decreases in renal blood flow or abnormal perfusion, typically a complication of conditions that cause hemodynamic abnormalities such as severe dehydration, hypotension, hypovolemia, shock, and so forth.[3,4] It does not initially cause morphologic abnormalities in the kidneys and can be reversible with the correction of hemodynamic changes, but it can lead to primary renal AKI due to renal ischemia if not corrected.[3,4]

Postrenal AKI typically develops when a blockage in urine outflow causes intranephron hydrostatic pressure to increase and prevent ultrafiltration at the glomerular tuft, thus preventing the creation of new urine.[4] A unique cause of postrenal AKI in birds and reptiles is egg binding, which can prevent the passage of urates, when the common endpoint, the urodeum, or the urinary and reproductive system is compressed by an egg. Renal AKI is a consequence of a disease process within the kidney itself.

CAUSES

There are many potential causes of AKI in animals with some variations among species groups. **Box 1** lists common causes for most domestic species while **Box 2** contains additional causes found in various exotic species. Many of the causes of AKI in domestic species apply to exotics as well, while some conditions are species specific. While the exact cause of AKI remains undetermined in many cases, it is important to make every effort to identify the etiology due to its potential influence on treatment and prognosis. Grading schemes for AKI have been developed for humans and for dogs and cats through the International Renal Interest Society (IRIS) (**Table 1**). This has not been applied to exotic animals. While similar grading schemes could be applied to exotic companion mammals (with adjustments made for species variation in serum creatinine measurements), an entirely different system would be needed for avian, reptile, and amphibian species as creatinine is not a reliable indicator of renal disease in these species. In addition, in avian, reptile, and amphibian species, the severity of disease does not always correlate with the elevation of bloodwork parameters.

DIAGNOSIS

History and Physical Examination

Many clinical signs of AKI are nonspecific, and most patients will have a history of illness of only hours to days. Obtain a thorough history including any previous medications or toxin exposure. Clinical signs may include lethargy, anorexia, nausea/vomiting (in species which are able to), diarrhea, melena, polydipsia, polyuria,

Box 1
Common causes of acute kidney injury in the dog and cat[2,3]

- Nephrotoxins
  - Organic Compounds
    - Ethylene glycol
    - Solvents
    - Pesticides
    - Heavy metals
      - Lead
      - Mercury
      - Arsenic
      - Bismuth
      - Zinc
  - Drugs
    - Antibiotics
      - Aminoglycosides
      - Cephalosporins
      - Tetracyclines
      - Sulfonamides
      - Penicillins
      - Vancomycin
      - Fluoroquinolones
    - Amphotericin B
    - Chemotherapeutics
      - Cisplatin and carboplatin
      - Doxorubicin
      - Methotrexate
    - Cyclosporine
    - Azathioprine
    - ACE-inhibitors
    - Mannitol, other diuretics
    - Allopurinol
    - Cimetidine
    - Methoxyflurane
    - Lipid-lowering drugs
    - Non-steroidal anti-inflammatory drugs
    - Penicillamine
    - Vitamin D analogs
    - Thiacetarsamide
  - Plants
    - Grapes and raisins
    - Lilies (cats)
  - Other Toxins
    - Envenomation (snake, bee, and so forth.)
    - Hemoglobin/myoglobin
    - Melamine/cyanuric acid
    - Radiographic contrast agents (possible)
    - Superphosphate fertilizer
    - Vitamin D-containing rodenticides

- Infectious
  - Bacterial pyelonephritis
  - Leptospirosis
  - Babesiosis
  - Leishmaniasis
  - Lyme Disease
  - Rocky Mountain Spotted Fever
  - Feline Infectious Peritonitis (FIP)

Ischemia
- Hypovolemia/dehydration
- Hypotension–including anesthesia
- Hyperviscosity
  - Hyperglobulinemia
  - Polycythemia
- Disseminated intravascular coagulation
- Renal vessel thrombosis
- Shock
  - Hemorrhagic
  - Septic
  - Traumatic
  - Burns
- Decreased cardiac output
- Heat stroke

Obstructive
- Calculi
- Mucous plugs/dried blood
- Neoplasia
- Blood clots
- Urethral or ureteral strictures

Other
- Systemic inflammatory response syndrome
- Hypercalcemia
- Pancreatitis
- Cardiac failure
- Hepatic failure
- Sepsis
- Amyloidosis
- Immune-mediated glomerulonephritis
- Urine leakage into the abdomen
- Neoplasia
  - Lymphoma
  - Adenocarcinoma
  - Sarcoma/hemangiosarcoma
  - Nephroblastoma

stranguria, hematuria, or oliguria/anuria.[2,43–49] Physical exam findings can include weakness, lethargy, signs of dehydration, hypothermia or fever, tachycardia or bradycardia, malodorous breath, oral ulcerations, hypersalivation, palpable renomegaly or abdominal pain, enlarged urinary bladder, and peripheral edema.[1,2,43] History of chronic kidney disease may be present. Remember many exotic patients are extremely adept at hiding their clinical signs of illness until disease is advanced. Some patients may be extremely critical at presentation, and even minimal restraint can be too much for them to handle. Some patients, especially avian patients, may need to have a hands-off approach taken until they are more stable. Some patients may also have progressed to a more chronic form of disease by the time they show signs.

Clinical Pathology

Initial laboratory evaluation should include a complete blood count, biochemistry profile, and, if possible, acid-base assessment, urinalysis, and urine culture. Leukocytosis may be present with pyelonephritis or other infectious agents, but a stress leukogram, leukopenia, hemoconcentration, or anemia may be present as well.[1,2,43] BUN or urea

Box 2
Additional common causes of AKI more specific to exotic species[9–42]

Ferrets
- Aleutians disease (parvovirus)
- Systemic coronavirus (ferret FIP-like disease)
- Bacterial nephritis and pyelonephritis
- Renal cysts (common in ferrets, rarely a cause of disease)
- Lymphoma, rarely other neoplasia
- Grape/raisin toxicity (anecdotal)
- Zinc or copper toxicity
- Obstructive
  - Urolithiasis–cysteine, struvite
  - Prostatomegaly/periprostatic cysts secondary to adrenocortical disease
  - Preputial neoplasia

Rabbits
- *Encephalitozoon cuniculi*
- Urolithiasis and urinary sludge–calcium carbonate or other calcium salts
- Bacterial nephritis and pyelonephritis
- Nephrocalcinosis and Vitamin D toxicity
- Neoplasia (nephroblastoma)
- Herniation of the urinary bladder through the inguinal ring
- Renal adipose deposition–secondary to anorexia, hepatic lipidosis, pregnancy toxemia

Guinea Pigs
- Urolithiasis–calcium carbonate
- Bacterial nephritis and pyelonephritis
- Excessive Vitamin D consumption

Chinchillas
- Urolithiasis–calcium carbonate
- Obstruction secondary to paraphimosis (fur ring), balanoposthitis

Mice
- Pyelonephritis
- Obstruction due to the infection of the preputial glands or bulbourethral glands
- *Klossiella muris*
- Hydronephrosis
  - Occurs more commonly in certain genetic strains
  - Obstruction secondary to the retrograde movement of seminal plugs in the urethra

Rats
- Hydronephrosis as with mice
- Nephrocalcinosis–dietary factors, strain related
- Pyelonephritis
- *Trichosomoides crassicauda*
- Neoplasia

Hedgehogs
- Pyelonephritis
- Neoplasia

Sugar Gliders
- Renal Klossiellosis–*Klossiella dulcis n.* sp
- Obstruction secondary to enlarged cloacal and paracloacal glands
  - Neoplasia
  - Hyperplasia/cysts
  - Impaction/infection
- Obstruction secondary to the self-mutilation of the penis
- Copper toxicity

Avian
- Neoplasia–primary and metastatic

- Nutritional
  - Excessive dietary calcium or Vitamin D3
  - Hypovitaminosis A
  - Iron storage disease
  - Renal lipidosis

Infectious
- Bacterial nephritis–ascending infection from cloaca, hematogenous spread
- Fungal nephritis
  - Aspergillosis–local invasion from air sac, hematogenous spread
  - Cryptococcosis
  - Microsporidiosis
- Parasitic
  - Coccidia (*Eimeria* spp.)
  - Cryptosporidiosis
  - Trematodes/cestodes
  - hemoparasites
- Viral
  - Polyomavirus
  - Adenovirus
  - Pigeon Paramyxovirus 1
  - Bornavirus
  - West Nile Virus

Toxin
- Capture myopathy and subsequent myoglobinuric nephrosis
- Vitamin D containing rodenticides–both primary and secondary (eating rodents that have been affected by toxicosis)
- Heavy Metal
  - Lead
  - Zinc
  - Mercury–especially mercury-containing fish
  - Arsenic
- Crude oil
- NSAIDs
  - Diclofenac
  - Ketoprofen
- Allopurinol–experimentally
- Aminoglycosides
- Garlic and onion
- Plant or fungal toxins on feed
- Obstructive–cloacolith, ureterolith (urate concretions), egg retention
- Trauma

Reptiles
- Infectious
  - Bacterial nephritis
  - Fungal nephritis
  - Microsporidia (particularly *Encephalitozoon pogonae*)
  - Viral
    - Inclusion body disease (Arenavirus)
    - Ranavirus (chelonians)
    - Picornavirus (tortoises)
    - Adenoviruses (lizards)
    - Herpesviruses (chelonians)
  - Parasitic
    - *Spironucleus (Hexamita)* protozoa
    - *Entamoeba invadens*
    - Intranuclear coccidia (tortoises)
    - *Cryptosporidium* sp. (rare)
    - *Klossiella* coccidia (boas)
    - *Myxosporidia* protozoa (chelonians)

- *Styphlodora renalis* and *S. horrida* trematodes (boas and pythons)
- Spirorchid flukes (aquatic chelonians)
- Urolithiasis–cloacal uroliths or ureteroliths causing obstruction
- Cold stunning (sea turtles)
- Hypovitaminosis A
- Hypervitaminosis D
- Neoplasia (renal adenocarcinoma)
- Aminoglycosides
- Excessive protein ingestion
- Severe dehydration–secondary to inappropriate husbandry

Amphibians
- Infectious
  - Bacterial nephritis–ascending infection or septicemia
  - Fungal nephritis
  - Viral
    - Ranavirus
    - Lucke's renal adenocarcinoma (herpesvirus)
  - Parasitic
    - Trematode flukes
    - Oligochaete worms
    - Myxozoa
    - Coccidia (various species)
    - *Entamoeba ranarum*, other protozoa
- Hypovitaminosis A
- Dehydration
- Urolithiasis/cystic calculi
- Toxin
  - Oxalate nephropathy (plant ingestion)
  - Heavy metals
    - Copper
    - Cadmium
    - Lead
    - Zinc
  - Volatile compounds in glue used for PVC piping
  - Water quality abnormalities
  - Numerous possibilities in free ranging amphibians

concentrations may be useful in amphibians and some reptilian species, but is not routinely measured in birds, and creatinine is not used in any of these species groups. Uric acid is the main nitrogenous waste product of birds and most reptiles, and its utility in the diagnosis of renal disease is discussed later in discussion. Other biochemical changes may include hyperphosphatemia, hypo- or hypercalcemia, hypo- or hypernatremia, hypo- or hyperkalemia, and metabolic acidosis.[1,2,43] Hyperkalemia is common with obstructive AKI or animals that are in the oliguric/anuric phase.[2]

In species groups with a cloaca (avian, reptile, and amphibian), urine and urates comingle with feces in the cloaca. Urinalysis can still be helpful, though contamination from feces must be considered in the results, and is discussed further with each group.

Tests to identify specific causes of AKI should be performed based on the clinical history and species. In domestic animals, these can include ethylene glycol or other toxin levels, testing for Leptospirosis or other infectious agents, serum cholecalciferol levels, and so forth.[2,43] Some exotics may be too small to obtain enough blood or urine for certain tests, some may be too weak to handle lab sampling on presentation, or it may be impractical to obtain certain tests from certain animals based on size or temperament. Additional testing will be discussed with each species group.

Table 1
International Renal Interest Society classification system for acute kidney injury[2]

Grade	Blood Creatinine (mg/dL)	Clinical Description
I	<1.6	Nonazotemic AKI: a. documented AKI: historical, clinical, laboratory, or imaging evidence of AKI, clinical oliguria/anuria, volume responsiveness[a] b. progressive nonazotemic increase in blood creatinine; ≥0.3 mg/dL within 48h c. measured oliguria (<1 mL/kg/h) or anuria over 6h
II	1.7–2.5	Mild AKI: a. Documented AKI and static or progressive azotemia b. Progressive azotemic increase in blood creatinine; >0.3 mg/dL within 48h, or volume responsiveness c. Measured oliguria (<1 mL/kg/h) or anuria over 6h
III IV V	2.6–5.0 5.1–10.0 >10.0	Moderate to severe AKI: a. Documented AKI and increasing severities of azotemia and functional renal failure

[a] Volume responsiveness is an increase in urine production to greater than 1 mL/kg/h over 6h and/or decrease in serum creatinine to baseline over 48h.

Diagnostic Imaging

Diagnostic imaging is useful in assessing renal disease in non-mammalian exotic patients. Given the kidney's position within the pelvis in most birds, reptile, and amphibians, ultrasound is often not the preferred modality for evaluating the kidneys, but radiographs and CT scans are popular options for analysis.

Cytology and Histopathology

A renal aspirate may be performed in cases where amyloidosis, lymphoma, or other neoplasia is suspected, but, again, can be difficult to obtain in these non-mammalian patients, based upon their kidneys' location.[2,43] In birds, coelioscopy can be performed to allow for biopsies of the kidneys. Histopathologic examination of the renal tissue will yield the most information about the chronicity of the disease process and may identify a certain cause, but in many cases it may not identify the cause, but only the result of the damage to the renal tissue.[2,43] Renal biopsy is indicated when the results would change the therapy or prognosis and benefits must outweigh the risks (anesthesia, bleeding, and so forth.). This is considered on a case-by-case basis and will be easier to obtain in some species than others.

TREATMENT

Treatment of AKI should be initiated as soon as possible and requires intensive patient monitoring. The goals of therapy are to preserve and restore renal hemodynamics, increase solute excretion, decrease the toxicity of nephrotoxic agents, maintain urine output, and correct fluid, acid-base, and electrolyte abnormalities.[1,2,43] Treatment is most successful during the initiation and extension phases of AKI, and the underlying cause must be identified and treated if possible.[1,2,43] Administration of nephrotoxic drugs should be discontinued. If pyelonephritis is suspected, or in endemic areas of certain infectious diseases, empiric therapy with antibiotics should be started. More specific therapies will be discussed with each species group.

Fluid Therapy

Intravenous (IV) fluid therapy is the mainstay of treatment for all animals with AKI. IV fluid therapy helps to correct dehydration, reverse azotemia, and correct electrolyte and acid-base abnormalities.[1,2,43] In many exotic species, IV catheterization is extremely difficult due to patient size, inability to visualize a vein (reptiles), or difficulty maintaining peripheral vein catheterization (birds), or the tendency of patients to chew or become tangled in fluid lines. If these small patients are extremely dehydrated or hypovolemic, a peripheral vein may not be visible. An alternative option in these animals is intraossesus (IO) catheterization; any therapies given IV can also be administered IO (**Fig. 1**). The preferred sites for IO catheterization are the ulna in birds and the proximal tibia or distal femur in reptiles and amphibians. Typically, in these debilitated patients, an IO catheter can be placed using local analgesia and either a spinal needle

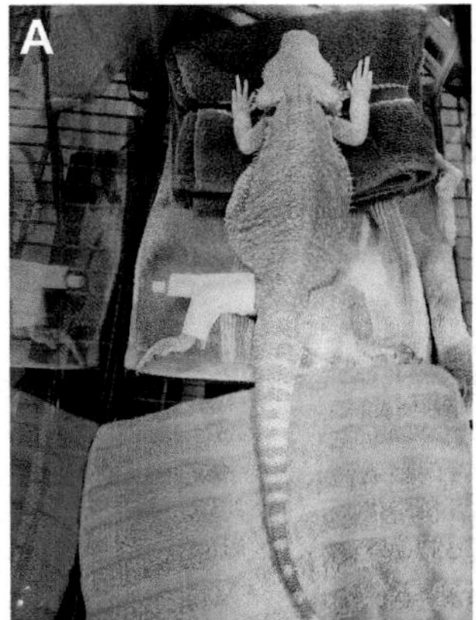

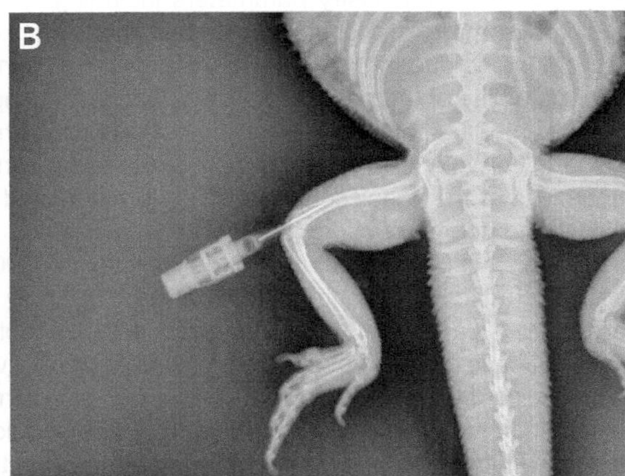

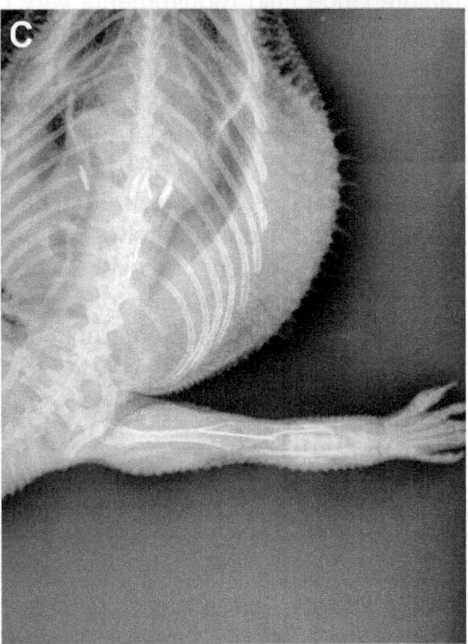

Fig. 1. (*A*) IO catheter placement in the proximal tibia of a bearded dragon (*Pogona vitticeps*) (*B* & *C*) catheter placement confirmed with two view (dorsoventral and lateral) radiographs (Photo courtesy Dr. Daniel Johnson.).

or hypodermic needle based on the size of the bone. Placement can be confirmed with 2 view radiographs, and the needle is covered with an IV port and secured to the limb with tape and either sutures or other bandage material. In certain situations, subcutaneous (SC) fluids may be necessary if IV or IO fluids cannot be administered; while this is commonplace in exotic species due to patient size, it is less ideal in cases of AKI. However, in some situations, risks of catheter placement outweigh the benefits. Sometimes a large bolus of SC fluids can be given to the patient while client discussions about therapy are taking place. This can help improve perfusion and blood pressure making IV catheterization easier.

Frequent monitoring is necessary to make adjustments in therapy and watch for volume overload. Monitoring parameters include: hydration status, body weight, urine output, mucous membrane color, capillary refill time, heart and respiratory rate, peripheral blood pressure, central venous pressure, packed cell volume and total protein, and serum chemistry parameters including renal values and electrolytes.[1,2,43] Again, in some exotic species, frequent monitoring of bloodwork parameters may be challenging due to the ability to obtain a blood sample on a repeated basis (small vein, instability of the patient, or size of patient limiting the maximum safe blood volume taken). Parameters excluding labwork should be monitored at least every 4 hours.

The initial volume of fluid to be administered can be calculated the same way regardless of the species involved. The formula used is based on the animal's body weight and degree of hydration:

Body weight (kg) x estimated % dehydration x 1000 = fluid deficit in milliliters.

Keep in mind for some tiny exotic patients, this may be a very small volume of fluids (example: 100g cockatiel or sugar glider with 8% dehydration would receive 8 mL). This should be replaced over 4-12 hours, but can be given more slowly in certain cases (such as cardiac disease to reduce the risk of volume overload. In addition to the deficit, the animal's normal maintenance fluids should also be given, and estimated ongoing fluid losses (such as from diarrhea, vomiting, and so forth.) should be accounted for as well. Maintenance fluid requirements vary by species (44–66 mL/kg/day for canine/feline).[2] Isotonic fluids such as Lactated Ringers (LRS), Plasma-Lyte A, or Normosol-R can typically be administered initially, but the type of fluid should be adjusted based on the patient's fluid and electrolyte status.[1,2] Urine output should be closely monitored (discussed later in discussion), and other parameters such as body weight, PCV/TS, and central venous pressure (CVP) can be used as well.[2,43] Fluid therapy should be continued until azotemia has resolved or stabilized, then fluid therapy can be tapered by approximately 25% per day.[2,43] Renal values have reached a plateau when there is no change over 24 hrs in a well-hydrated patient.[43] Abrupt discontinuation of fluids can lead to rapid dehydration, especially from post-obstructive or therapeutic diuresis. Some animals may become polyuric with recovery from AKI, and fluid therapy must be adjusted to account for this as well.

Urine Output Monitoring

Measuring urine output is one of the most important, but often most neglected, aspect of monitoring animals with AKI. Urine output monitoring is extremely important when tapering fluids, as output should diminish by a corresponding degree to which fluids are tapered; if not, the kidneys are unable to regulate fluid balance adequately.[1] Placement of an indwelling urinary catheter is the most accurate method for monitoring urine volume. In exotic animal medicine, an indwelling catheter cannot be used in birds, reptiles, or amphibians because of their anatomy. For animals in which catheterization is not practical, absorbent pads can be placed under the patient to estimate urine volume. The pads are weighed before and after use and the urine volume is calculated from the difference. One gram equals approximately one milliliter of urine produced.[2] Alternatively, patients can be housed on a grate off the cage floor so urine can be collected. Body weight monitoring can also be helpful. Urine output monitoring is not commonplace in avian, reptile, and amphibian patients currently, but utilizing some of these techniques can help a clinician be cognizant of this important aspect of AKI assessment.

Management of oliguria or anuria

Once the patient has been rehydrated, urine output should rapidly increase. Oliguria in small animal patients is defined as urine output <1 mL/kg/hr in a well-hydrated, normotensive patient, with anuria meaning no urine production (<0.08 mL/kg/h).[2] Relative oliguria describes a patient producing 1-2 mL/kg/h of urine despite higher infusion volumes of IV fluids.[2] If urine production is not sufficient, first the patient's hydration status should be reassessed, being sure to account for insensible losses, ongoing losses, volume of urine produced, and so forth. and recalculate fluids for the next four hours.[2,50–53] If the patient is well hydrated, specific therapy to increase urine flow is the next step in the treatment of oliguria/anuria. There is currently no evidence that these medications (described later in discussion) improve the outcome in human or veterinary AKI patients, but it is thought that if a patient is able to respond to these medical interventions, their kidney injury is likely less severe and, as such, they tend to have a better prognosis.[43] Animals that remain oliguric/anuric for 6-12 hrs after medical intervention should be considered as failing to respond.[43] At that point renal replacement therapy (dialysis) is the only option.[43]

The loop diuretic furosemide is the initial drug of choice. While this drug may increase urine output, reduce tubular obstruction, and improve renal blood flow, it does not increase GFR or improve outcome or survival rates in patients with AKI.[2] An initial dose of 2 mg/kg IV is suggested, and if effective, urine output typically increases within 20-40 minutes. If the initial dose fails to increase urine production, escalating doses up to 4-6 mg/kg can be administered at hourly intervals and the effective doses continued every 6-8 hours.[1,2] Alternatively, a loading dose of 0.66 mg/kg IV followed by a constant rate infusion (CRI) of 0.5-1.0 mg/kg/h can be used, and has been shown to be more effective at producing diuresis in normal dogs.[1,53,54] Dosing of furosemide for exotic species is typically extrapolated from small animal medicine, and no studies exist documenting which protocol is preferred. In exotics where IV administration is not possible, intramuscular (IM) administration is useful and effective, but there are species considerations (discussed later in discussion).

Mannitol is an osmotic diuretic that increases renal blood flow, GFR, and tubular fluid flow and acts as a free radial scavenger.[43] In the past it has been recommended as well, but use has fallen out of favor as studies have not shown mannitol to be any more effective than volume expansion alone, and it can contribute to circulatory overload.[1,43,53]

Fenoldopam is a specific dopamine D_1 receptor agonist used to treat emergency hypertension in humans and has gained popularity for use in oliguric or anuric AKI because of its effect on systemic vasodilation and promotion of diuresis. It has an extremely high affinity for the feline D_1 receptor compared to dopamine.[55] A study in healthy cats using a 2h infusion of fenoldopam at 0.5 μg/kg/min documented an increase in urine output, sodium excretion, fractional excretion of sodium and creatinine clearance within 6h that lasted for at least 24h.[55] However, one study of critically ill cats and dogs with AKI that received fenoldopam showed no improvement in survival to discharge, length of hospital stay, or improvement in renal biochemical parameters when compared with patients with AKI not receiving fenoldopam.[56] The recommended dosage range is 0.1–1 μg/kg/min as a constant rate infusion.[43] No literature exists on the use of fenoldopam in exotics other than in lab animal medicine describing use in rats, mice, or rabbits for extrapolation to human use.

Dopamine as a low-dose CRI was used in the past to increase urine output, but numerous studies in humans along with those in small animal patients, have shown no benefit in patients with AKI. Its use can also result in serious adverse effects such as tachyarrhythmias, vasoconstriction, and hypertension; as such it is no longer recommended for therapy in AKI.[2,43] Dopamine usage in exotic animal patients has mainly been restricted to use in managing hypotension during anesthesia. In rabbits, dopamine and phenylephrine at dog and cat doses have not been found to be effective.[57,58]

Correction of acid-base and electrolyte abnormalities

Metabolic acidosis is common in animals with AKI. Mild metabolic acidosis typically corrects with IV fluid therapy alone. Sodium bicarbonate IV therapy (isotonic solutions only) is typically reserved only for severe cases (pH < 7.1) as this therapy itself has significant risks, including volume overload, pulmonary edema, hypertension, hypernatremia, and cerebrospinal fluid acidosis.[1,2,53] Bicarbonate therapy is rarely used in exotics other than in species large enough to obtain repeated blood samples so that monitoring can be performed. Dosing is extrapolated from domestic species.

Moderate to severe hyperkalemia may occur if the animal is oliguric or anuric, which can lead to life-threatening cardiac arrhythmias. Urine production must be ensured, and mild to moderate hyperkalemia may resolve with IV fluid therapy alone. Severe hyperkalemia may need additional therapy such as calcium gluconate to protect the heart, dextrose, regular insulin, terbutaline, or sodium bicarbonate.[2,53] Hypokalemia may occur from excessive urinary loss, inadequate intake, or GI loss. Potassium may be added to IV fluids and continued orally if needed. Calcium gluconate may be given IV for hypocalcemia, but care must be taken to evaluate both calcium and phosphorus levels to avoid the risk of dystrophic mineralization. Disorders of calcium and phosphorus are common with reptile patients, so care must be taken to evaluate this closely in these patients, in particular. Historically the calcium x phosphorus product was used to assess the risk of soft tissue mineralization.

Treatment of other uremic complications

Vomiting is extremely common with AKI in domestic species. The cause is multifactorial, but ulceration of the GI tract can occur as a result of uremia. Antiemetics such as maropitant, metoclopramide, or ondansetron may be useful. Histamine receptor antagonists such as famotidine and cimetidine or proton-pump inhibitors such as omeprazole, pantoprazole, or esomeprazole may be beneficial as well. Sucralfate is a mucosal protectant for esophageal or gastric ulcers. Dosing is empirical for most exotic species and listed in **Box 3**.

Hypertension is common with AKI and may be exacerbated by IV fluid therapy. Volume overload must be addressed if that is the case. In cases of hypertension secondary to AKI, the calcium channel blocker amlodipine may be used, but caution must be used not to induce hypotension and decrease renal perfusion.[2,43] ACE inhibitors such as enalapril or benazepril should be avoided due to their negative effect on GFR.[2,43]

Animals with AKI are typically anorexic. In domestic species, placement of a feeding tube allows enteral nutrition, or parenteral nutrition can be given if enteral nutrition is not an option.[2,43] For exotic patients, lack of food intake can lead to its own life-threatening complications (gastrointestinal stasis in herbivores, hypoglycemia in small

Box 3
Dosages of medications useful in patients with AKI.[2]

Dosages provided are for canine/feline patients and may be extrapolated to exotics in cases where pharmacokinetic studies for the species are not available.

Metoclopramide 0.1-0.5 mg/kg IV, IM, SQ q8h or 0.01-0.02 mg/kg/h IV CRI

Maropitant 1 mg/kg IV or SQ q24 h up to 5 days

Ondansetron 0.1-0.2 mg/kg SQ q8h or 0.5 mg/kg loading dose IV then 0.5 mg/kg/h IV CRI

Famotidine 0.5-1 mg/kg IV, SQ, PO q12-24h

Ranitidine 1-2 mg/kg IV, SQ, IV q8-12h**no longer available

Cimetidine 5-10 mg/kg IV, PO q6-8h

Omeprazole 0.5-1 mg/kg PO q12 h

Pantoprazole 1 mg/kg IV q12-24h

Esomeprazole 1 mg/kg IV, SQ q12 h

Sucralfate 250-500 mg PO q8-12h

Amlodipine 0.2-0.4 mg/kg PO q24 h

patients, and so forth.). Syringe feeding or gavage feeding via tube is typically easily accomplished in most exotic patients making the use of feeding tubes less necessary, unless a patient is unable to swallow.

The unique physiology of avian, reptile, and amphibian patients necessitates additional drug therapies, which may be useful. These will be discussed in each corresponding section.

Renal replacement therapy

RRT can be considered for patients that remain oliguric or anuric despite appropriate medical therapy, those with refractory hyperkalemia or acid-base disturbances, removal of certain toxins, or for volume overload.[43] These therapies include peritoneal dialysis (PD), hemodialysis (IHD), and continuous renal replacement therapy (CRRT), or even kidney transplantation in cats. While PD can be performed at many 24 hr referral centers, it requires specialized equipment, is labor-intensive, and necessitates experience and understanding of the technique. IHD and CRRT are only available at certain facilities, and data is limited on these therapies in veterinary medicine. There are no reports of RRT in exotic patients other than as lab animal models, other than one report in rabbits.[59–62]

PROGNOSIS

The prognosis for AKI in all species is guarded to poor overall. Reported mortality rates for all causes in canine/feline patients is 45-75%, though prognosis can vary based on the cause.[1,2,43] Degree of azotemia is not predictive of outcome, but factors that confer a poorer prognosis include lack of urine production, hypocalcemia, hyperphosphatemia, anemia, and other organ involvement such as sepsis, pancreatitis, and so forth.[1,2,43] Survival with RRT can be 44-60%which sounds favorable, but without this therapy, these animals would not have survived.[43,63–65] Despite appropriate therapy, residual kidney disease or incomplete recovery is common and affects about 50% of patients that survive an acute event.[43,66]

Unfortunately, no statistics exist on reported outcomes for exotic species with AKI, however, it can be assumed that survival rates would be similar to lower than domestic species. There are limitations in exotic animal medicine that affect treatment, such as patient size affecting the ability to treat with IV/IO fluids or obtain repeated blood samples for monitoring, and RRT is not an option for exotics at this time. Exotic patients are also extremely adept at hiding their clinical signs of illness until disease is advanced, so these patients are often in critical condition before presenting to the veterinarian, making them more difficult to treat.

AVIAN ACUTE KIDNEY INJURY

Anatomy and Physiology

While there are some similarities of AKI in avian species to mammals, there are many differences as well in anatomy, exam findings, diagnosis, and treatment options. There can also be differences between various groups of birds, such as psittacines vs. birds of prey. Birds possess a cloaca which is the common opening between the GI tract, urinary tract, and reproductive tract. It is made of 3 compartments–the coprodeum (most cranial where feces is stored), the urodeum (contains openings of the ureters and reproductive tract), and the proctodeum (caudal segment that communicates with the vent). The kidneys are positioned in the renal fossae, bony depressions within the synsacrum in the caudal coelomic cavity. The kidneys are made of 3 divisions, and the lumbar and sacral nerve plexuses run through the renal parenchyma. This can result in neurologic dysfunction of the legs with various renal diseases. Avian kidneys contain 2 types of nephrons: mammalian, or those with a loop of Henle (looped nephrons), and reptilian, those without (loopless nephrons).[67] The majority are the loopless nephrons which secrete uric acid.[67] There is some potential to concentrate urine with the looped nephrons, but since the majority are loopless, typically avian patients do not make concentrated urine.[67]

The renal portal system is found in most non-mammalian classes including birds, reptiles, amphibians, and fish. The renal portal system constitutes a ring formed by the cranial and caudal renal portal veins ventral to the kidneys. This ring of vessels receives blood from the GI tract, pelvic region, and legs. This blood passes through the renal parenchyma before returning to the renal veins, common iliac veins, and the caudal vena cava (CVC).[67,68] The renal portal system is involved in the secretion of urates into the blood so that uric acid can be excreted by the kidneys in birds.[67] The proportion of venous blood that enters the kidney tissue depends on the action of the renal portal valve.[68] This is a smooth muscle sphincter with both sympathetic and parasympathetic innervation, that lies within each common iliac vein.[68] Under sympathetic stimulation the valves relax and open, diverting blood to the common iliac veins and CVC, thereby bypassing the kidney tissue and increasing venous return directly to the heart.[67,68] When the valves are closed, blood flows to the parenchyma of the kidney.[67,68] The coccygeomesenteric vein drains the mesentery of the hindgut into the hepatic and/or renal portal veins. Colitis may serve as a source of infectious agents, toxins, and inflammatory products to the avian kidney if blood flow draining the colon is diverted into the renal vasculature.[37]

GFR is similar in birds to mammals and is most dependent on hydration status. A decrease in GFR can be a sign of renal disease or an appropriate response to water restriction. There have been limited studies investigating renal blood flow in birds; however, there seems to be the autoregulation of renal blood flow over a wide range of systemic blood pressures.[67] Birds also have a unique ability to maintain renal blood flow even with severe hemorrhage or other hemodynamic alterations.[67–69] The major end-product of nitrogen catabolism in birds is uric acid. Uric acid accounts for about 70% to 80% of the nitrogen excreted in ureteral urine, along with minor amounts of creatinine, amino acids, and urea.[70] These waste products are not eliminated by glomerular filtration, but by active secretion into the proximal tubules.[69] As the concentration of urates secreted into the lumen increases past its solubility limit, there is the potential for crystal formation in the proximal tubule.[67] This potential has important implications for clinicians because normal patient hydration provides a GFR sufficient to reduce the risk of possible sludge formation or obstruction. Maintaining adequate levels of dietary vitamin A also helps to keep the reptilian portion of the avian kidneys healthy by reducing the incidence of squamous metaplasia, which could also cause plugging.[67] While drinking is important for most birds (an estimated 5% body weight per day), many species can maintain their water intake through their food, particularly carnivores and frugivores.[67] As body mass decreases, drinking rate increases.[67] The kidney filters a large volume of fluid daily, with up to 11 times the total body water filtered in a 100-g bird. Most (approximately 95%) of this volume is reclaimed by tubular reabsorption. Birds can concentrate their urine using mammalian (looped nephrons). For this reason, avian urine can range from dilute to hyperosmotic. Further concentration of the urine can occur by retroperistalsis into the coprodeum and large intestine, where a single layer of columnar epithelium can reabsorb water.[67,69] The movement of ureteral fluid of urine and urates is controlled by the tonicity of the fluid within the GI tract.[67] Some species also possess salt glands near the nasal cavity or orbits which can also regulate plasma osmolality. Birds do not have a urinary bladder; the ureters empty into the urodeum and the urine, urates, and feces are excreted together (with few exceptions, such as ratites),.

Physical Examination and Clinical Signs

Birds with renal disease often present with nonspecific symptoms such as lethargy, weakness, staying at the bottom of the cage rather than on a perch, sitting with feathers fluffed up and eyes closed, and decreased appetite (**Fig. 2**). Some patients will exhibit polyuria and polydipsia, discoloration of the urates, regurgitation, and dehydration. If the kidneys are enlarged, such as in cases of neoplasia, there can be coelomic enlargement, dyspnea secondary to air sac compression, or paresis of

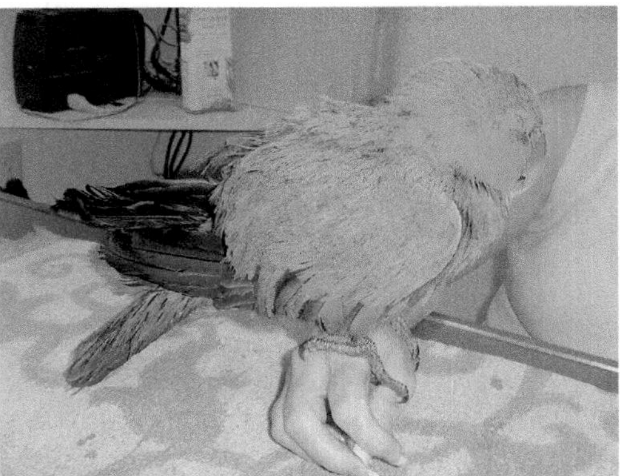

Fig. 2. Eclectus parrot (*Eclectus roratus*) demonstrating clinical signs of "sick bird syndrome." The patient is fluffed, quiet, keeping its eyes closed, having trouble perching, and anorexic all of which could be signs of AKI or any underlying illness. (Photo courtesy Dr. Daniel Johnson.)

a hind limb secondary to sciatic nerve compression.[37] Birds with AKI will likely still have a normal body condition while weight loss is very common with chronic renal disease.

Diagnosis

Assessment of renal function in birds is difficult because clinical signs are often nonspecific and can be subtle or absent until the disease is advanced. Lack of sensitive and specific biomarkers can make diagnosis challenging, as while a variety of biochemical alterations may occur, not many are specific for renal disease. Often multiple tests are needed to confirm a diagnosis.

Birds are uricotelic with 70-90% of their total nitrogenous waste being secreted as uric acid (UA).[69,71] As such, this is the value most often used to screen birds for renal disease. The excretion of UA is 90% dependent on tubular secretion and largely independent of urine flow.[71] Blood UA concentrations are only mildly affected by hydration status but reflect the functional capacity of the renal proximal tubules.[37,71] Although plasma UA can be useful as a screening tool for advanced renal disease, UA level does not increase significantly until there is extensive renal tubular damage.[37,71] It has been estimated that renal function must be less than 30% of its original capacity before hyperuricemia develops.[69,71] Even though dehydration should not play a big role in hyperuricemia, clinically it seems to in psittacine birds as noted by many authors.[37,71] It is standard of care to repeat fasting UA concentrations on well-hydrated birds before a suggestion of renal disease is made.[37,71] Birds with persistent hyperuricemia after fluid therapy and/or fasting raise suspicion for some form of renal disease.[37] In birds of prey, UA production is directly related to the amount of protein consumed and transient increases are noted following high-protein meals.[69]

If the plasma concentration of uric acid exceeds the solubility of uric acid, it will start to precipitate leading to gout. Two forms of gout can occur, articular and visceral. In joints and along tendons, once a seed of uric acid is deposited, it acts as a crystallization point resulting in a growing deposit known as tophi (**Fig. 3**). Visceral gout typically occurs secondary to acute renal tubular failure and renal deposition of UA. These birds develop anuria resulting in a rapid increase in blood UA concentration and deposition of uric acid on many visceral surfaces. Visceral gout is often rapidly fatal.

Electrolyte, mineral, and protein levels can vary in birds with renal disease, but the effect of renal disease on these values has been poorly studied in birds.[37,69,71]

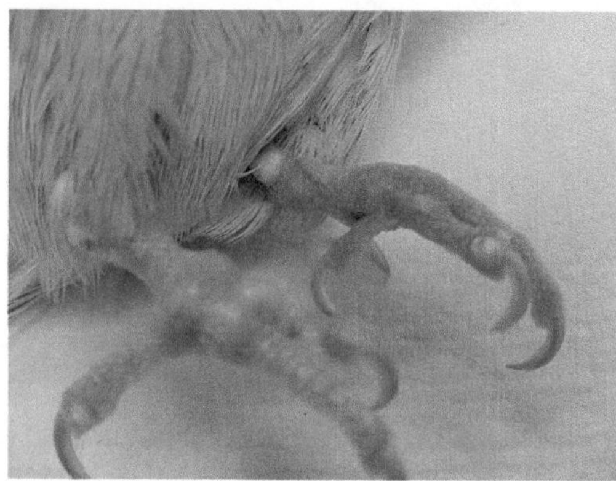

Fig. 3. Gout tophi visible in multiple joints of the feet of a budgerigar (*Melopsittacus undulatus*). (Photo courtesy Dr. Daniel Johnson.)

Minimal investigation into other blood work abnormalities (acid-base status, lactate measurement, and so forth.) have been done as well. While hypoproteinemia can be associated with renal failure, few studies have evaluated serum protein in birds with renal disease.[69,71] Also current analytical methods for albumin do not accurately report avian albumin levels, so serum/plasma protein electrophoresis is recommended for more accurate quantification.[69,71] Possible findings with renal failure can also include hyponatremia, hyperkalemia, hypocalcemia, and hyperphosphatemia.[37,69] Some hematologic changes can be observed, but again are nonspecific for renal disease. These can include anemia, heterophilia, monocytosis, and/or lymphopenia.[37,69]

The tubular marker N-acetyl-B-d-glucosaminidase (NAG) is a marker of tubular dysfunction found in both plasma and urine.[71,72] NAG may be useful as a marker of kidney injury before increases in uric acid or other parameters are noted. Recently NAG has been evaluated in pigeons (*Columba livia domestica*) and Hispaniolan Amazon parrots (*Amazona ventralis*) to evaluate normal ranges and the effect of gentamicin-induced renal disease on pigeons.[72] It needs to be investigated in larger sample sizes and a wider variety of avian species to t determine if it will be a useful marker of renal disease.[71,72] Because so many renal diseases in birds are chronic, the usefulness of acute injury markers may be lower than it is in humans and other mammals.[71]

The use of urine gamma-glutamyl transferase (GGT) as a means to screen for early renal disease prior to hyperuricemia is increasing.[73] No published studies have evaluated urine GGT use in birds, but one author uses it routinely.[73]

Urinalysis can be performed in birds and is indicated in cases of polyuria. Free-catch samples are collected in a clinical setting, and can be done so from a bare cage floor or with wax paper used as cage lining to prevent absorption. Since urine is eliminated with feces, samples are easily contaminated so bacteria seen on exam must be accounted for. Avian urine is usually clear, a cloudy sample can indicate crystals, casts, or cells.[69] Urates are typically white to off-white. Green or yellow urates (biliverdinuria) can indicate liver disease. Red, blue, or purple tinged urates or feces can be seen with the ingestion of berries or other pigment-containing foods. Hemoglobinuria may be seen with heavy metal toxicity and causes the urine and/or urates to be dark red, pink, or brown.[69,74] Specific gravity can vary for reasons discussed above, but is typically 1.005 to 1.020 in polyuric birds though this has low clinical relevance.[69,74] Urine dipsticks may be used, but only pH, protein, glucose, ketones, blood, and urobilinogen are useful. Urine pH is typically 6.5-8 and is lower in carnivores and higher in omnivores/herbivores as with other species.[69,74] Zero to trace protein levels are expected, but positive protein levels are seen with fecal contamination, hematuria, hemoglobinuria, and possible renal dysfunction.[74] However, because differences exist between mammals and birds in regards to proteinuria, this is not always a consistent finding with renal disease.[69] Glucose, ketones, and blood should all be negative. Glucose and ketones may be seen with diabetic patients. Nonhemolyzed trace blood may be from fecal or cloacal contamination.[74] Positive urobilinogen may indicate fecal contamination, severe liver disease, or intravascular hemolysis.[74] Urine sediment exam may be difficult to interpret as the urate crystals obscure other findings, and methods to remove them may damage other cells.[69] Normal urine is free of casts, but even if present, their significance is controversial.[69] Red blood cells may be significant, especially in higher numbers, but may also come from the digestive or reproductive tracts or the cloaca itself. White blood cells are never normal and can indicate infection or urinary compromise.[74] WBC and bacteria can originate from the cloaca or GI tracts.[74]

Diagnostic imaging can be useful in some cases of renal disease in birds. Radiographs are often taken first, and barium or other contrast agents can be given to differentiate the GI tract from the kidneys and gonads as many structures are superimposed. Radiography can detect increased opacity, renomegaly, or calcification.[75,76] Contrast urography can be performed but is challenging in birds because of differing anatomy within the kidneys to mammals and the clearance of the contrast agent is so rapid, the bird must be positioned on the film before the contrast is given.[75,76] Urography is contraindicated with dehydration or severe renal dysfunction, so typically is not used in cases of AKI.[75] Ultrasonography can be attempted but is challenging as the air sac system disrupts the sound waves and prevents penetration.[75] However, in birds with a distended coelom, this improves transducer coupling and improves image quality, thus the kidneys can be seen more easily.[75] Ultrasonography can identify neoplasia, renal cysts, hemorrhage, and possibly areas of hypercalcification or severe gout, along with changes in echogenicity which can indicate nephritis.[75]

More advanced imaging modalities include endoscopy, scintigraphy, and CT or MRI. Endoscopy carries the distinct advantage of being able to visualize the kidneys to help determine the abnormality along with collect biopsies of targeted areas.[75,77] However, this obviously requires full anesthesia, which is a higher risk in patients with AKI, along with the risk of bleeding when biopsies are obtained.[75,77] Scintigraphy is only used in research because of the challenge of sampling pure ureteral urine.[78] CT has become more commonplace in recent years and is advantageous because of the ability to assess the kidneys three-dimensionally without the superimposition of surrounding structures.[75,78] MRI is not used as often as CT because it typically requires a longer scanning time and is extremely loud, making anesthetic monitoring extremely challenging, especially in a sick avian patient.[75,78] Protocols for CT are well described.[78,79] Enlargement of the kidneys is easily detected with CT along with calcifications, neoplasia, and blood flow and changes in tissue density when using contrast.[78,79]

Causes

Multiple causes of AKI in birds are possible and are outlined in **Box 2**. These are in addition to those affecting domestic species, as birds can suffer AKI for some of the same reasons. Primary neoplasia of the kidney is the most common form of neoplastic disease of the kidney and can present acutely as the enlargement of the kidney and can compress the sciatic nerve, leading to paresis or paralysis (especially in budgerigars) or compression of coelomic structures causing air sac compression and dyspnea.[38,80] Metastatic mineralization of the kidney has been reported secondary to diets containing excess calcium fed to nestlings or hand fed babies, adult cockatiels and budgerigars, or laying hen diets fed to birds that are not laying (roosters).[38] Hypovitaminosis A can contribute to renal disease by inducing squamous metaplasia of the renal epithelium.[38,80] While viral diseases such as polyomavirus and adenovirus can cause AKI and renal lesions on histopathology, typically the birds present with symptoms consistent with the viral infection, not kidney disease.[38,80] Bacterial nephritis can occur from bacteria spreading from the cloaca up the ureters into the kidneys or by hematogenous spread.[38,80] The fungal infection Aspergillosis can invade from the abdominal air sac into the kidney.[38,80,81] Parasitic infections of the kidney are more common in wild birds and a review is found in Phalen.[38,80]

Myoglobinuric nephrosis occurs after exertional rhabdomyolysis (capture myopathy) or severe crushing injuries in birds.[38] Hemoglobinuric nephrosis occurs in birds with intoxications that cause hemolysis, including heavy metal toxicity such as acute lead and zinc ingestion or ingestion of crude oil, cadmium, mercury, or arsenic.[38,80,82,83] Vitamin D containing rodenticides are toxic to birds directly, but poisoned rodents can be consumed by birds of prey, causing intoxication in them as well.[38] Aminoglycosides have caused fatal renal disease in birds characterized by tubular necrosis but these drugs are rarely used now.[84,85] Nonsteroidal anti-inflammatories have the potential to be nephrotoxic following short or long term treatment. The most commonly used NSAID in birds is meloxicam, and studies show when used at recommended dosages for the species (some species require lower doses such as pelicans), meloxicam does not cause renal disease.[86–88] Ketoprofen has been suspected of causing renal failure.[89] Diclofenac has been used widely in cattle, and when these animals die, vultures feeding on carcasses develop renal failure.[38,90] This has resulted in up to a 95% population decline in some species of vultures.[90] Ingestion of numerous toxic plants could cause could cause renal disease, but this seems to be rare in captive birds.

Obstructive processes are less common in birds. Urolithiasis, which is seen in chickens, is also likely to be caused by excess dietary calcium.[38,80,91] Uroliths partially or completely obstruct the ureters causing tubule dilation, loss of nephrons, and ultimately renal failure.[38,80,92] This has been reported in a parrot as well.[93] Cloacoliths or eggs that are lodged in the cloaca can also put pressure on the sciatic nerves and the kidneys causing paresis or paralysis and/or acute kidney injury.

Trauma to the kidney is rare because it is protected within the renal fossae of the synsacrum. However, the author has had two cases of known kidney trauma in which the patient recovered. In one case, the patient was a chicken attacked by a hawk that suffered a puncture wound over the dorsum just cranial to the hip and lateral to the spine resulting in penetration into the coelomic cavity and air sac rupture. After 3-4 days of management, urates and urine started leaking out of the wound onto the patient's back. Further diagnostic testing to evaluate the extent of the injury to the kidney was declined, and the wound eventually healed and the patient made a full recovery, though the degree of internal damage is unknown. In another case, a pekin duck (*Anas platyrhynchos domesticus*) presented with signs of AKI, and on radiographs there was a piece of metal evident in the kidney (**Fig. 4**). After stabilization on IV fluids and supportive care, exploratory surgery was performed and the metal and surrounding granuloma was removed. The patient made a full recovery. The metal was recognized as piece of fencing material that the patient had ingested which had migrated out of the GI tract into the coelomic cavity and lodged adjacent to the kidney.

Clinical Management

As in mammalian patients, fluid therapy is one of the most important treatments when managing AKI in birds. Because uric acid is eliminated by active tubular secretion, fluid is needed to flush the suspension through the kidneys, otherwise it will accumulate and lead to gout. Fluid therapy is discussed extensively in Stacey Leonatti Wilkinson article, "Urine Output Monitoring and Acute Kidney Injury in Mammalian Exotic Animal Critical Care," of this edition. Fluid selection is based on biochemical analysis, electrolyte levels, and acid-base status but if that status is not known, in avian patients typical balanced isotonic crystalloid solutions such as Lactated Ringers can be used.[80] Fluids can be administered by PO, SC, IV, or IO routes depending on the patient's status. Fluids are often administered by gavage with liquid oral nutrition for patients that are not in shock or debilitated. Subcutaneous fluids can be administered easily in the inguinal or interscapular regions, and 20-30 mL/kg can be administered in one location (**Fig. 5**). Care must be taken to avoid inadvertent administration into an air sac. Some avian patients are so debilitated at presentation that any handling can

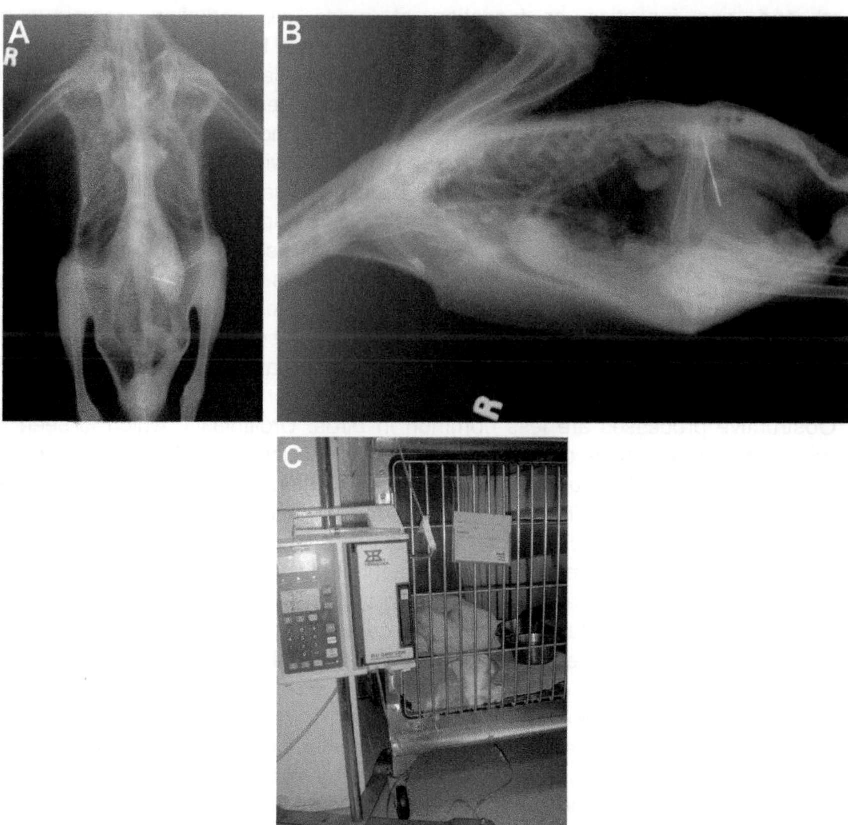

Fig. 4. Ventrodorsal (*A*) and lateral (*B*) radiographs of a Pekin duck (*Anas platyrhynchos domesticus*) demonstrating a metallic foreign body that appears to be lodged in the kidney. This patient presented for clinical signs and biochemical abnormalities consistent with AKI. (*C*) the same patient hospitalized on IV fluids with a catheter in the medial metatarsal vein.

be extremely detrimental or even fatal. While IV/IO fluids are ideal in cases of AKI, the benefit of placing a catheter or obtaining a blood sample must be weighed against the risk of doing so. Often with extremely ill birds, patients can be given a bolus of SC fluids then placed in an incubator with heat and supplemental oxygen if needed until they are more stable for handling and diagnostics.

IV or IO fluids can be beneficial in certain AKI cases, but the choice depends on many factors.[80,94] (**Fig. 6**) IV catheters may be placed for initial fluid therapy but are very difficult to keep stable in an avian patient that is not extremely debilitated or sedated, and the patient must be supervised as fatal hemorrhage can occur if the catheter is disrupted by the patient.[94] IV catheters can be placed in patients as small as cockatiels and up using 24-26g catheters in the jugular, basilic, or medial metatarsal veins.[94] The medial metatarsal can only be used in larger birds, but can be secured with tape only and is an excellent choice for waterfowl.[94] Other IV catheters typically need to be sutured in place and covered with a bandage.[94] IO catheters can be placed quickly, are more stable and reliable, are easier to maintain, larger fluid boluses can be given, and can be placed in smaller patients, but placement is more

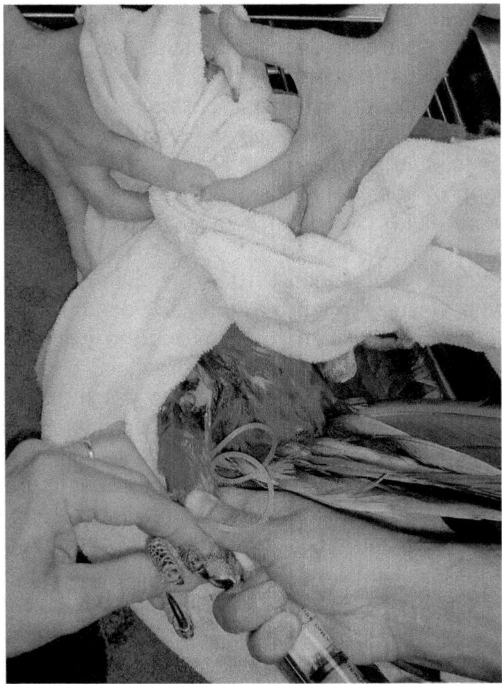

Fig. 5. Greenwing macaw (*Ara chloropterus*) receiving SC fluid therapy in the inguinal region.

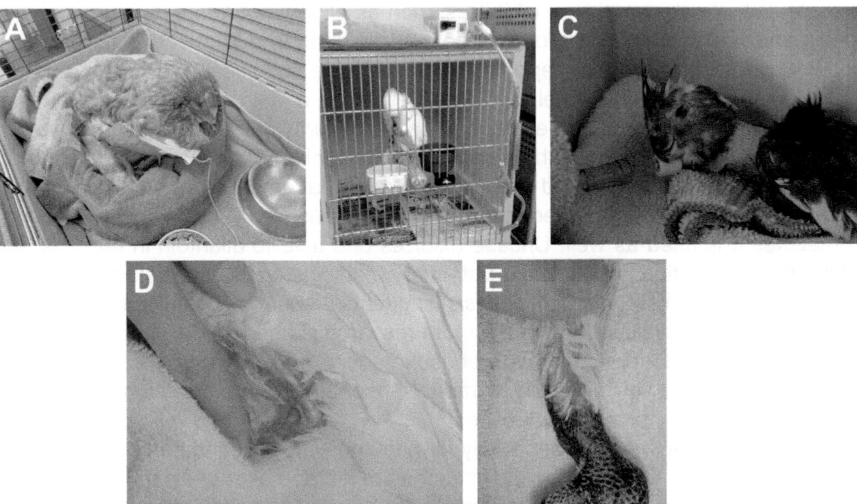

Fig. 6. Various IV/IO catheter options in birds: (*A*) Domestic chicken (*Gallus gallus*) receiving IO fluid therapy through a catheter in the ulna (Photo courtesy Dr. Daniel Johnson) (*B*) Umbrella cockatoo (*Cacatua alba*) receiving IV fluid therapy through a catheter in the ulnar vein (photo courtesy Angela Lennox) (*C*) cockatiel (*Nymphicus hollandicus*) with a jugular catheter (photo courtesy Angela Lennox) (*D*) ulnar vein where it crosses over the medial aspect of the elbow (Photo courtesy Dr. Daniel Johnson) (*E*)) medial metatarsal vein. (Photo courtesy Dr. Daniel Johnson.)

painful.[80] IO catheters are typically placed in the distal ulna or the proximal tibiotarsus; the humerus and femur should be avoided because they are pneumatic bones and fluids administered would enter the respiratory system.[94] IO catheters are typically placed with sedation and local anesthetic. E-collars are extremely stressful for birds and should be avoided if possible. Fluid therapy is generally continued until the blood uric acid level drops to either normal or mildly elevated levels (10–20 mg/dL) and the bird is showing signs of improvement (eating, more active, and so forth.). Lower amounts of parenteral fluids are given if overhydration is either suspected or a concern.

Measuring urine output is not practical in birds because of the elimination of urine in combination with other wastes through the common cloaca. The author typically monitors urine output more subjectively by maintaining the patient on paper towels or newspaper so that the amount of urine being produced can be visualized around each dropping as it soaks into the paper. Trying to weigh urine-soaked bedding to calculate the volume produced can be attempted but is often impractical in avian patients because of the small volumes produced. If urine needs to be collected, the patient can be set up over a bare cage floor or over wax paper to prevent absorption. In the author's experience, true anuria seems to be rare in birds and fluid therapy alone seems to stimulate diuresis, making urine production stimulation with furosemide uncommon, though it can be used if needed.

In addition to fluid therapy, other treatments and supportive care will be needed for avian patients with AKI. As mentioned previously, all sick birds typically will benefit from being housed in a warm incubator with increased humidity and supplemental oxygen if needed. Nutritional support in the form of gavage feeding will be necessary in patients that are anorexic. Many resources and commercial diets (such as EmerAid products, Lafeber Co., Cornell, IL) are available for this. Essential fatty acid supplements (omega-3 supplementation) seem to be beneficial for avian patients with renal disease.[37,80] Xanthine oxidase inhibitors such as allopurinol decrease uric acid synthesis and are widely used though research information documenting its benefit is scant and toxicity has been reported in at least one species.[37,80,95] In the author's experience, it does seem to help patients feel better, and it can be useful in lowering the uric acid level, though it does depend on the severity of the patient's disease process at presentation. The xanthine dehydrogenase inhibitor colchicine is used for its antigout activity in humans and has been used to treat amyloidosis and renal fibrosis in small animals.[37] No controlled study has been published on its use in birds, though sometimes it is used as well. Uricase oxidizes uric acid to allantoin in humans, and while little information is available in veterinary medicine on its use, a study in pigeons and red-tailed hawks (*Buteo jamaicensis*) suggests it could be useful in birds to lower uric acid levels as well, though much more research is needed.[96] Phosphate binders can be used with documented hyperphosphatemia, though hyperphosphatemia due to AKI typically resolves with fluid therapy. Phosphate binders are often only needed once chronic kidney disease develops.

Analgesia is often needed, especially for patients with gout and nerve compression from renal masses. Often cage modifications are needed as these patients may have difficulty ambulating. On initial admission to the hospital, usually patients will be set up on the floor of a cage with soft towels to rest against and a low perch if they are able to perch, with shallow food and water bowls on the floor easily accessible. Opioids can be used in the hospital, and various options such as gabapentin, low-level laser therapy, or local analgesia, can be used as well. While NSAIDs should typically be avoided in cases of AKI, if an avian patient survives the acute insult and now needs chronic management for kidney disease and arthritis pain or neuropathic pain, NSAIDs (typically meloxicam) can be used judiciously with a discussion with the owner based on risk/benefit for quality of life. Articular gout and renal neoplasia both carry a poor prognosis and euthanasia must be considered when quality of life cannot be maintained. GI ulceration is rarely described in birds with renal disease, and chronic anemia cannot be managed the same as in mammals due to the structure of avian erythropoietin.[80] Dialysis has not been described in birds, and coelomic dialysis is not possible because of the abdominal air sacs.[80] The insoluble nature of uric acid also makes dialysis unrealistic. Renal transplantation is unrealistic given the anatomy and placement of the avian kidney.[80]

Specific therapies are indicated based on the underlying cause of AKI. Many bacteria have been reported to cause nephritis in birds, and because of the possibility of ascending infection from the cloaca, antibiotics are often used in cases of AKI. Culture and sensitivity from blood sampling or biopsy is ideal, but, while pending, choose antibiotics that have renal penetration (trimethoprim-sulfamethoxazole, fluoroquinolones) and treatment should likely be continued for 4-6 weeks.[37,80] While various viral infections can affect the kidneys, polyomavirus is the most likely to result in clinical renal disease. There is no specific treatment, only supportive care. Renal coccidiosis caused by *Eimeria* spp. is the most common form of renal parasitism, though others reported include cryptosporidiosis, trematodes, cestodes, and hemoparasites.[80] Treatment depends on the organism being targeted, and most parasitic diseases are diagnosed in outdoor birds. While Aspergillosis is most often a respiratory pathogen, systemic involvement can occur as can local invasion from an abdominal air sac directly to the kidney, leading to kidney dysfunction.[81] Treatment is often needed for months and can involve IV and PO medications along with endoscopic debridement and topical therapy. Amphotericin B is recommended IV as initial first-line therapy, and while this drug has been associated with nephrotoxicity in mammals, this has not been documented in birds.[80] Treatment for Aspergillosis is beyond the scope of this article and is documented elsewhere.

Toxicities have various treatments. Heavy metal toxicity, a potential cause of AKI, can be treated with chelation using calcium disodium salt of EDTA (CaEDTA) given parenterally. Nephrotoxiticity has been documented with CaEDTA in humans but never in birds, though the use of fluids and different treatment regimens are recommended to help avoid this possibility. For ingested toxins, if ingestion is recent, crop lavage or endoscopic removal can be performed, along with the administration of activated charcoal and supportive therapy for the specific toxin. For Vitamin D3 toxicity, fluid therapy is the main treatment of choice as steroid use to stimulate calciuresis is not recommended in birds due to the potential for severe side effects.

Obstructive cloacoliths can be crushed and removed with forceps via the cloaca with or without endoscopic assistance,[97] and in a case with reported ureteroliths, surgery was necessary.[93]

No effective treatment for neoplasia exists as surgical removal is nearly impossible due to the anatomy and placement of the avian kidney.[80] Case reports of adjunctive treatment including chemotherapy and radiation exist, but have not been extensively evaluated in birds, and so far, have not yielded a good clinical response. Palliative care for these tumors focusing on analgesia is typically chosen.

REPTILIAN ACUTE KIDNEY INJURY

Anatomy and Physiology

Reptiles have paired kidneys each connected to the cloaca by a ureter, similar to birds. In lizards, the kidneys are located within the pelvic canal, while they are located in the caudal coelom in most other reptiles. Most lizards and all chelonians possess a urinary bladder while bearded dragons (*Pogona vitticeps*), some monitors, snakes, and crocodilians do not. If present, the bladder is connected to the ventral urodeum by a urethra; as such, the contents of the bladder are never sterile. The bladder also functions as a site of fluid storage and reabsorption in times of low water availability, and the bladder, colon, and cloaca can be important sites of sodium excretion and water resorption.[39,98] Some species (iguanids and sea turtles) possess extrarenal salt excreting glands as well. Glomeruli in reptilian kidneys contain far fewer nephrons than avian kidneys, and thus lack some functions of the avian renal system.[39] Reptiles also lack a loop of Henle, so urine cannot be concentrated above the osmolality of plasma. Reptiles possess a renal portal system whereby blood flow from the caudal end of the body may supply the renal tubules (but not the glomeruli) before reaching systemic circulation. This can potentially affect the renal excretion of certain medications and increase harmful side effects of others.[39,99] Pharmacokinetic studies have shown that some medications have variable levels of absorption whether they are given in the cranial or caudal half of the body. In most cases, these effects are not clinically significant, though there are some anesthetics that produce greater sedative effects when given in the cranial half of the body. This seems to be due more in part to the hepatic portal system than the renal portal system. Even though with most drugs there is no significant difference, it remains common practice to avoid injections in the caudal half of the body for medications with possible renal side effects (eg, aminoglycosides).[39,99,100] There is limited experimental research on hypovolemia and its effects on cardiovascular measurements in reptiles. While hypovolemia and lack of perfusion is a common cause of AKI in mammals, this effect is unknown in reptiles. It is suspected that because of the renal portal system, during periods of dehydration and prolonged hypovolemia, blood from the hind limbs and tail traverses to the afferent renal portal veins, preserving renal perfusion.[101]

The kidneys eliminate nitrogenous wastes resulting from protein metabolism. Protein metabolism results in ammonia, which must be filtered from the blood into the urine to prevent toxic levels that cannot be tolerated by the brain (a process that requires large amounts of water) or converted to a less toxic compound that can remain in the bloodstream.[39,40] Reptiles vary in their excretion of different nitrogenous waste products as either ammonia, urea, or uric acid depending on access to water, with aquatic animals producing more ammonia and terrestrial species producing mainly uric acid.[39,40] During dehydration, ultrafiltrate's flow through the kidneys may be severely reduced or even absent, allowing uric acid to precipitate or crystallize in kidney tubules or glomeruli, causing gout.[39]

Physical Examination and Clinical Signs

As in other exotic animals, reptiles are also extremely adept at hiding clinical signs of illness until disease is advanced. Thus, in reptiles, true AKI is often extremely hard to recognize or diagnose until chronic changes to the kidneys are present. Clinical signs of AKI in reptiles are often nonspecific such as lethargy, reduced appetite, weight loss, and signs of dehydration, such as sunken eyes and thick, ropy saliva.[39] Often animals are weak and recumbent rather than sitting up in a normal posture. Although polyuria and polydipsia are not as common as in mammals, reptiles can exhibit these signs, especially with acute renal failure.[40] In lizards, a common sign is tenesmus or constipation as enlarged kidneys can compress the distal colon, making it difficult to pass feces.[40] (**Fig. 7**) Enlarged kidneys may be palpated cranial to the pelvic rim or on internal digital cloacal palpation in large lizards.[40] Some conditions may result in hypoalbuminemia and edema, especially in the pharyngeal area.[39,40,102] A foul odor to the oral

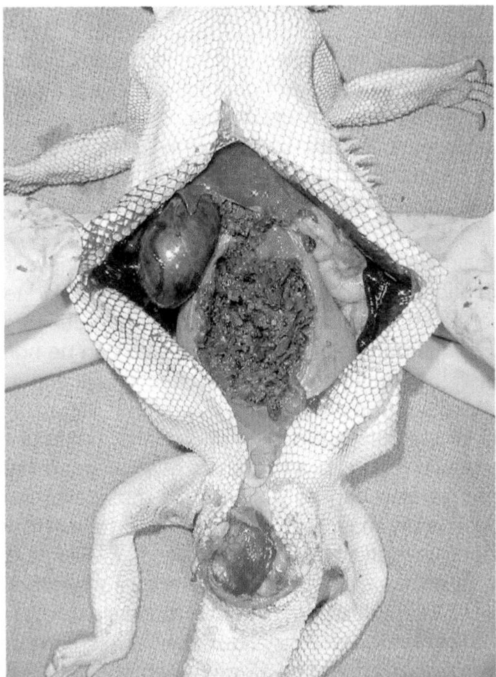

Fig. 7. Necropsy photo demonstrating marked renomegaly secondary to renal adenocarcinoma in a bearded dragon (*Pogona vitticeps*). Note the marked distension and impaction of the colon secondary to renomegaly obstructing the pelvic canal.

cavity, difficulty swallowing, and/or gulping motions may be seen as well.[39] The eyes may appear swollen with enlarged scleral or iridial blood vessels that may be associated with hypertension.[39] The presence of multiple swollen joints often is indicative of articular gout (**Fig. 8**). If renal secondary hyperparathyroidism is present, signs of hypocalcemia are seen, including weakness, tremors, or seizures, though bony changes typically would only occur later in disease.[40,103]

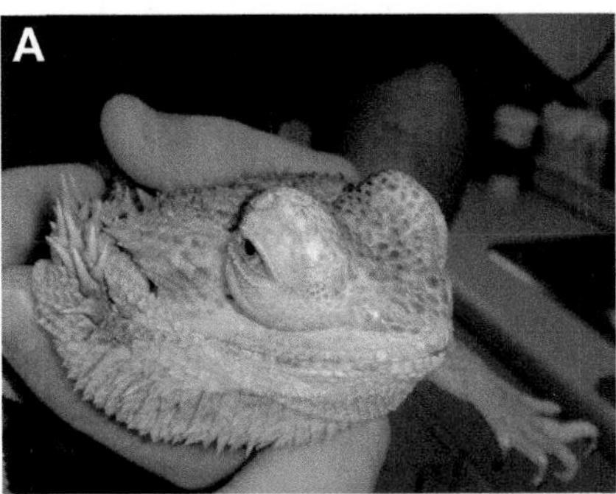

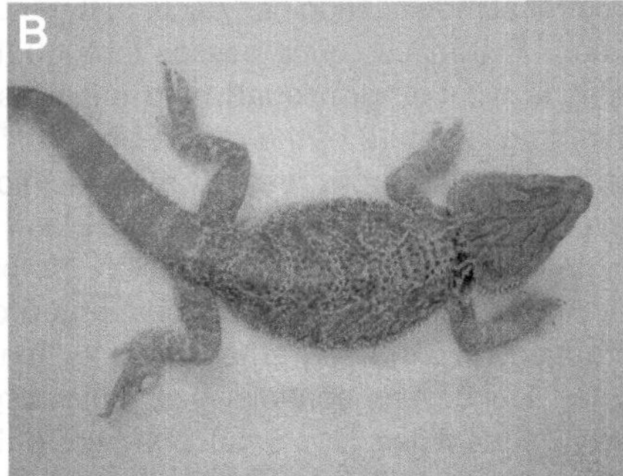

Fig. 8. (*A*) Bearded dragon (*Pogona vitticeps*) with swollen eyes. This clinical sign can often be seen with kidney disease in reptiles. (Photo courtesy Dr. Daniel Johnson.). (*B*) Multiple swollen joints consistent with articular gout in a bearded dragon (*Pogona vitticeps*) (Photo courtesy Stacey Wilkinson).

Diagnosis

Assessment of renal function in reptiles is difficult because clinical signs are often nonspecific and can be subtle or absent until the disease is advanced. While several biochemical alterations may occur, many are not specific for renal disease. In reptiles, significant organ damage must occur before some parameters will become elevated, and it is not uncommon to have severe disease in a patient with normal bloodwork. Other factors such as age, gender, season, and reproductive status can affect blood parameters as well.[40,104]

Uric acid is the main waste product produced by the kidneys in most squamates, and persistent elevations are often indicative of severe kidney injury (acute or chronic).[39,105] Hyperuricemia can also result from severe dehydration and reduction in renal blood flow,[105] although elevations in uric acid can be normal after a meal in carnivorous reptiles.[40,105] Creatinine is not produced in high enough quantities in reptiles to be useful in the diagnosis of renal disease.[39,40,105] Serum urea nitrogen is a significant nitrogenous waste product in most chelonians and is of greater importance than uric acid in aquatic species, and trends can be more helpful than a single value.[39,100,106] Ammonia also can be a significant metabolite in many aquatic reptiles.[39,105] Hypoalbuminemia may be present and lead to edema, though this seems to occur less commonly in reptiles than in mammals.[39,102] Elevated phosphorus levels are common with renal disease, and can be accompanied by either hypo- or hypercalcemia. The optimum calcium:phosphorus ratio in reptiles is 1.5-2:1, and a reduction or inversion of this ratio is common with renal disease.[39,40,107] If the calcium phosphorus product is > 55-70 mg/dL, tissue mineralization can occur.[39,40] AST, CK, LDH, and GGT are present in small amounts in the reptilian kidney, but are nonspecific markers of renal disease.[39,105] They tend to be elevated acutely, so may be present with AKI but normal with CKD. Hyponatremia and hyperkalemia may occur from AKI or dysfunction of the cloaca, colon, or bladder.[39,105] 90% of potassium excretion occurs via the kidney, so a decreased renal function can lead to hyperkalemia and metabolic acidosis.[105] Hyperchloremia can occur with dehydration, AKI, or disorders of the salt glands.[39,105] Elevations in PCV usually indicate dehydration.[39,104] Non-regenerative anemia can occur as in other species later in disease.[39,104] An elevated white blood cell count may indicate infection or inflammation, but the absence of a leukocytosis or leukopenia does not rule infection in or out.[39]

Urinalysis may be helpful but carries several limitations. Because reptiles lack a loop of Henle, they are unable to concentrate urine above the concentration of plasma. Postrenal modification can occur in the bladder, colon, and cloaca depending on species.[39,98] Because urine passes through the cloaca, it is not sterile. Cystocentesis is difficult without ultrasound, and urine leakage post sampling is possible given the thin, fragile nature of the reptile bladder.[39,40] As in other species, urine pH tends to be alkaline in herbivores and more acidic in omnivores and carnivores.[39,40] Protein levels are typically zero to trace, and blood should only be present in samples obtained by cystocentesis or expression.[39,40] Ketones, nitrite, and leukocytes have not been evaluated in reptiles, and bilirubin and urobilinogen are not useful because they are produced in extremely small amounts, if any.[39,40] On sediment examination, erythrocytes, leukocytes, epithelial cells, microorganisms, spermatozoa, crystals, and casts may be identified.[39,40] Small numbers of leukocytes and epithelial cells can be present, but reptile urine is mostly acellular.[39,40] *Spironucleus* (formerly *Hexamita*) should always be of concern if identified as this protozoa can ascend the urinary tract and infect the kidneys.[39,108] The significance of casts and crystals is unclear, but, in one study, casts were seen in tortoises with renal disease and not in healthy tortoises.[109]

The kidneys and urinary bladder in most reptiles cannot normally be seen on plain radiography. In lizards, renomegaly may be identified as a soft tissue mass extending cranially from the pelvic canal.[110] (**Fig. 9**) This can lead to constipation or dystocia.[110] Uroliths or soft tissue mineralization, most often of the great vessels or lining of the stomach, can be seen on radiographs. While IV urography can be used as in other species, this may be contraindicated in cases of AKI due to potential nephrotoxic effects, though this theory may be changing due to recent evidence in humans.[111] IV contrast agents should be given in the cranial half of the body to avoid abnormalities caused by the renal portal system if injected into the tail vein.

Other imaging modalities can be used as well, and a more detailed description can be found in other sources.[39,40] Ultrasonography is more useful in squamates than chelonians. Apply alcohol to the skin to fill in the spaces between the scales and then ultrasound gel. In large lizards, the probe can be placed cranial to the hind limb and angled caudally, or at the base of the tail and angled cranially. In chelonians the probe can be placed in the prefemoral fossa and angled caudally and dorsally, being careful of entrapment in large specimens. Conditions such as mineralization, urolithiasis, abscesses, and/or neoplasia can be visualized.[39,40] CT or MRI can be very useful to provide imaging of the kidneys, especially in large chelonians.[39,40] Nuclear scintigraphy has been evaluated and normal images developed for green iguanas (*Iguana iguana*).[112] Iohexol clearance studies have been evaluated in green iguanas and Kemp's ridley sea turtles (*Lepidochelys kempii*) as a method for estimating GFR and renal function.[107,113] Iohexol is excreted exclusively by glomerular filtration, and the plasma clearance can be calculated by measuring the plasma iohexol level over time after a single IV injection.[107] The patient must be fasted and well hydrated, so this is likely most useful after the initial stabilization of AKI.

Endoscopy allows the visualization of the kidneys along with the ability to take samples or administer treatments. Typically, coelioscopy is rapid to perform, so anesthesia is brief.[107] This technique is well described in other sources.[40,111,114] Renal biopsy is the gold standard for definitive diagnosis, devising a treatment plan, and assessing prognosis. Biopsy samples obtained by endoscopy are easier to obtain and less invasive, but surgical biopsies can be performed as well, most easily in snakes. In lizards only the cranial pole of the kidney is accessible surgically, or a

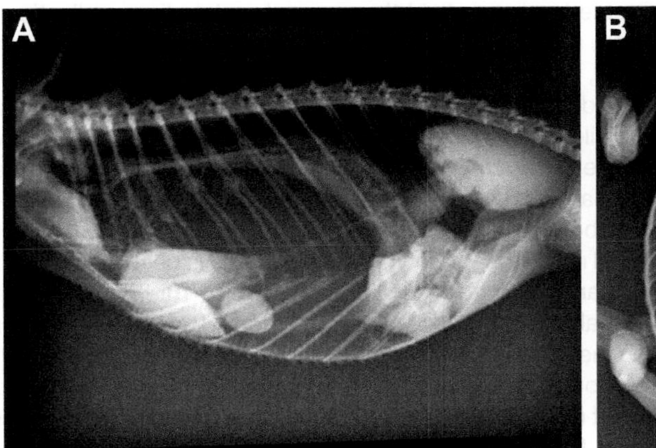

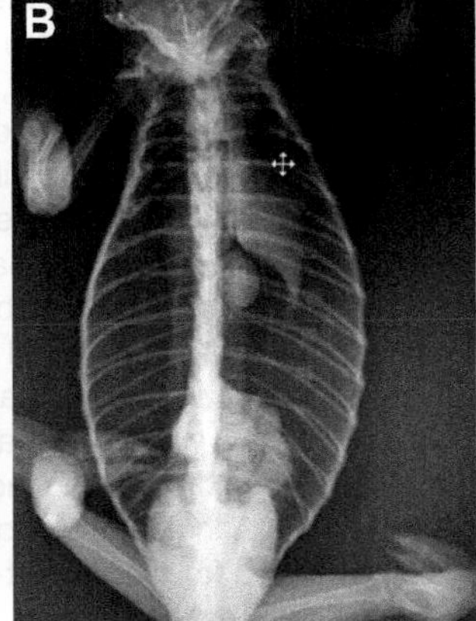

Fig. 9. Lateral (*A*) and dorsoventral (*B*) radiographs of a veiled chameleon (*Chamaeleo calyptratus*) with AKI. Marked renomegaly with mineralization is visible (Photos courtesy of Katherine Baine Tindell).

cut-down technique has been described where a biopsy can be obtained between the rear leg and base of the tail to access the caudal pole of the kidney.[39] Ultrasound-guided biopsies are not as easily performed in reptiles and carry a significant risk of hemorrhage or damage of other structures. Cost, patient condition, anesthetic risk, and turnaround time for results may limit the usefulness of biopsy in reptiles with AKI.

Articular and visceral gout are common sequelae of AKI. Visceral gout can be visualized as a grey or white sheen within the oral mucosa, or over the surfaces of organs seen during endoscopy. If joint swelling is present, an aspirate can be obtained and examined cytologically. Typically, the material will grossly be thick, white, and pasty or gritty, and on microscopic examination, uric acid crystals are non-staining, linear, needle-like crystals that can be confirmed using a polarizing filter.[39,40]

Causes

A variety of causes of renal disease exist in reptiles, with some more likely to cause AKI than others. Causes are listed in **Box 2**, in addition to causes affecting domestic animals. Chronic subclinical dehydration is suspected to be a major contributing factor in the development of chronic renal disease, and is common in reptile patients when owners do not provide the right habitat, proper humidity, or provide water properly for the species kept.[39,98] But, even before CKD develops, chronic dehydration may predispose a reptile to renal compromise or inability to recover from an acute insult.[41] Similarly, improper temperatures can predispose to renal disease because renal metabolism requires a preferred temperature for uric acid secretion from the proximal renal tubules to the ureters.[39,98] Other nutritional issues such as hypocalcemia, hypovitaminosis A, hypervitaminosis D_3, or high protein diets can also cause renal damage or lead to gout.[39,40,42,106,115] Various infectious causes such as bacterial or fungal infections, microsporidia (specially *Encephalitozoon pogonae*), viral, and parasitic (especially *Spironucleus*) infections can affect renal cells as well.[39–42,108,115] Other causes include toxins, trauma, urolithiasis, and neoplasia.[39–42,115–117]

Clinical Management

Because reptiles tend to present late in the course of disease, prognosis of AKI is often guarded to poor. Initial stabilization of reptile patients is similar to other species, with the main distinction being to first warm the patient to its preferred optimum temperature zone so that it will be able to absorb fluid therapy and metabolize medications given. Most all sick reptiles are somewhat dehydrated, and fluid therapy can be given PO, SC, intracoelomically (IC), IV, or IO. Refer to Stacey Leonatti Wilkinson article, "Urine Output Monitoring and Acute Kidney Injury in Mammalian Exotic Animal Critical Care," for more detailed information on fluid therapy in reptiles. Shallow warm water soaks can also be helpful as in many species, fluid uptake through the cloaca can occur, and the urinary bladder, colon, and cloaca are sites of fluid regulation. Debilitated patients must be supervised and have the head propped up out of water. Most IV catheterization will require a cut down procedure; this is described for the cephalic vein of large lizards and the jugular vein of snakes (**Fig. 10**). In lizards, the ventral coccygeal vein or ventral abdominal vein can also be considered but are harder to maintain since they are on the ventral aspect of the patient (**Fig. 11**). The jugular vein is most useful in chelonians, though sometimes sedation must be employed in order to extend the head for placement (**Fig. 12**). IO catheters are placed in the distal femur or proximal tibia most commonly, but the distal humerus or the bridge of the shell in chelonians can be used as well though are less reliable (see **Fig. 1**). Fluid rates for reptiles are lower than other species.[39,40] Recent work in measuring plasma osmolality in reptiles indicates that even though their plasma osmolality is higher than mammals,

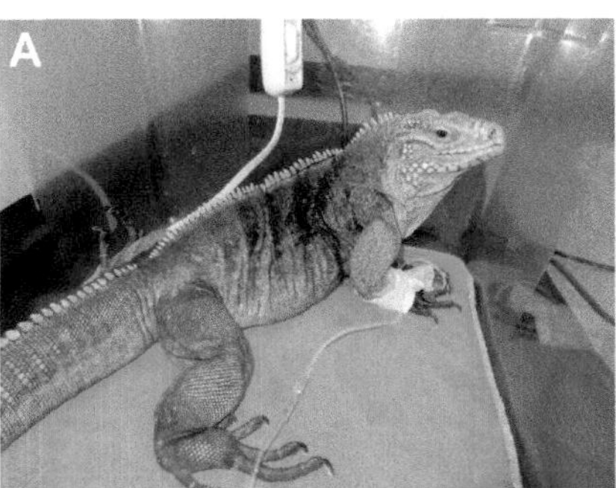
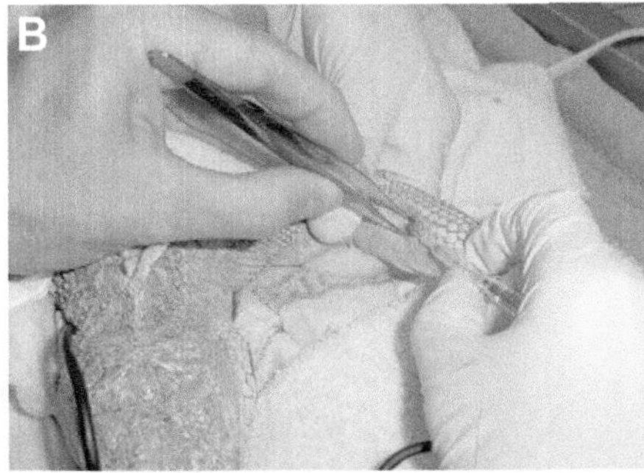

Fig. 10. (*A*) Grand Cayman blue iguana hybrid (*Cyclura lewisi* hybrid) receiving IV fluid therapy through a cephalic vein catheter placed via cut-down procedure (photo courtesy Stacey Wilkinson) (*B*) cephalic cut-down in a green iguana (*Iguana iguana*) (Photo courtesy Dr. Daniel Johnson.).

balanced electrolyte solutions clinically work well for reptiles and as such, "reptile ringers" has fallen out of favor.[118,119] Fluid therapy can be adjusted based on electrolyte abnormalities, acid-base status, and so forth. as in other species.

Measurement of urine output in reptiles can be done, but is often not as easily accomplished as in mammalian species because of the elimination of urine in combination with other waste through the cloaca. Also, most reptiles do not pass droppings every day. Urine output can be visualized by maintaining the patient on paper towels, newspaper, or absorbent pads, but trying to weigh urine-soaked bedding to calculate urine volume is less practical because of patient size and small volumes of urine being produced. If urine needs to be collected, the patient can be set up over a bare cage floor or over wax paper to prevent absorption. If needed, in larger patients with a bladder, urinary catheterization can be performed under endoscopic guidance to measure urine output and guide fluid therapy in critical patients.[40] For anuric patients, furosemide can be given to stimulate urine production.[39,40] Diuretic use is controversial because theoretically, loop diuretics such as furosemide should not work because

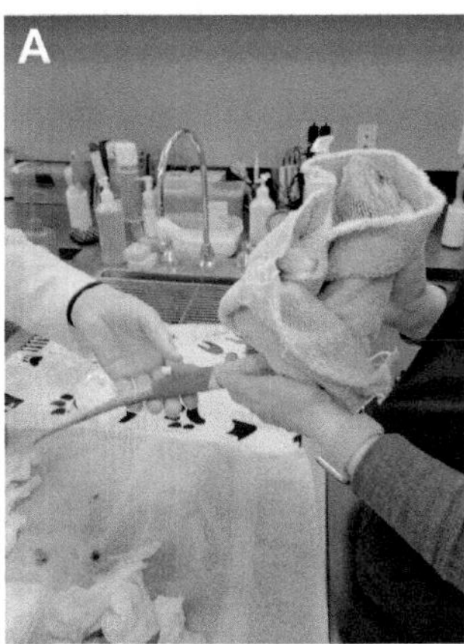
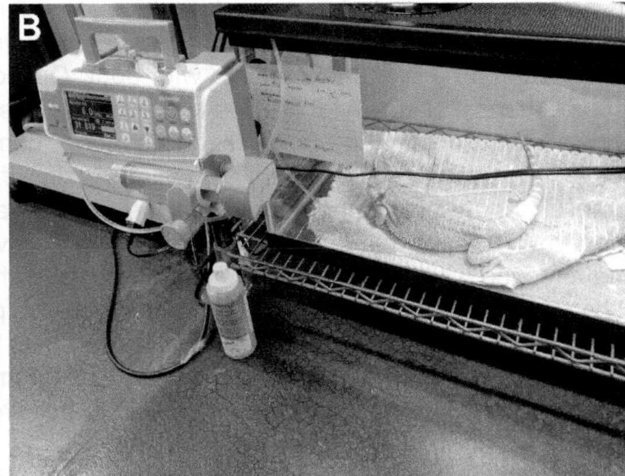

Fig. 11. (*A*) IV catheter placement in the ventral coccygeal vein of a bearded dragon (*Pogona vitticeps*) (*B*) The same patient receiving IV fluid therapy through the catheter via a syringe pump (Photo courtesy Dr. Daniel Johnson.).

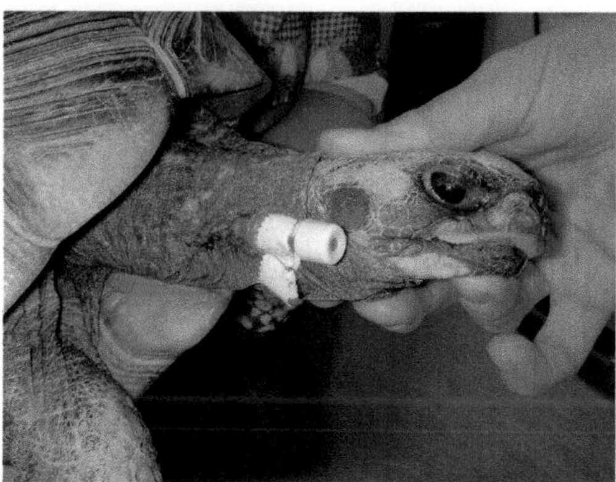

Fig. 12. Jugular IV catheter placement in a yellow-footed tortoise (*Chelonoidis denticulata*) (Photo courtesy Dr. Daniel Johnson.).

reptiles lack a loop of Henle and the ability to concentrate urine. Clinically however, they do seem to help and recent research suggests there may be other mechanisms by which furosemide produces a diuretic effect in reptiles.[120]

Other medications are used, as in birds and mammals, to help increase supportive care and address underlying causes. Significant elevations in uric acid (>25 mg/dL) may lead to gout.[39] As in birds, allopurinol can be used to help decrease hepatic production of uric acid and anecdotally it helps patients feel better. Other medications that help prevent tubular reabsorption of uric acid, such as probenecid or sulphapyrazole, could be used as well, but there is significantly less experience with these medications in reptiles and doses range widely.[39,40] Hyperphosphatemia can be treated with phosphate binders, such as aluminum hydroxide. Calcium gluconate can be given IM, IV, or IO if needed and oral calcium given once the animal stabilizes. Proper UVB lighting for the species should be provided to aid in Vitamin D_3 production and calcium absorption, as the kidney plays a significant role in vitamin D synthesis. Antibiotics, antifungal medications, and antiparasitics can be used depending on the underlying cause. Reptiles tend to take longer to recover from most disease processes, so antibiotics (ideally based on culture) typically will need to be given for at least 4-6 weeks or longer. Metronidazole tends to be effective for protozoal infections. Analgesics should be used for patients with gout. Opioids, especially pure mu-agonist drugs, are most effective for reptiles. Other therapies such as calcitriol, erythropoietin, appetite stimulants, GI protectants, and so forth. commonly used in mammals have not been investigated in reptiles. For ingested toxins, if ingestion is recent, endoscopic removal can be performed, along with the administration of activated charcoal and supportive therapy for the specific toxin. Obstructive cloacoliths can be crushed and removed with forceps via the cloaca, with or without endoscopic assistance.[121] Other uroliths can be removed surgically when the patient is stable. Renal tumors can typically be easily surgically removed in snakes, but this is extremely difficult or impossible in lizards and chelonians, due to anatomy. Minimal reports of chemotherapy exist, and those typically have yielded poor results. Renal transplantation or dialysis has not been investigated in reptiles.

Most reptiles can go prolonged periods of time without eating, so in cases of true AKI, fluid therapy and other treatments are prioritized over nutritional therapy. Nutritional support in the form of syringe feeding or tube feeding may be implemented according to species requirements in order to support malnourished patients, or those that are not regaining a normal appetite with treatment. As in other species, dietary considerations include the reduction of protein and phosphorus along with increasing water intake.[39,40] Please see this edition's article on nutritional support in exotic animal critical care for further information.

CLINICS CARE POINTS

- Monitoring blood and urine parameters are different than mammals–UA (instead of BUN & Crea), different UA parameters
- Be conscious of the amount of blood that can be taken at once or over time in small patients
- Numerous causes of AKI exist–attempt to determine the cause so specific treatment can be initiated
- IO catheters are commonly needed due to difficulty placing or maintaining AN IV catheter
- IV/IO fluid therapy can be challenging in small or active patients–monitor lines closely for chewing, becoming tangled or occluded, and so forth.
- Monitor for signs of fluid overload similar to mammalian species–body weight, PCV/TS, hydration status, urine output, mucous membrane color, capillary refill time, heart and respiratory rate, peripheral blood pressure if possible
- Monitor urine output by collecting urine from the cage or weighing bedding, cannot place an indwelling catheter in these species
- Watch for post-obstructive diuresis and correct if needed, though this is also not common in avian and reptilian patients
- Furosemide can be used to stimulate urine output despite species differences
- Syringe or gavage feeding and other supportive care (heat, and so forth.) will likely be needed
- Warm reptiles to POTZ before initiating treatment
- Swollen joints often indicate articular gout

SUMMARY

Acute kidney injury can occur in any species, and there are many clinical signs, causes, diagnostics, and treatment options that are conserved across species groups. However, there are many differences in anatomy and physiology along with management challenges that are present in avian and reptile species that are not dealt with in dogs and cats. Patient size often limits the amount of diagnostic testing and certain treatment options. Exotic patients tend to hide their clinical signs of illness–as such, they are often presented when the disease is more advanced and any handling or stress can often be fatal, limiting the amount of testing and treatment that can be done initially. The prognosis for AKI is guarded in exotic species, as in domestic animals, but if the disease is identified and treated swiftly, patients can often recover, though sometimes permanent kidney damage remains. More advanced therapies and testing options being used for humans, dogs, and cats need further research in exotic animals.

DISCLOSURE

The author declares no conflicts of interest.

REFERENCES

1. Langston C. Acute kidney injury. In: Ettinger SJ, Feldman EC, Cote, editors. Textbook of veterinary internal medicine: diseases of the dog and cat. 8th ed. St. Louis: Elsevier; 2017. p. 4650–85.
2. Ross L. Acute kidney injury in dogs and cats. Vet Clin North Am Small Anim 2022;22:659–72.
3. Monaghan K, Nolan B, Labato M. Feline acute kidney injury: 1. Pathophysiology, etiology, and etiology-specific management considerations. J Feline Med Surg 2012;25:775–84.
4. Claus MA. Pathophysiology of AKI. Proc International Veterinary Emergency and Critical Care Symposium. 2017.
5. Han SJ, Lee HT. Mechanisms and therapeutic targets of ischemic acute kidney injury. Kidney Res Clin Pract 2019;38:427–40.
6. Okusa MD, Portilla D. Pathophysiology of acute kidney injury. In: Chertow GM, Marsden PA, Skorecki K, et al, editors. Brenner and rector's the kidney. 11th edition. St. Louis: Elsevier; 2019. p. 906–39.
7. Faubel S, Edelstein CL. Mechanisms and mediators of lung injury after acute kidney injury. Nat Rev Nephrol 2016;12:48–60.
8. Doi K, Rabb H. Impact of acute kidney injury on distant organ function: recent findings and potential therapeutic targets. Kidney Int 2016;89:555–64.
9. Di Girolamo N, Huynh M. Disorders of the urinary and reproductive systems in ferrets. In: Quesenberry KE, Orcutt CJ, Mans C, et al, editors. Ferrets, rabbits, and rodents: clinical medicine and surgery. 4th ed. St. Louis: Elsevier; 2021. p. 39–54.
10. Garbin M, Pablo LS, Alexander AB. Management of hyperkalemia and associated complications in a ferret (*Mustela putortius furo*) with urinary obstruction requiring surgery. J Exot Pet Med 2021;39:4–7.
11. Reavill DR, Lennox AM. Disease overview of the urinary tract in exotic companion mammals and tips on clinical management. Vet Clin Exot Anim Pract 2020; 23:169–93.
12. Pacheco RE. Cysteine urolithiasis in ferrets. Vet Clin Exot Anim Pract 2020;23: 309–19.
13. Hanak EH, Di Girolamo N, DeSilva U, et al. Composition of ferret uroliths in North America and Europe: 1055 Cases (2010-2018). Abstract, presented at: Exotics Conference with AAZV, Saint Louis, MO. 2019.
14. Minnesota Urolith Center. Cystine rising: Ferreting out the cause. In: Minnesota Urolith Center image of the month. 2018. Available at: https://vetmed.umn.edu/urolith-center/image-of-month/cystine-rising-ferreting-out-cause. Accessed November 29, 2022.
15. Nwaokorie EE, Osborne CA, Lulich JP, et al. Epidemiology of struvite uroliths in ferrets: 272 cases (1981-2007). J Am Vet Med Assoc 2011;239:1319–24.
16. Nwaokorie EE, Osborne CA, Lulich JP, et al. Epidemiological evaluation of cystine urolithiasis in domestic ferrets (*Mustela putorius furo*): 70 cases (1992–2009). J Am Vet Med Assoc 2013;242:1099–103.
17. Powers LV, Winkler K, Garner MM, et al. Omentalization of prostatic abscesses and large cysts in ferrets (*Mustela putorius furo*). J Exot Pet Med 2007;16: 186–94.
18. van Zeeland YRA, Lennox A, Quinton JF, et al. Prepuce and partial penile amputation for treatment of preputial gland neoplasia in two ferrets. J Small Anim Pract 2014;55:593–6.

19. Di Girolamo N, Toth G, Selleri P. Prognostic value of rectal temperature at hospital admission in client-owned rabbits. J Am Vet Med Assoc 2016;248:288–97.
20. Di Girolamo N, Selleri P. Disorders of the urinary and reproductive systems (rabbit). In: Quesenberry KE, Orcutt CJ, Mans C, et al, editors. Ferrets, rabbits, and rodents: clinical medicine and surgery. 4th ed. St. Louis: Elsevier; 2021. p. 201–19.
21. Tschudin A, Clauss M, Codron D, et al. Water intake in domestic rabbits (*Oryctolagus cuniculus*) from open dishes and nipple drinkers under different water and feeding regimes. J Anim Physiol Anim Nutr 2011;95:499–511.
22. Clauss M, Burger B, Liesegang A, et al. Influence of diet on calcium metabolism, tissue calcification and urinary sludge in rabbits (*Oryctolagus cuniculus*). J Anim Physiol Anim Nutr 2012;96:798–807.
23. Kunzel F, Fisher P. Clinical signs, diagnosis, and treatment of *Encephalitozoon cuniculi* infection in rabbits. Veterinary Clin North Am Exot Anim Pract 2018; 21:69–82.
24. Graham JE, Garner MM, Reavill DR. Benzimidazole toxicosis in rabbits: 13 cases (2003 to 2011). J Exot Pet Med 2014;23:188–95.
25. Wong AD, Gardhouse S, Rooney T, et al. Associations between biochemical parameters and referral centre in pet rabbits with urolithiasis. J Small Anim Prac 2021;62:554–61.
26. Martorell J, Bailon D, Majo N, et al. Lateral approach to nephrotomy in the management of unilateral renal calculi in a rabbit (*Oryctolagus cuniculus*). J Am Vet Med Assoc 2012;240:863–8.
27. Rhody JL. Unilateral nephrectomy for hydronephrosis in a pet rabbit. Veterinary Clin North Am Exot Anim Pract 2006;9:633–41.
28. Rembeaux H, Langlois I, Burdick S, et al. Placement of ureteral stents in three rabbits for the treatment of obstructive ureterolithiasis. J Small Anim Pract 2021;62:489–95.
29. Pizzi R. Cystoscopic removal of a urolith from a pet guinea pig. Vet Rec 2009; 165:148–9.
30. Wenger S, Hatt JM. Transurethral cystoscopy and endoscopic urolith removal in female guinea pigs (*Cavia porcellus*). Veterinary Clin North Am Exot Anim Pract 2015;18:437–46.
31. Lewis TT, Lennox AM. Nonsurgical removal of urethral uroliths using a self-retaining retractor with elastic stays in female guinea pigs (*Cavia porcellus*): 16 Cases (2006-2019). J Exot Pet Med 2021;36:11–5.
32. Pignon R, Mayer J. Guinea pigs. In: Quesenberry KE, Orcutt CJ, Mans C, et al, editors. Ferrets, rabbits, and rodents: clinical medicine and surgery. 4th ed. St. Louis: Elsevier; 2021. p. 270–97.
33. Higbie CT, DiGeronimo PM, Bennet RA, et al. Semen-matrix calculi in a juvenile chinchilla (*Chinchilla lanigera*). J Exot Pet Med 2019;28:69–75.
34. Martel-Arquette A, Mans C. Urolithiasis in chinchillas: 15 cases (2007-2011). J Small Anim Pract 2016;57:260–4.
35. Frohlich J. Rats and Mice. In: Quesenberry KE, Orcutt CJ, Mans C, et al, editors. Ferrets, rabbits, and rodents: clinical medicine and surgery. 4th ed. St. Louis: Elsevier; 2021. p. 345–67.
36. Johnson-Delaney C. Sugar gliders. In: Quesenberry KE, Orcutt CJ, Mans C, et al, editors. Ferrets, rabbits, and rodents: clinical medicine and surgery. 4th ed. St. Louis: Elsevier; 2021. p. 385–400.

37. Echols MS. Evaluating and treating the kidneys. In: Harrison GJ, Lightfoot TL, editors. Clinical avian medicine. 1st ed. Palm Beach: Spix Publishing; 2006. p. 451–92.
38. Phalen D. Diseases of the avian urinary system. Veterinary Clin North Am Exot Anim Pract 2020;23:21–45.
39. Divers SJ, Innis CJ. Urology. In: Divers SJ, Stahl SJ, editors. Mader's reptile and amphibian medicine and surgery. 3rd ed. St Louis: Elsevier; 2019. p. 624–48.
40. Wilkinson SL, Divers SJ. Clinical management of reptile renal disease. Veterinary Clin North Am Exot Anim Pract 2020;23:151–68.
41. Johnson JG III, Watson MK. Diseases of the reptile renal system. Veterinary Clin North Am Exot Anim Pract 2020;23:115–29.
42. Reavill DR, Schmidt RE. Urinary tract disease of reptiles. J Exot Pet Med 2010; 19:280–9.
43. Monaghan K, Nolan B, Labato M. Feline acute kidney injury: 2. Approach to diagnosis, treatment, and prognosis. J Feline Med Surg 2012;25:785–93.
44. Yerramilli M, Farace G, Quinn J, et al. Kidney disease and the nexus of chronic kidney disease and acute kidney injury: the role of novel biomarkers as early and accurate diagnostics. Vet Clin N Am Small Anim 2016;46:961–93.
45. Cobrin AR, Blois SL, Kruth SA, et al. Biomarkers in the assessment of acute and chronic kidney diseases in the dog and cat. J Sm Anim Pract 2013;54:647–55.
46. Paes-Leme FO, Souza EM, Paes PR, et al. Cystatin C and Iris: advances in the evaluation of kidney function in the critically ill dog. Front Vet Sci 2021;8:1–5.
47. Montesinos A, Ardiaca M, Bonvehi C, et al. Plasma levels of symmetric dimethylarginine in domestic ferrets *(Mustela putorious furo*) with and without renal disease. Proc Intern Conf Avian Herp Exot Mammal Med 2017;444.
48. Toporek AH, Semler MW, Self WH, et al. Balanced crystalloids versus saline in critically ill adults with hyperkalemia or acute kidney injury: secondary analysis of a clinical trial. Am J Respir Crit Care Med 2021;203:1322–5.
49. Hansen B. Fluid overload. Front Vet Sci 2021;8:668–88.
50. Langston CA. Effects of IV fluids in dogs and cats with kidney failure. Front Vet Sci 2021;8:659–60.
51. Yerram P, Karuparthi P, Misra M. Fluid overload and acute kidney injury. Hemodial Int 2010;14:348–54.
52. Barsant JA. Urinary tract catheterization and nosocomial infections in dogs and cats. In: Proceedings of the ACVIM Forum. 2010. p.445-447.
53. Langston C. Managing fluid and electrolyte disorders in kidney disease. Vet Clin North Am 2017;47:471–90.
54. Adin DB, Taylor AW, Hill RC, et al. Intermittent bolus injection versus continuous infusion of furosemide in normal adult greyhound dogs. J Vet Intern Med 2003; 17:632–6.
55. Simmons JP, Wohl JS, Schwartz DD, et al. Diuretic effects of fenoldopam in healthy cats. J Vet Emerg Crit Care 2006;16:96–103.
56. Nielsen LK, Bracker K, Price LL. Administration of fenoldopam in critically ill small animal patients with acute kidney injury: 28 dogs and 34 cats (2008–2012). J Vet Emerg Crit Care 2015;25:396–404.
57. Huynh M, Pignon C. Assessment and care of the critically ill rabbit. Veterinary Clin North Am Exot Anim Pract 2016;19:379–409.
58. Gladden JN, Lennox AM. Emergency and critical care of small mammals. In: Quesenberry KE, Orcutt CJ, Mans C, et al, editors. Ferrets, rabbits, and rodents: clinical medicine and surgery. 4th ed. St. Louis: Elsevier; 2021. p. 595–608.

59. Dziuk E, Siekierzynski M. Experimental model of peritoneal dialysis. Acta Physiol Pol 1973;24:465–72.
60. Gotloib L, Crassweller P, Rodella H, et al. Experimental model for studies of continuous peritoneal dialysis in uremic rabbits. Nephron 1982;31:254–9.
61. Zunic-Bozinovski S, Lausevic Z, Krstic S, et al. An experimental, non-uremic rabbit model of peritoneal dialysis. Physiol Res 2008;57:253–60.
62. Wojick K, Berube D, Barr J III. Clinical technique: peritoneal dialysis and percutaneous peritoneal dialysis catheter placement in small mammals. J Exot Pet Med 2008;17:181–8.
63. Cooper RL, Labato MA. Peritoneal dialysis in cats with acute kidney injury: 22 cases (2001–2006). J Vet Intern Med 2011;25:14–9.
64. Diehl SH, Seshadri R. Use of continuous renal replacement therapy for treatment of dogs and cats with acute or acute-on-chronic renal failure: 33 cases (2002–2006). J Vet Emerg Crit Care 2008;18:370–82.
65. Langston CE, Cowgill LD, Spano JA. Applications and outcome of hemodialysis in cats: a review of 29 cases. J Vet Intern Med 1997;11:348–55.
66. Worwag S, Langston CE. Acute intrinsic renal failure in cats: 32 cases (1997–2004). J Am Vet Med Assoc 2008;232:728–32.
67. Orosz SE, Echols MS. The urinary and osmoregulatory systems of birds. Veterinary Clin North Am Exot Anim Pract 2020;23:1–19.
68. Fitzgerald BC, Beaufrère H. Cardiology. In: Speer BL, editor. Current therapy in avian medicine and surgery. St. Louis: Elsevier; 2016. p. 252–328.
69. Scope A, Schwendenwein I. Laboratory evaluation of renal function in birds. Veterinary Clin North Am Exot Anim Pract 2020;23:47–58.
70. Tsahar E, Del Rio CM, Izhaki I, et al. Can birds be ammonotelic? Nitrogen balance and excretion in two frugivores. J Exp Biol 2005;208:1025–34.
71. Vergneau-Grosset C, Beaufrère H, Ammersbach M. Clinical biochemistry In:Advances in clinical pathology and diagnostic medicine. In: Speer BL, editor. Current therapy in avian medicine and surgery. St. Louis: Elsevier; 2016. p. 486–501.
72. Wimsatt J, Canon N, Pearce RD, et al. Assessment of novel avian renal disease markers for the detection of experimental nephrotoxicosis in pigeons (*Columbia livia*). J Zoo Wildl Med 2009;40:487–94.
73. Echols MS. Avian Renal Disease: Part I and II. Proc American Board of Veterinary Practitioners Conference. 2012.
74. Lane RA. Avian urinalysis a practical guide to analysis and interpretation. In: Rosskopf WJ, Woerpel RW, editors. Diseases of cage and aviary birds. Baltimore: Williams and Wilkins; 1996. p. 783–94.
75. Krautwald-Junghanns ME, Konicek C. Diagnostic imaging of the avian urinary tract. Veterinary Clin North Am Exot Anim Pract 2020;23:59–74.
76. Krautwald-Junghanns M-E, Pees M, Reese S, et al. Diagnostic imaging of exotic pets. Hannover (Germany): Schlütersche Verlagsgesell; 2011. p. 26, urinary tract), p. 32 (urography), p. 54–63 (computed tomography), p. 64–9 (MRI), p. 122–35 (urogenital tract.
77. Taylor M. Endoscopic examination and biopsy techniques. In: Ritchie BW, Harrison GJ, Harrison LR, editors. Avian medicine. Principles and applications. Lake Worth: Wingers Publishing; 1994. p. 327–54.
78. van Zeeland Y, Schoemaker N, Hsu E. Advances in diagnostic imaging. In: Speer B, editor. Current therapy in avian medicine and surgery. St Louis: Elsevier; 2016. p. 531–49.

79. Echols MS. Comuted tomography basics and artifacts. Proc of Exotics Con 2022;319.
80. Cojean O, Larrat S, Vergneau-Grosset C. Clinical management of avian renal disease. Veterinary Clin North Am Exot Anim Pract 2020;23:75–101.
81. Greenacre CB, Latimer KS, Ritchie BW. Leg paresis in a black palm cockatoo (*Probosciger aterrimus*) caused by aspergillosis. J Zoo Wildl Med 1992;23: 122–6.
82. Degernes LA. Toxicities in waterfowl. Sem Avian Exot Pet Med 1995;4:15–22.
83. Leighton FA. The toxicity of petroleum oils to birds. Environ Res J 1993;1: 92–103.
84. Flammer K, Clark CH, Drewes LA, et al. Adverse effects of gentamicin in scarlet macaws and galahs. Am J Vet Res 1990;51:404–7.
85. Marshall KL, Craig LE, Jones MP, et al. Quantitative renal scintigraphy in domestic pigeons (*Columba livia domestica*) exposed to toxic doses of gentamicin. Am J Vet Res 2003;64:453–62.
86. Montesinos A, Maria Ardiaca M, Carles Juan-Sallés C, et al. Effects of meloxicam on hematologic and plasma biochemical analyte values and results of histologic examination of kidney biopsy specimens of African grey parrots (*Psittacus erithacus*). J Avian Med Surg 2013;29:1–8.
87. Pereira ME, Werther K. Evaluation of renal effects of flunixin meglumine, ketoprofen and meloxicam in budgerigars (*Melopsittacus undulatus*). Vet Rec 2007; 160:844–6.
88. Sinclair KM, Chuch ME, Farver TB, et al. Effects of meloxicam on hematologic and plasma biochemical analysis variables and results of histologic examination of tissue specimens of Japanese quail (*Coturnix japonica*). Am J Vet Res 2012; 73:1720–7.
89. Mulcahy DM, Tuomi P, Larsen RS. Differential mortality of male spectacled eiders (*Somateria fischeri*) and king eiders (*Somateria spectabilis*) subsequent to anesthesia with propofol, bupivacaine, and ketoprofen. J Avian Med Surg 2003;17:117–23.
90. Oaks L, Gilbert M, Virani MZ, et al. Diclofenac residues as the cause of vulture population decline in Pakistan. Nature 2004;427:630–3.
91. Blaxland JD, Borland ED, Siller WG, et al. An investigation of urolithiasis in two flocks of laying fowls. Avian Pathol 1980;9:5–19.
92. Mallinson ET, Rothenbacher H, Wideman RF, et al. Epizootiology, pathology, and microbiology of an outbreak of urolithiasis in chickens. Avian Dis 1983;28:25–43.
93. Dennis P, Bennett R. Ureterotomy for removal of two ureteroliths in a parrot. J Am Vet Med Assoc 2000;217:865–8.
94. Lichtenberger M, Lennox A. Critical care. In: Speer BL, editor. Current therapy of avian medicine and surgery. 1st ed. Saint Louis: Elsevier; 2016. p. 582–8.
95. Lumeij JT, Sprang EP, Redig PT. Further studies on allopurinol-induced hyperuricaemia and visceral gout in red-tailed hawks (*Buteo jamaicensis*). Avian Pathol 1998;27:390–3.
96. Poffers J, Lumeij JT, Redig PT. Investigations into the uricolytic properties of urate oxidase in a granivorous (*Columba livia domestica*) and in a carnivorous (*Buteo jamaicensis*) avian species. Avian Pathol 2002;31:573–9.
97. Beaufrère H, Nevarez J, Tully TN. Cloacolith in a blue-fronted amazon parrot (*Amazona aestiva*). J Avian Med Surg 2010;24:142–5.
98. Dantzler WH. Renal function (with special emphasis on nitrogen excretion). In: Gans C, Dawson WR, editors. Biology of the reptilia, vol 5, Physiology A. London: Academic Press; 1976. p. 447–503.

99. Perry SM, Mitchell MA. Routes of administration. In: Divers SJ, Stahl SJ, editors. Mader's reptile and amphibian medicine and surgery. 3rd ed. St Louis: Elsevier; 2019. p. 1130–8.
100. Holz P, Barker IK, Burger JP, et al. The effect of the renal portal system on pharmacokinetic parameters in the red-eared slider (*Trachemys scripta elegans*). J Zoo Wildl Med 1997;28:386–93.
101. Holz PH. The reptilian renal portal system – a review. Bull Assoc Reptil Amphib Vet 1999;9:4–9.
102. Miller HA. Urinary diseases of reptiles: pathophysiology and diagnosis. Semin Avian Exot Pet Med 1998;7:93–103.
103. Boyer TH, Scott PW. Nutritional diseases. In: Divers SJ, Stahl SJ, editors. Mader's reptile and amphibian medicine and surgery. 3rd ed. St Louis: Elsevier; 2019. p. 932–50.
104. Heatley JJ, Russell KE. Hematology. In: Divers SJ, Stahl SJ, editors. Mader's reptile and amphibian medicine and surgery. 3rd ed. St Louis: Elsevier; 2019. p. 301–18.
105. Heatley JJ, Russell KE. Clinical chemistry. In: Divers SJ, Stahl SJ, editors. Mader's reptile and amphibian medicine and surgery. 3rd ed. St Louis: Elsevier; 2019. p. 319–32.
106. Massry SG, Fadda GZ. Chronic renal failure is a state of cellular calcium toxicity. Am J Kidney Dis 1993;21:81–6.
107. Hernandez-Divers SJ. Renal evaluation in the green iguana (*Iguana iguana*): assessment of plasma biochemistry, glomerular filtration rate, and endoscopic biopsy. J Zoo Wildl Med 2005;36:155–68.
108. Juan-Salles C, Garner MM, Nordhausen RW, et al. Renal flagellate infections in reptiles: 29 cases. J Zoo Wildl Med 2014;45:100–9.
109. Kolle P. Urinalysis in tortoises. Proc ARAV 2000;111–3.
110. Holmes SP, Divers SJ. Radiography - lizards. In: Divers SJ, Stahl SJ, editors. Mader's reptile and amphibian medicine and surgery. 3rd ed. St Louis: Elsevier; 2019. p. 491–502.
111. McDonald J, McDonald R, Comin J, et al. Frequency of acute kidney injury following intravenous contrast medium administration: a systematic review and meta-analysis. Radiology 2013;267(1):119–28. Available at: https://www.ncbi.nlm.nih.gov/pubmed/23319662.
112. Greer LL, Daniel GB, Shearn-Bochsler VI, et al. Evaluation of the use of technetium Tc99m diethylenetriamine pentaacetic acid and technetium Tc99m dimercaptosuccinic acid for scintigraphy imaging of the kidneys in green iguanas (*Iguana iguana*). Am J Vet Res 2005;66:87–92.
113. Kennedy A, Innis C, Rumbeiha W. Determination of glomerular filtration rate in juvenile Kemp's ridley turtles (*Lepidochelys kempii*) using Iohexol clearance, with preliminary comparison of clinically healthy turtles vs. those with renal disease. J Herpetol Med Surg 2012;22:25–9.
114. Divers SJ. Diagnostic endoscopy. In: Divers SJ, Stahl SJ, editors. Mader's reptile and amphibian medicine and surgery. 3rd ed. St Louis: Elsevier; 2019. p. 604–14.
115. Zwart P. Renal pathology in reptiles. Veterinary Clin North Am Exot Anim Pract 2006;9:129–59.
116. Garner MM, Hernandez-Divers SM, Raymond JT. Reptile neoplasia: a retrospective study of case submissions to a specialty diagnostic service. Veterinary Clin North Am Exot Anim Pract 2004;7:653–71.

117. Keller KA. Urolithiasis (cystic calculi and cloacal uroliths). In: Divers SJ, Stahl SJ, editors. Mader's reptile and amphibian medicine and surgery. 3rd ed. St Louis: Elsevier; 2019. p. 1355–6.
118. Dallwig RK, Mitchell MA, Acierno MJ. Determination of plasma osmolality and agreement between measured and calculated values in healthy adult bearded dragons (*Pogona vitticeps*). J Herpetol Med Surg 2010;20:69–73.
119. Guzman DS-M, Mitchell MA, Acierno M. Determination of plasma osmolality and agreement between measured and calculated values in captive male corn snakes (*Pantherophis [Elaphe] guttatus guttatus*). J Herpetol Med Surg 2011;21:16–9.
120. Parkinson LA, Mans C. Effects of furosemide administration to water-deprived inland bearded dragons (*Pogona vitticeps*). Am J Vet Res 2018;79:1204–8.
121. Mans C, Sladky KK. Endoscopically guided removal of cloacal calculi in three African spurred tortoises (*Geochelone sulcata*). J Am Vet Med Assoc 2012;240:869–75.

Nutritive Support for Critical Exotic Patients

La'Toya V. Latney, DVM, DECZM, Dip ABVP (Reptile/Amphibian), CertAqV

KEYWORDS

- Body condition score • Clinical nutrition • Energy requirements • Metabolism
- Malnutrition

KEY POINTS

- Nutritional support should be administered to critical exotic patients shortly after cardiovascular stability is achieved.
- Commercial supportive care diets have been evaluated and used with success in invertebrates, fish, herptile, small mammals, and avian patients.
- Measures for malnutrition including loss of adipose tissue, muscle girth, and biochemical analyte markers should be monitored to qualify metabolic derangements.

INTRODUCTION

In domestic small animal medicine, it has been estimated that up to 50% of hospitalized patients are malnourished.[1] With the difficulty of achieving appropriate husbandry for exotic animal patients far exceeding that of dogs and cats, unsurprisingly, exotic animal practitioners manage high caseloads of critical patients that also suffer from malnutrition. The metabolic, physiologic, and anatomic diversity of exotic companion species make it incredibly challenging to estimate or generalize nutritive requirements for several species. The National Resource Council[2–4] has provided accessible nutrient requirements for animals reared for research and food production; however, these requirements are derived to support production efficiencies and food conversion for harvest, not longevity. This review will serve to give very basic guidelines on clinical nutritional support, with attention to how species-specific anatomy influences clinical intervention. An overview of malnutrition, guidelines for body condition score (BCS) and nutritional assessment, recommendations for enteral and parenteral support, clinical techniques, risks, and guidelines for monitoring are provided and adapted based on metabolic and anatomical considerations.

Pathophysiology of Malnutrition and Comorbidities that Impact Nutritional State

Although there are different species-specific responses to fasting, the general components of energy usage follow a similar pattern. During short-term fasting and

Avian and Exotic Medicine & Surgery, The Animal Medical Center, 510 East 62nd Street, New York, NY 10065, USA
E-mail address: latoya.latney@amcny.orgo

Vet Clin Exot Anim 26 (2023) 711–735
https://doi.org/10.1016/j.cvex.2023.05.009 vetexotic.theclinics.com
1094-9194/23/© 2023 Published by Elsevier Inc.

physiologically or environmentally-induced fasts (brumation, estimation, hibernation, gravidity/pregnancy), stored glycogen is used as the compensatory energy source. In periods of protracted fasting, stress, and illness, glycogen and lipid stores are depleted quickly and a catabolic shift to accelerated proteolysis occurs.[5] When protein catabolism is initiated, the body experiences a negative nitrogen balance and net protein loss, which can compound the challenges faced by a critically ill patient. The primary consequences of malnutrition, outlined in **Box 1**, threaten the conserved and compensatory metabolic processes clinicians rely on to effectively stabilize and treat debilitated patients. A lack of adequate nutrient intake results in the same metabolic consequences for invertebrates and vertebrates. It negatively influences the patient's nitrogen balance, accelerates the risk and progression to a catabolic state, and this state is (1) energetically demanding and (2) difficult to reverse once initiated.[5]

The largest clinical barrier to providing and sustaining nutritive support include diseases that result in *protein intolerance*, *protein loss*, and *any disease that prevents ingestion and digestion of normal diet items*, see **Table 1**. Management of comorbidities is beyond the scope of this article; however, a review of the taxa-based anatomic considerations may offer exotic practitioners' insight on how to improve recovery in patients with a negative energy balance.

Water Loss: Challenges to Nutritive Recovery and Special Anatomic Considerations

Water is arguably the most important nutrient for any species; any disease that compromises hydration implicitly affects the gastrointestinal tract. The large amount of anatomic and physiologic variability in exotic animal patients makes assessing patient's hydration status difficult for exotic animal practitioners. The costs of integumentary, respiratory, and urinary system water loss, in addition to digestive losses, have a profound impact on hydration, and subsequently on the absorption of critical macronutrients and micronutrients.

As the largest organ of the body, the integument harbors major variations among invertebrates, semiaquatic vertebrates, herptile, and avian species. Compared with mammals, it is dynamically modified to prevent evaporative water loss. The amphibian integument cofunctions as the respiratory system and as a major osmoregulatory organ. For piscine species, the integument and gills also function in osmoregulation. To prevent severe water loss, a relative environmental humidity of greater than 70% is required for most captive amphibians to thwart the risk of desiccation; however, many species have variations in lipid content in their skin, making some species near waterproof.[6] Most amphibians show a range of behavioral adaptations to prevent loss, conserve, and absorb water; therefore, natural husbandry of the species should be closely reviewed to guide treatment approaches. Comparatively, disease and/or desiccation of the amphibian skin could mirror the same impacts seen in mammals with severe renal impairment. *Batrachochytrium dendrobatidis*, a fungal pathogen

Box 1
Primary disease conditions caused by malnutrition

Primary Consequences of Malnutrition

- Gastrointestinal dysmotility
- Loss of the gastrointestinal mucosal barrier
- Lack of albumin production
- Altered drug metabolism
- Loss or dysregulation of nutrient, electrolyte, and water absorption
- Visceral autonomic dysfunction or compromise

Table 1
Causes of protein imbalances in critical exotic patients

Protein Intolerance	Protein Loss	Prevention of Intake or Digestion
• Hepatic encephalopathy • Hyperuricemia	• Gastrointestinal disease (malabsorption/maldigestion) • Pancreatic disease • Protein-losing enteropathies • Traumatic, toxic, and other endocrine-induced hepatopathies • Mobilization of physiologic lipid stores for reproduction • Anorexia due to reproduction in invertebrate, piscine, and herptile species • Seasonal anorexia • Protein-losing nephropathies • Severe skin disease, burns, or wounds • Chylothorax • Cachexia secondary to neoplastic disease	• Pain • Dental disease • Respiratory disease • Reproductive disease • Orthopedic disease • Renal disease

responsible for the worldwide extirpation of amphibians, causes death by overwhelming replication in the integument. This subsequently leads to the catastrophic failure of homeostatic mechanisms that control sodium and potassium transport, hastening a rapid progression to electrolyte and toxin-induced cardiac arrest when left untreated.[7]

Decreases in ambient humidity can severely affect the hydration of arthropods. Severe dehydration in theraphosids causes immobilization due to insufficient open circulatory flow, which functions as a hydraulic necessity for ambulation.[8–10] Scorpions are unique in that they have the lowest metabolic rates and lowest evaporative cuticular and respiratory water loss in comparison to other arthropods as adapted "sit and wait" hunters, yet activity alone can cause up to 30% of all evaporative water lost attributed to respiratory water loss in times of stress.[11] As nocturnal crustaceans, terrestrial hermit crabs avoid temperature extremes by drinking water at night and by storing water within their shells. Shell water can account for 30% to 50% of the crab's weight, and it is used as a reservoir to replace evaporative losses.[8] Xeric reptiles, often thought to have a higher tolerance for water loss, suffer from severe evaporative loss if not afforded burrows or hides that provide appropriate humidity clines. Some varanid lizards have high metabolic rates higher than other squamates, and yet, up to 70% of their total body water loss can be evaporative, and approximately 85% to 90% of their water intake comes from consumed prey.[12–14]

The respiratory tract of avian and reptile possess tidal volumes far greater than that of mammals and paired with unidirectional air flow mechanism to maximize oxygen absorption, it becomes clear that respiratory evaporative losses can become substantial, especially in patients with respiratory disease. Avian reptiles however are seen as the convergent example of minimizing evaporative water loss like mammals as a functional characteristic of endothermy.[15] Nitrogenous waste excretion, water, and electrolyte resorption varies greatly between invertebrates, piscine, herptile, and avian species when compared with mammals that rely heavily on advanced renal mechanisms. Knowledge of nonmammalian evolutionary adaptations may influence or change fluid therapy delivery and management, as cutaneous, colonic, and cloacal water absorption are recognized as natural methods that may be used to support euhydration in a hospital setting.

The comparative gastrointestinal tract volume of herbivores and omnivores across all taxa follow an evolutionary similarity whereby gastrointestinal volume is larger than that of carnivores and can account for up to 40% to 61% of total body weight.[16] Foregut and hindgut fermentation requires large fluid volumes to maintain liquefied ingesta. The high metabolic rate of the small herbivorous mammals' function by way of a higher daily fluid requirement for maintenance (100–150 mL/kg/d) than noted for cats and dogs. Relative to lagomorphs, hystricomorphic and non-xeric myomorphic rodents,[16] the fluid requirements of carnivorous and insectivorous mammals are not as high herbivores; however, rapid gastrointestinal fluid loss due to diarrhea in companion ferrets, hedgehogs, and sugar gliders is a common emergency presentation.[17]

Goal for Addressing Nutrition in Critical Patients

Exotic animal practitioners face nutrition-based challenges in practice that starkly highlight why its impact cannot be overlooked in emergency medicine (**Box 2**). The main goal of nutritional support is to optimize protein synthesis, preserve lean body mass, and reduce or prevent metabolic derangements.[5] Once a patient has been hemodynamically stabilized, nutritional support should be implemented as soon as possible to reverse a negative energy balance to prevent those at-risk for entering a catabolic state. Therefore, it is imperative for exotic animal practitioners to have a reliable way to measure the BCS to aid in the nutritional assessment for several captive species.

NUTRITIONAL ASSESSMENT

Initial Assessment

BCS is derived from evaluating the girth of prominent muscle bodies and qualifying adipose tissue reserve. The measures of BCS for exotic patients vary based on species and anatomy. Further information about nutritional assessment and recommendations are available for numerous species, produced by the American Zoo and Aquarium Association's Nutritional Advisory Group, and are free to access at https://nagonline.net/3877/body-condition-scoring. When metabolic wasting occurs, an initial body loss of subcutaneous fat stores is appreciated in most mammals. Additional areas of critical adipose tissue loss may occur in the periorbital sinuses, retroperitoneal space, abdominal or coelomic mesentery, coelomic fat body loss, and in squamates, coccygeal fat body loss (**Fig. 1**A, B). In mammals, cachexia measurements are qualified by the initial loss of lean body mass, usually noted in the epaxial, gluteal, scapular, and temporal muscles. In porcine pets, prominence of the ribs, spine, and hip bones are noted.[18,19] Often these are the first muscle bodies to

Box 2
Benefits of nutritional support in critical patients

Nutritional Support in Critical Patients[1]

- Decreased morbidity and mortality
- Improved tolerance to invasive procedures
- Shortened hospitalization periods
- Decreased incidence of infections
- Earlier ambulation
- Hastened wound healing
- Reduced complications

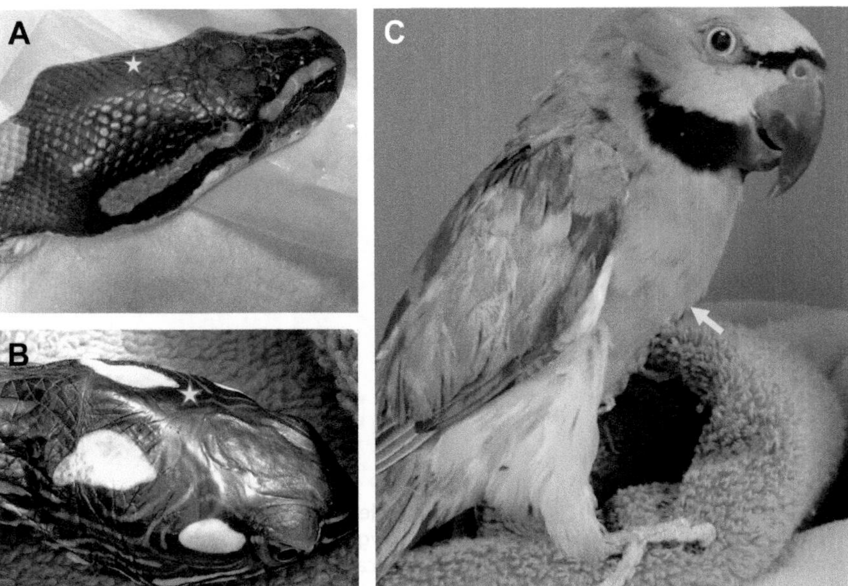

Fig. 1. Decreased temporal musculature (*yellow star*) in (*A*) *Python regius*, (*B*) *Trachemys scripta scripta*, and (*C*) reduced pectoral musculature (*yellow arrow*) resulting in a prominent keel in *Psittacula alexandri*.

experience detectable losses when a patient is cachectic or impending cachexia.[20] In avian species, loss of pectoral musculature can result in a prominent keel, and these changes can occur quickly due to intrinsic high metabolic rate (**Fig. 1**C).[21]

The body plan for reptiles is highly diverse; therefore, as a rule, the author uses periorbital fat reserves and muscles of *adductor mandibularis* or *pseudotemporalis* as a predictive measure for all reptiles as a first assessment (see **Fig. 1**A,B; **Fig. 2**B: Pic of bearded dragon and snakes and turtle). Muscle bodies and adipose tissue reserves that occur distal to the head become very specific to species, based on evolutionary design, ambulation style, and relies on their ability to engage in species-specific repertoire of natural behaviors (**Fig. 2**A–C). In most amphibians, significant pygostyle and hindlimb muscle loss can be appreciated in cachectic patients.[22] For piscine species such as goldfish and koi, the appearance of a concave coelomic shape can indicate poor BCS (**Fig. 2**D).[23,24] In theraphosids, appreciable girth changes can be noted in the opisthosoma (**Fig. 3**).[9,10]

For many captive pets, obesity is a significant comorbidity. If the patient's BCS indicates that obesity is a concern, precautions should be taken to monitor for radical shifts in metabolic status due to rapid autolysis of fat and the accumulation of lactate and ketone bodies in mammals (**Fig. 4**A, B). When blood samples are unavailable for acid–base screening, the author uses urine chemistry monitoring as a proxy for changes in blood pH, to evaluate for hydration changes, and to evaluate for protein loss, glucose loss, and ketonuria in mammalian species.

Measures of Malnutrition

Malnutrition is often defined as an in imbalance of nutrients, both nutrient deficiencies and nutrient excesses. In human medicine, a validated, subjective global assessment is used to qualify nutrient loss and nutritional status via evaluation of muscle wasting,

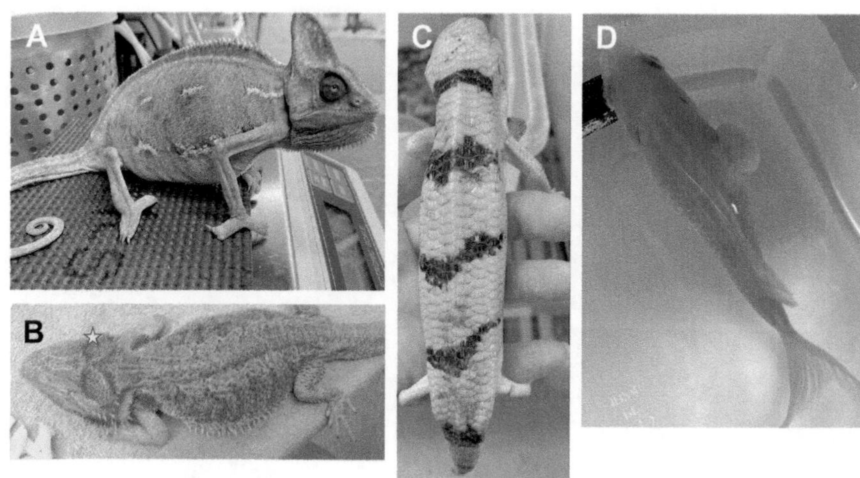

Fig. 2. (*A*) Forelimb, hindlimb, and coccygeal muscle wasting in *Chamaeleo calyptratus*, (*B*) Temporal muscle wasting (*yellow star*), and coccygeal muscle wasting in *P vitticeps*, (*C*) Prominent spine in *Tiliqua* sp, and (*D*) coelomic concavity (*blue arrow*) in a *Carassius auratus* with neoplasia.

loss of subcutaneous tissue, edema or ascites, and integument quality.[20] Measurement of catabolic products can be used to assess nutritional state, including blood urea nitrogen (BUN) monitoring during 24 hours. Laboratory indicators of malnutrition include hypoalbuminemia, decreased BUN levels, hypocholesterolemia, anemia, and lymphopenia. Physical examination findings and laboratory measures can be critically evaluated by veterinarians to determine the severity of a patient's malnutrition and to what degree their current illness will interfere with metabolic energy needs.

INDICATIONS FOR INTERVENTION

An inability to meet the resting energy requirements (RER) for a patient dictates the need for intervention.[25] Treating malnutrition and preventing its development in critical

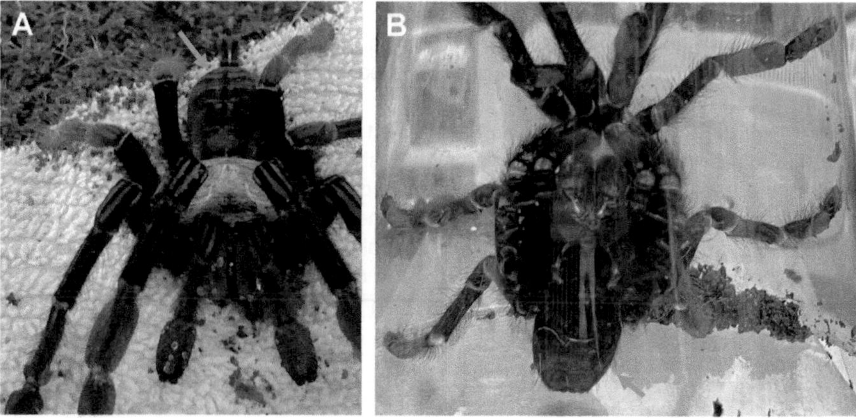

Fig. 3. (*A*) Reduced girth of the opisthosoma (*blue arrow*) of a dehydrated *Cyriopagopus* sp tarantula suffering from diarrhea. (*B*) Ventral view of the reduced opisthosoma (*blue arrow*).

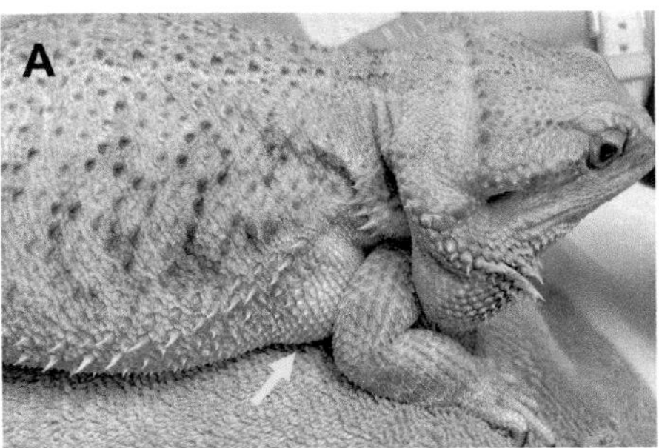

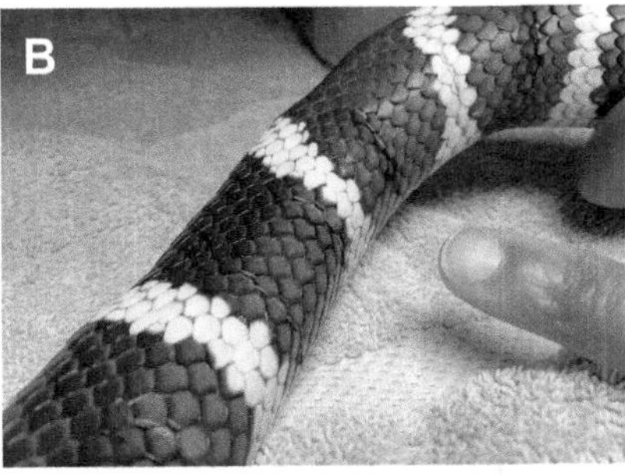

Fig. 4. (*A*) Obese *P vitticeps*, note fat deposition in pectoral girdle (*yellow arrow*). (*B*) Tubular shape and indentations noted during ambulation in an obese *Lampropeltis getula californiae*.

patients serve as the major goals for providing nutrition. In cats and dogs, the RER can be calculated by allometric formulas such as follows: RER = 70 × (body weight in kg)$^{0.75}$. Estimations in body weight loss can also be used as a guideline to start treatment for malnutrition, for example, 10% loss of body weight in 3 to 5 days for adult cat and dogs, and 5% loss for pediatric patients.[25] In order to provide safe nutritive support to exotic patients, it is recommended that one start with 10% to 20% of the RER the first day and gradually increase during the next few days by increments of 10% to 25% until 100% RER is reached.[26] This approach ensures that protein intake is optimized and can be metabolized. **Table 2** reviews basic RER, reported caloric requirements, minimal protein, fat, fiber, and carbohydrate requirements reported for captive exotic companion animals. The RER has traditionally been multiplied factor by an illness or metabolic factor; however, in efforts to avoid overfeeding and complications, nutritionists instead recommend monitoring for declines in body weight or body condition as the prompt to reassess and modify the nutritional plan (eg, increasing the number of calories provided by 25%).[5] Several commercial supportive care diets have been evaluated in the literature and are available for independent review.[27–30] Many commercial diets can be used to help ensure diet appropriate protein sources for several species (**Fig. 5**).

Considerations for Diet Preparation

Commercial diets designed for longevity and critical nutrition support are readily available for companion avian and small mammal species. For nonparrot avian species, amphibian, herptile, piscine, and invertebrate patients, options are limited and require extrapolatory use of commercial diets and/or diet preparation of native prey. Although advances in nutrition research continue to help elucidate the needs of the exotic companion pets, exotic animal veterinarians often have limited access diet items that are vitamin-stable and micronutrient and macronutrient balanced for many different species.

Commercially reared rodent and invertebrate prey species do not have compositions that reflect the optimal nutritive profile required for the captive animals that consume them.[28–30] Therefore, the author often injects (frozen-thawed) smaller sized feeder rodents with water and supportive care diet to alter their nutritive profile before offering them to self-eating carnivores. Modifying invertebrate nutrient composition requires that a water source for rehydration and a gut-loading diet be provided before patient consumption.[22,30]

Table 2
Summary of reported disease concerns, basic energy requirements, monitoring recommendations, and supplemental diet guidelines for companion exotic patients

Invertebrates	Diseases of Concern	BMR/RER/MER	Nutritional Pearls	Monitoring Recommendations	Diet Guidelines/Supplementation	Resources
Terrestrial Invertebrates	Beetles, Crickets, roaches: viral disease, bacterial disease Hermit crabs: shell fractures, limited access to healthy water (fresh and salt) Arachnids (old and new world): Parasitic disease, dehydration, exoskeleton fractures/molting emergencies Scorpions: dehydration, exoskeleton fractures/molting emergencies Hissing Cockroaches: obesity, constipation	Unknown for most groups *Paraphysa* sp fed *Tenebrio molitor* worms, to maintain weight, 1 larva per 3 d = 0.193 kcal/d		A healthy arthropod will not typically lose more than 10% of its body weight during a fast Theraphosids: Inability to extend limbs = severe dehydration Molting emergencies Expulsion of nematodes in feces, or presence of nematodes near fangs Cockroaches: severe cuticular distension	Unknown. Most use critical care formulas and baby foods that mirror normal diet intake, feed 0.5%–1% body weight at a time, once weekly Provide safe sources of hydration daily	8–10,52–54

Piscine Species	Diseases of Concern	Energy Requirements (RER/MER)	Nutritional Pearls	Monitoring Recommendations	Diet Guidelines/Supplementation	Resources
Freshwater Fish	Obesity, poor nutrient balance in water quality	Varies, however less energy than vertebrates dietary energy/protein ratio that supported best performance of goldfish (9.7 kcal/g) or 29% protein	Ingredients should have vitamin-stabilized components. Best protein source recommended is fishmeal	Fecal production, position in water column, signs of positive or negative buoyancy, changes in behavior with conspecifics and caretaker	General diet: 29%–42% protein, 10%–20% fat, 5%–25% carbohydrates/fiber with carnivorous cold-water fish having the starch digestive intolerable, to warm water omnivorous and herbivorous species with high starch digestive tolerance	23,24,55–58

					Betta fish: 35% animal or plant protein Goldfish: 29% protein Oscar: spirulina 55 g/kg of the diet supplementation show to improve performance and bloodwork values Goldfish: 4 feedings daily increased growth performance	
Marine fish	Obesity, nutrient defects secondary to poor water quality Lack of species-specific dietary requirements		Ingredients should have vitamin-stabilized components. Best protein source recommended is fishmeal	Fecal production, position in water column, signs of positive or negative buoyancy, changes in behavior with conspecifics and caretaker	General Diet: 29%–42% protein, % fat, 10%–20% fat, 5%–25% carbohydrates/ fiber with carnivorous cold-water fish having the starch digestive intolerable, to warm water omnivorous and herbivorous species with high starch digestive tolerance	23,24

Companion Mammals	Diseases of Concern	Energy Requirements (RER/MER)	Nutritional Pearls	Monitoring Recommendations	Diet Guidelines/ Supplementation	Resources
Mice	Skin disease (parasitism, autoimmune), respiratory disease			Offer frequent feedings to meet metabolic demands, hypoglycemia can occur quickly	Diet: 14%–16% protein, 5% fat, <20% fiber	17
Rats	Respiratory disease, subclinical renal disease		GI Transit time: 2–4 h and is dependent on food particle size Urine output: 13–23 mLs/h USG: 1.022–1.050	Offer frequent feedings to meet metabolic demands, hypoglycemia can occur quickly, monitor urine chemistry for signs of ketoacidosis in obese patients	Diet: 14%–16% protein, 5% fat, <20% fiber	17

(*continued on next page*)

Table 2 (*continued*)						
Companion Mammals	**Diseases of Concern**	**Energy Requirements (RER/MER)**	**Nutritional Pearls**	**Monitoring Recommendations**	**Diet Guidelines/ Supplementation**	**Resources**
Gerbils	Ovarian disease, skin disease				Diet: 22% protein, 5% fat, <20% fiber	17
Hamsters	Liver Disease, Cardiac disease, endocrinopathies, Neoplasia, Uterine disease,		Urine output: 13–23 mLs/h USG: 1.022–1.050 GI Transit time: 2–4 h and is dependent on food particle size		Diet: 14%–17% protein, 5% fat, <20% fiber	17
Guinea Pigs	Ovarian disease, obesity, dental disease, cardiac disease, gastrointestinal ileus, endocrinopathies		GI Transit time: 20 h (8–30 h)		Diet: 18%–20% protein, NA % fat, 10%–20% fiber Ascorbic Acid: 10–25 mg/kg daily, dosing above 150 mg/kg daily induces osteoarthritis	16,17,66
Chinchillas	Dental disease, obesity, subclinical cardiac disease, peracute metabolic disease, gastrointestinal ileus		Urine Output: 3–4 mL/kg/h USG: like rabbits GI transit: 12–15 h	Monitor urine output, monitor glucose and ketone production in critical patients that are obese	Diet: 16%–20% protein, NA % fat, 15%–35% fiber	17

Rabbits	Dental disease, obesity, orthopedic disease, gastrointestinal ileus, primary GI disease	400 kJ(kg) 0.75	USG: pH 8–9, 1.005–1.020	L-Lactate: 5-7 mmol/L is normal (Langlois 2014) L-Lactate <3.3 mmol/L sustained for >24 h = ↑MM in rabbits (Ardiaca 2016) True hyponatremia 2.3 OR (death) in rabbits with Na <129 mEq/L in ill rabbits (Bonvehi 2014) Anorexia + BUN >24.74 (Zoller 2019) 3 times higher odds of not surviving within 15 d of presentation, as compared with BUN 14	Diet: 16%–20% protein, 1.5%–2% fat, <15% carbohydrates/ 16%–25% fiber	17
Sugar gliders	Obesity, trauma, diabetes, dental disease	130 g require between approximately 76 kJ and 147 kJ (18 kcal–35 kcal)		Lethargy, inappetence, refusal of protein based sources (esp invertebrate prey)	Diet: 6%–14% protein, 19%–25% fat, % carbohydrates/fiber (	17,59
Hedgehogs	Obesity, gastrointestinal disease, neoplasia		GI Transit time: 12–16 h		Diet: 30%–50% protein, 10%–20% fat	17,60
Ferrets	Gastrointestinal disease (insulinoma, bacterial and viral disease), neoplasia, trauma	200–300 kcal/kg/d	GI transit: 2.5–3.6 h (meat), 1 h (liquid) Urine output: 2–3 mLs/h USG: >1.040 pH 6, trace protein common	Color, consistency, and frequency of defecation. Color changes my sign enteric viral or bacterial small or large bowel disease, tarry stools may indicate gastric ulceration. Given the rapid GI transit, diarrhea results in rapid and compounding hypoalbuminemia and hypovolemia	Diet: 30%–35% protein, 20%–30% fat, minimal carbohydrates (<30%), low fiber	17

(*continued on next page*)

Table 2
(continued)

Companion Mammals	Diseases of Concern	Energy Requirements (RER/MER)	Nutritional Pearls	Monitoring Recommendations	Diet Guidelines/ Supplementation	Resources
Suids	Obesity, severe orthopedic disease, bite wound trauma, severe dehydration, fecoliths (Hobbs 2021), dietary indiscretion	Piglet: 7–9 kg/d Adult: 23–36 kg/d		BCS monitoring, joint and hoof health secondary to obesity, consistency of stools	Diet: 12% protein, 2% fat, 10%–15% fiber	18,19,61

Herptiles	Diseases of Concern	Energy Requirements (RER/MER)	Nutritional Pearls	Monitoring Recommendations	Diet Guidelines/ Supplementation	Resources
Amphibians	Hypovitaminosis A, Poor nutrition, obesity, viral bacterial and fungal skin disease	Caloric requirement per 24 h in kcal, whereby BM is body mass in grams at 25C Anuran $0.02\ (BM)^{0.84}$ Salamander $0.01(BM)^{0.80}$ Caecilian $0.01(BM)^{1.0}$		Changes in coelomic girth may signify organomegaly, effusion, or gravidity Monitor limbs, femoral patches and pygostyle Can transilluminate femoral vasculature or abdominal vein in many species without direct handling to estimate perfusion	Diet: 25%–60% protein, 30%–60% fat, <10% fiber	22,62

Chelonians	Reproductive disease, respiratory pathogens, Hypocalcemia, trauma/fractures, inappropriate diet, reproductive disease, skin disease		Fractures require prolonged protein support to build dermal bone and epidermal beta keratin	Any fractures involving the thoracic girdle and/or pelvic girdle could impact respiration.	Herbivores Diet: 15%–35% protein, <10% fat, 50%–75% carbohydrates (of which is 15%–40% fiber) Omnivores: 15%–40%, 5%–40%, 20%–75% Carnivores (Mata Mata): Diet: 25%–60% protein, 30%–60% fat, <10% carbohydrates/fiber	
Lacertilians	Reproductive disease, Trauma, bacterial, viral and fungal pathogens, Hypocalcemia, obesity, inappropriate diet			Cachexia: Prominent lateral processes of the coccygeal vertebrae Loss of temporalis musculature Monitor colonic health closely and treat for any condition that compromises colonic health as a measure of critical importance	Herbivores Diet: 15%–35% protein, <10% fat, 50%–75% carbohydrates/(of which is 15%–40% fiber that is, *Iguana iguana*: <20%, 3% fat Omnivores: 15%–40%, 5%–40%, 20%–75% that is, *Pogona vitticeps* 41%–50% protein, 14%–27% fat Carnivores: Diet: 25%–60% protein, 30%–60% fat, <10% carbohydrates/fiber	29
Serpentes	Fractures, neurologic disease, bacterial, fungal and viral disease, inappropriate diet		When the regains normal feeding, inject prey with small volume of water to improve hydration, Inject pinkies with a balanced carnivore diets to provide appropriate calcium and micronutrient support	Loss of epaxial musculature and prominent ribs	Carnivores: Diet: 25%–60% protein, 30%–60% fat, <10% carbohydrates/fiber	29

(*continued on next page*)

Table 2
(continued)

Herptiles	Diseases of Concern	Energy Requirements (RER/MER)	Nutritional Pearls	Monitoring Recommendations	Diet Guidelines/ Supplementation	Resources
Crocodilians	Infectious diseases (viral-zoonotic, bacterial), trauma, conspecific resource hoarding-diet/ nutrition				Diet: 13%–15% protein, 3%–4% fat, % carbohydrates/ fiber Plant-based nutrition has been studied and used with success	36

Avian Species	Diseases of Concern	Energy Requirements (RER/MER)	Nutritional Pearls	Monitoring Recommendations	Diet Guidelines/ Supplementation	Resources
Columbiformes	Parasitism, fungal and viral infectious disease, trauma	MER = 2× BMR BMR = 78 W0.75		Frequent feedings daily are required to meet MER	Diet: 11%–18% protein, 4.5%–12.7% fat,	63
Passerines	Trauma, inappropriate diet, nutritional deficits in calcium and vitamin A	MER = 2× BMR BMR = 129 W0.75	MR 60% higher than birds in any other taxa	Frequent feedings daily are required to meet MER	Diet: 14% protein	21,64
Parrots	Reproductive disease, hypocalcemia, obesity, cardiovascular disease, orthopedic disease	Tropical Species: BMR [kcal/d] = 73.6W0.73 BMR [kJ/d] = 308W0.73 Temperate climates (Australia New Zealand): BMR is 21% higher than tropical species	Cannot synthesize several amino acids, arginine, lysine, and methionine. During breeding or molting, higher protein needs with critical amino acids may need to be provided in increased amounts in supportive care diet	Frequent feedings daily are required to meet MER	Varies by family however for nonlorikeets Diet: 6.8%–11% protein-maintenance, up to 20% in some species for growth Water requirement of adult parrots (ranging from 48 to 295 g) to be approximately 2.4% of body weight	21,46

Galliformes	Hypocalcemia, obesity, orthopedic disease, reproductive disease	MER = 2× BMR BMR = 78 W0.75		Frequent feedings daily are required to meet MER	Diet: 13%–15% protein	46
Anseriformes	Heavy metal toxicity, obesity, orthopedic disease, reproductive disease	MER = 2× BMR BMR = 78 W0.75		Frequent feedings daily are required to meet MER	Diet: 11%–20% protein	46,65

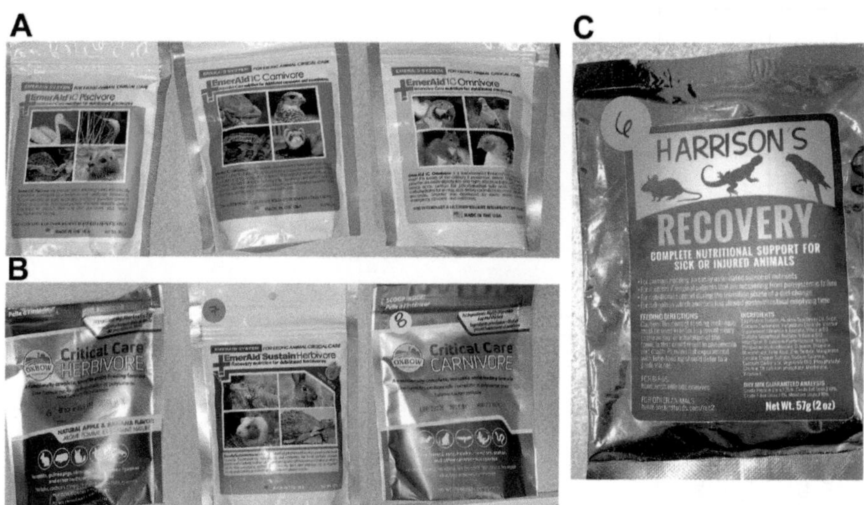

Fig. 5. Veterinary critical care diets designed for exotic companion animals (*A*) EmerAid, (*B*) Oxbow food line, and (*C*) Harrison's avian recovery diet.

The digestibility of insect feeders and absorption of novel nutrient sources are being evaluated in companion insectivores. Black soldier fly larvae (*Hermetia illucens*) are a staple food item in aquaculture[31] and has become a popular herptile feeder item given it's naturally high calcium content.[32] In mountain chicken frogs (*Leptodactylus fallax*), the soldier fly larval exoskeletons were not digested and passed intact from the digestive tract.[33] In leopard geckos (*Eublepharis macularius*) fed gut-loaded larvae and unsupplemented larvae, the nutrients of the gut-loaded prey seemed to be digested; however, the calcium-rich exoskeleton usually remained intact after passage through the GI tract, and serum calcium values depreciated over time in treated geckos.[32] As captive leopard geckos present often suffer from hypovitaminosis A,[34] safe supplementation measures have been evaluated. In one study that evaluated β-carotene assimilation in leopard geckos, oral supplementation with carrot juice (0.1 mL per 50 g of body weight) orally once a week (equivalent to 2 μg β-carotene per gram of body weight) resulted in higher liver levels of vitamin A than oral supplementation of cod liver oil (0.1 mL per 50 g of body weight [equivalent to 2 UI retinyl ester per gram of body weight]) orally once a week.[35]

A reevaluation of the natural diet items of native crocodilians has been explored,[36] given that farmed American alligators (*Alligator mississippiensis*) can thrive on plant-protein based diets with no deleterious effects on overall health[37] and further studies have revealed that plant compounded diets can be effectively used in the same species.[38] These studies remind us that estimations for digestibility and bioavailability cannot be generalized, and whenever possible, it is important to revisit the literature for guidance on nutritional support in captive herptiles.

CLINICAL TECHNIQUES

Enteral Support

Supportive care feedings can largely be provided by frequent syringe feeding for mammalian, invertebrate, most herptile patients (**Fig. 6**), and tube feedings can be provided to avian, chelonian, serpent, and piscine patients (**Fig. 7**). Contraindications

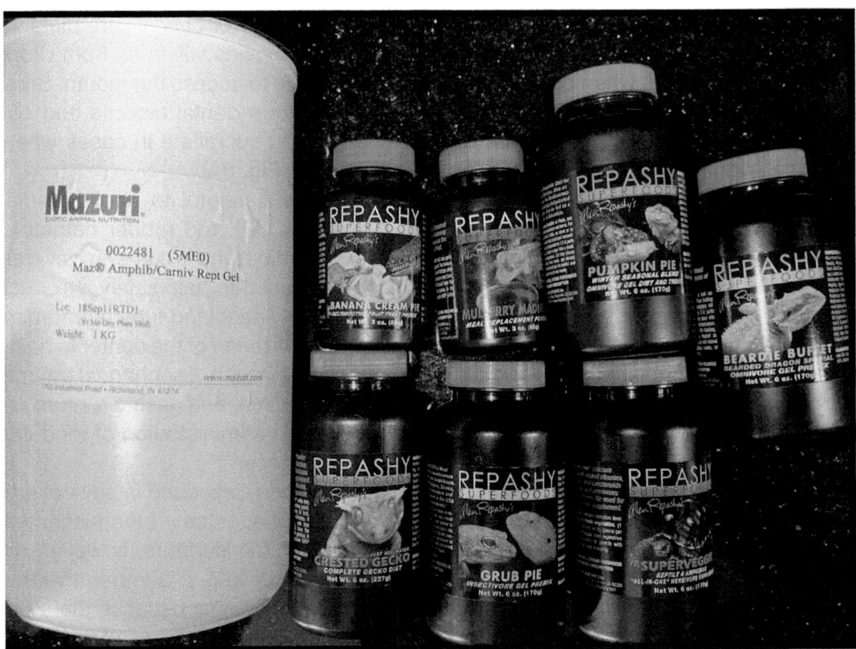

Fig. 6. Veterinary critical care diets designed for exotic companion herptile and insectivore species made by Mazuri (*left*) and Repashy (*right*).

to syringe feedings and/or tube feedings include patients that cannot maintain a normal head position at rest to prevent aspiration and protect their airways. Severe dental or oral disease, head trauma, cranial vault fractures, cervical trauma, esophageal trauma, gastrointestinal blockage, and/or frequent regurgitation/vomiting are also contraindications for both syringe and tube feeding.[26]

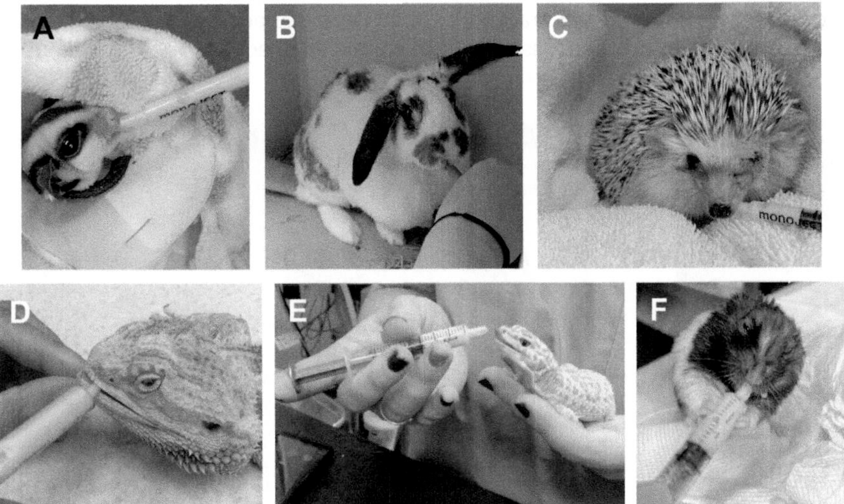

Fig. 7. Assisted syringe feeding in (*A*) *Petaurus breviceps*, (*B*) *Oryctolagus cuniculus*, (*C*) *Atelerix albiventris*, (*D*) *P vitticeps*, (*E*) *Eublepharis macularius*, and (*F*) *Meriones unguiculatus*.

Invertebrate patients can be syringe fed offered water and/or critical care diets via gelco catheter. Often dehydrated and debilitated theraphosids will drink from drops from the catheter tips when positioned between the fangs to access the mouth. Small syringes are recommended for herbivores recovering from dental disease and oral pain. The author uses a 1:1 mixture of lidocaine gel and sucralfate in cases where oral ulceration may limit food intake due to topical pain (**Fig. 8**A).

When administering tube feedings, the author finds it helpful to apply a small amount of sterile lubricant to metal gavage tubes (**Fig. 8**B), red rubber catheters, and silicone feeding tubes to prevent esophageal irritation and trauma in severely dehydrated patients. Often silicone tubes (**Fig. 8**C) are used to help safely introduce liquid diets into the stomach of patients while reducing irritation and tube entrapment in esophageal folds. Silicone tubes also allow direct visualization of the contents being expelled from the tube and into the distal esophagus or stomach. Esophageal trauma, aspiration pneumonia, accidental intratracheal administration, and gastric rupture are risks associated with tube feeding. The risk of accidental administration of food into the swim bladder of physostomous fish is rare but can occur.[23]

Nasogastric tube placement in small mammals has been described in several articles, which are available for independent review.[26] Esophagostomy tube placement has been historically reviewed in mammals and turtles in the literature; however, the same principles can be applied for placement in lizards as well. It is imperative that tube placement be confirmed before the instillation of food items because there is a risk of tube migration during placement, and the author has often witnessed this occur in cat and dog patients (**Fig. 9**). Additional risks include tube leakage/dislodgment, tube clogging with food material, overfeeding and subsequent regurgitation, and loss of airway protection, which can potentiate aspiration events. A recipe for unclogging feeding tubes with one-fourth of a teaspoon of pancreatic enzymes and 325 mg sodium bicarbonate in 5 mL water has been described as most effective for use in cats and dogs.[39] A detailed how to review of esophagostomy tube placement in several species is available.[40]

Parenteral Support

In cases where it is safe and practical to obtain vascular access, parenteral nutrition can and has been used successfully in many exotic species.[17,25,41] Indications for

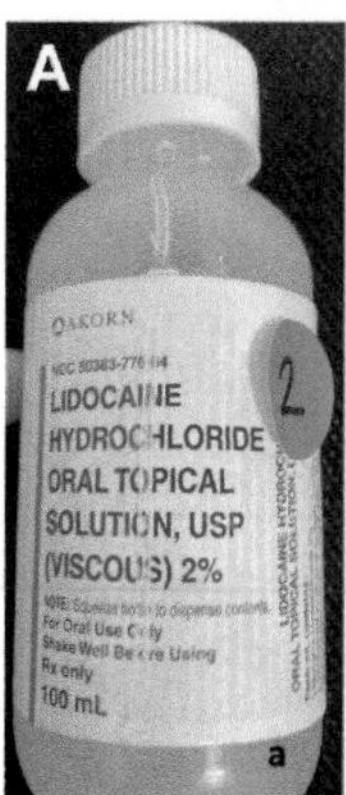

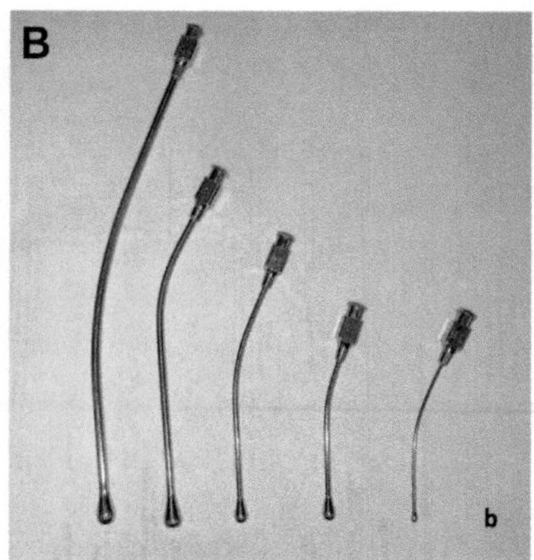

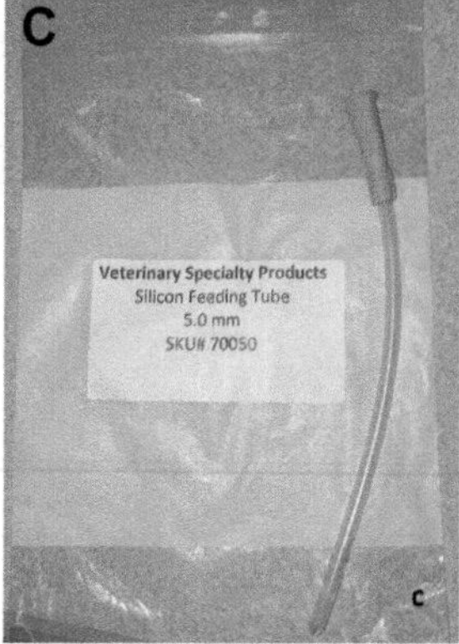

Fig. 8. (*A*) Viscous 2% lidocaine gel for oral use. (*B*) Avian gavage tubes of various sizes. (*C*) Silicone feeding tubes, available in several sizes up to 5.0 mm diameter.

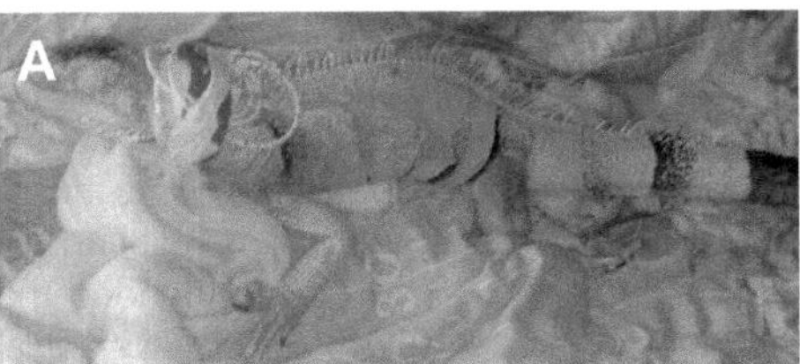

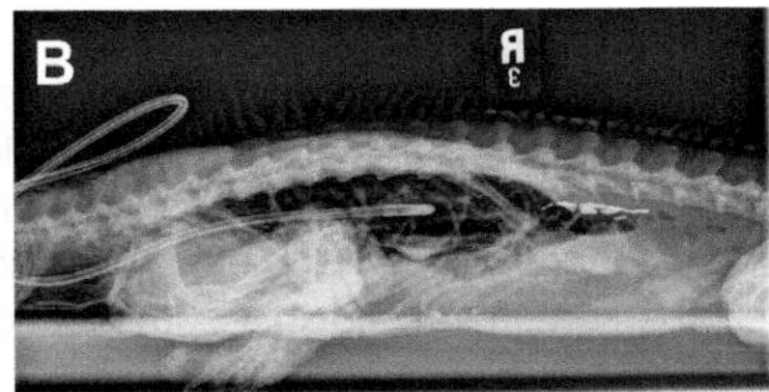

Fig. 9. (*A*) Elderly *Iguana iguana* with esophagotomy tube. (*B*) Lateral radiograph confirming tube placement with Iohexol administration.

parenteral support include the inability to meet 50% of RER with enteral methods alone. Vascular access should be maintained with a dedicated central line that is a long, aseptically placed, nonthrombogenic catheter. This line must be monitored daily.[25] In some cases, a peripherally inserted central venous catheter can be used for TPN. Parenteral support should be short acting; support is usually less than 1, or at most 2, weeks in cats and dogs. Parenteral nutrition also requires 24-hour nursing care and point of care access to biochemistry evaluation, which limits exotics practitioners' use largely to animals hospitalized at facilities with overnight care.

All nonprotein calories can be provided by dextrose solutions; however, this does not address protein demand, and patients are at a greater risk for hyperglycemia. Lipid emulsions are iso-osmolar and provide a more concentrated form of calories. In small animal medicine, patients receiving parenteral nutrition should receive 50% of goal nutrients the first day as a constant rate infusion over 24 hours, and if that is well tolerated, they can receive 100% of their target nutrition the following day.[25] Adjustments for exotic species should consider metabolic rates to avoid exacerbating preexisting conditions. Additionally, lipid emulsions have also been reported to successful in treating toxicosis in a variety of exotic animal species (**Table 3**).[42–44]

COMPLICATIONS

In addition to the aforementioned physical complication risks for any supportive feeding regimen, refeeding syndrome is the major metabolic risk that can worsen patient outcomes. Refeeding syndrome is a life-threatening metabolic complication that may occur in patients after prolonged anorexia or in certain catabolic states. During

Table 3
Toxicoses treated by lipid emulsion therapy

Species	Toxicity	Reference
Bearded dragon (*P vitticeps*)	Ivermectin Toxicosis: 2 mL/kg intravenously over 10 min followed by a constant rate infusion (CRI) of 0.25 mL/kg/min for 60 min of a 20% lipid emulsion	DeMel et al,[42] 2022
Loggerhead Sea turtles (*Caretta caretta*) Kemp's Ridleys Sea turtles (*L kempii*) Juvenile Green Sea turtles (*Chelonia mydas*)	Brevetoxicosis: 25 mg/kg 20% lipid emulsion intravenously at 1 mL/min, single dose	Perrault et al,[43] 2021
Domestic goose (*Anser anser domesticus*)	Oleander toxicosis: 20% lipid emulsion intravenously at 0.25 mL/kg/min for 2 h	Lubian et al,[44] 2021

the reintroduction of feeding, a rapid shift of key intracellular electrolytes from the vascular to the intracellular space causes life-threatening hypokalemia, hypophosphatemia, or hypomagnesemia.[25,26] This electrolyte abnormality can occur within days of resuming enteral feeding. At-risk patients should be fed conservative amounts initially and monitored closely and electrolyte abnormalities corrected via parenteral or enteral replacement. To avoid this complication in unique species, it is recommended that 0.5% to 1% body weight be fed to poikilotherms, and 1% to 1.5% body weight be fed as a maximum to mammals at the onset of supportive care feedings.[26]

RECOMMENDED MONITORING

Body weight reassessment should be performed to monitor for nutritive and fluid resuscitation gains. In most endothermic patients, this means routinely weighing patients a minimum of 2 to 3 times daily, and sometimes more frequently in avian patients, who can suffer from rapid changes due to an extremely high metabolism.[45] Monitoring losses can be performed with minimal disruption to the patient. It is recommended to monitor urinary losses, by weighing absorbent pads (1 mL = 1 g) when applicable. Approximating gastrointestinal losses can be extremely helpful, especially for patients who are experiencing diarrhea. This is often monitored via body weight change. Additionally, minimizing evaporative losses should be a priority.

Clinical diagnostics, when feasible and available, identify rapid metabolic changes. A hematocrit tube can be spun to characterize hydration, monitor for changes in serum characterization and even evaluate for the presence of severe lipemia. Severe lipemia will limit accurate biochemistry analyte evaluation in all species, especially when using tabletop laboratory chemistry analyzers.[46] BUN and creatinine monitoring, albumin, and cholesterol/lipid monitoring can be performed on mammals that can tolerate minimal blood loss without further compromise. Acid–base parameters help screen for emergent and/or ongoing causes for metabolic derangements.

Point-of-care diagnostic parameters routinely used in small animal critical care include evaluation of lactate, electrolytes, BUN, body temperature, total protein, glucose, acid–base derangements, oxygen carrying capacity (packed cell volume), and ultrasonographic presence of effusions. Lactate, BUN, and sodium have been studied to assess survival predictability in rabbits (*Oryctolagus cuniculus*) and are summarized in **Table 2**. Rabbits that present as an acute abdomen due to true mechanical obstructions often have elevated blood glucose levels greater than 300 mg/dL.

Glucose monitoring in several species is vital to ensuring that metabolic needs are being met. Several studies have revealed that handheld glucometers require adjustment factors for ferrets (*Mustela putorius furo*),[47] rabbits,[48] Prairie dogs (*Cynomys ludovicianus*),[49] and Kemp's Ridley Sea turtles (*Lepidochelys kempii*)[50] as single point glucose readings on these devices are inaccurate; therefore, monitoring for trends is recommended if a laboratory analyzer is not immediately available.

Noninvasive diagnostic tests are preferred and may be the only option for many clinicians faced with patient fragility and limited sample availability. The author uses urinary pH and urinalysis from opportunistic samples obtained while monitoring for urinary losses. In rabbits that do not have existing glomerular or renal interstitial disease, urine pH changes when blood pH shifts occur.[51] The presence of catabolic products can be quantified in the urine, and urine pH trends can be followed during the course of treatment. This is in addition to evaluating for markers of renal health, hydration improvements, and protein loss in animals suffering from renal disease. Water quality assessment, dissolved oxygen monitoring when feasible, and evaluation of fecal losses should also be monitoring in hospitalized aquatic species to (1) qualify response to treatment and (2) to help prevent iatrogenic bioaccumulation of metabolic byproducts in a hospital enclosure.

Supportive feedings via syringe feeding, tube feedings, and/or via esophagostomy tube feedings can be discontinued, and only begin when the patient can consume approximately 75% of its RER without much coaxing.[5]

SUMMARY

Nutritive support for exotic patients should be implemented as soon as possible in critical patients. Reassessment of body condition, weight, and diagnostic monitoring for protein absorption, tolerance, and reduction of catabolic loss is recommended to help guide restorative therapy. Several critical care diets are available based on digestive strategy; however, feeder rodent and live invertebrate prey require modifications to improve nutritive quality. Fluid requirements and evaporative water loss can vary based on taxa; ectoderms suffer evaporative losses at a greater magnitude than endotherms. Enteral and parenteral nutrition strategies can be appropriate for patients, with natural history and anatomic and physiologic differences considered as much as possible.

CLINICS CARE POINTS

- Handheld glucometers have been shown to be inaccurate for many exotic species (eg, ferrets, rabbits, sea turtles, and praire dogs) and should be used to monitor trends only if laboratory analyzer measurements are immediately unavailable.
- Lactate, BUN, and sodium have been studied to assess survival predictability in rabbits, whereby L-lactate less than 3.3 mmol/L for greater than 24 hours, anorexia associated with BUN greater than 24.74 mg/dL, and true persistent hyponatremia (<129 mEq/L) has been associated with increased mortality over time.
- The bioavailability of feeder insects can vary based on the digestive capability of the insectivore, as reported in Leopard geckos and Mountain chicken frogs fed black soldier fly larva.
- Parental nutrition has been successfully used exotic animal medicine. Lipid emulsions require central line, single-use catheters that can be monitored with 24-hour nursing care. Lipid emulsions are iso-osmolar, can be used to achieve 50% of the RER, and has successfully treated plant and drug toxicoses in a variety of exotic animal species.

DISCLOSURE

The author has nothing to disclose and is unaware of any conflicts of interest.

REFERENCES

1. Eirmann L, Michel KE. Enteral Nutrition. In: Silverstein D, Hopper K, editors. Small animal critical care. 2nd edition. St. Louis: Saunders; 2014. p. 53–7.
2. National Research Council. Nutrient requirements of poultry: ninth revised edition. Washington, DC: The National Academies Press; 1994. https://doi.org/10.17226/2114 (Chickens, turkeys, geese, ducks, Japanese quail, bob white quail).
3. National Research Council (US). Subcommittee on laboratory animal nutrition. Nutrient requirements of laboratory animals. Fourth Revised Edition. Washington (DC): National Academies Press (US); 1995. PMID: 25121259. (Mice, rabbits, guinea pigs, gerbils, voles).

4. National Research Council. Nutrient requirements of fish and shrimp. Washington, DC: The National Academies Press; 2011. https://doi.org/10.17226/13039.
5. Chan DL, Freeman LM. Nutrition in critical illness. Vet Clin North Am Small Anim Pract 2006;36(6):1225–41.
6. Withers PC, Hillman SS, Drewes RC. Evaporative water loss and skin lipids of anuran amphibians. J Exp Zool 1984;232(1):11–7.
7. Salla RF, Rizzi-Possignolo GM, Oliveira CR, et al. Novel findings on the impact of chytridiomycosis on the cardiac function of anurans: sensitive vs. tolerant species. PeerJ 2018;6:e5891. Available at: https://www.ncbi.nlm.nih.gov/pmc/articles/PMC6228586/.
8. Marnell C. Tarantula and hermit crab emergency care. Vet Clin North Am Exot Anim Prac 2016;19(2):627–46.
9. Pellett S, Bushell M, Trim SA. Tarantula husbandry and critical care. Companion Animal 2015;20(2):119–25.
10. De Voe RS. Captive invertebrate nutrition. Vet Clin North Am Exot Anim Prac 2009;12(2):349–60.
11. Gefen E. The relative importance of respiratory water loss in scorpions is correlated with species habitat type and activity pattern. Physiol Biochem Zool 2011;84(1):68–76.
12. Thompson GG, Withers PC. Evaporative water loss of Australian goannas. Amphibia-Reptilia 1997;18(2):177–90.
13. Maslanka MT, Frye FL, Henry BA, et al. Nutritional Considerations. In: Warwick C, Arena PC, Burghardt GM, editors. Health and welfare of captive reptiles. Cham: Springer International; 2023. https://doi.org/10.1007/978-3-030-86012-7_14. p447–85.
14. Thompson GG, Bradshaw SD, Withers PC. Energy and water turnover rates of a free-living and captive goanna, Varanus caudolineatus (Lacertilia: Varanidae). Comp Biochem Physiol A 1997;116(2):105–11.
15. Eto EC, Withers PC, Cooper CE. Can birds do it too? Evidence for convergence in evaporative water loss regulation for birds and mammals. Proc. R. Soc. B: Biol Sci 2017;284(1867):20171478. Available at: https://royalsocietypublishing.org/doi/full/10.1098/rspb.2017.1478.
16. Grant K. Rodent Nutrition Digestive Comparisons of 4 Common Rodent Species. Vet Clin Exot Anim 2014;17:471–83.
17. van Zeeland Y, Schoemaker NJ. Nutrition and Fluid Therapy (Small Mammal). In: Graham JE, Doss GA, Beaufrere H, editors. Exotic animal emergency and critical care medicine. 1st Edition. Hoboken: Wiley-Blackwell; 2021. p. p109–21.
18. Tynes VV. Potbellied pig husbandry and nutrition. Vet Clin North Am Exot Anim Prac 1999;2(1):193–208.
19. Carr J, Wilbers A. Pet pig medicine : The normal pig. In Pract 2008;30:160–6.
20. Elliot DA. Nutritional Assessment. In: Silverstein D, Hopper K, editors. Small animal critical care. 2nd edition. St. Louis: Saunders; 2014. p. 856–9.
21. Koutsos EA, Matson KD, Klasing KC. Nutrition of birds in the order Psittaciformes: a review. J Avian Med Surg 2001;15(4):257–75.
22. Latney L, Clayton LA. Updates on amphibian nutrition and nutritive value of common feeder insects. Vet Clin North Am Exot Anim Pract 2014;17:347–67.
23. Hoppes LA, Koutsos KA. Nutrition and Nutritional Support. In: Clayton LA, Hatfield K, editors. Clinical guide to fish medicine. Hoboken: John Wiley & Sons; 2021. p. p67–96.
24. Corcoran M, Roberts-Sweeney H. Aquatic Animal Nutrition for the Exotic Animal Practitioner. Vet Clin North Am Exot Anim Prac 2014;17:333–46.

25. Michel KE, Eirmann L. Parenteral Nutrition. In: Silverstein D, Hopper K, editors. Small animal critical care. 2nd edition. St. Louis: Saunders; 2014. p58-62.
26. Briscoe J, Latney LV, Caitlin. Nutritional support in exotic pet species. In: Chan DL, editor. Nutritional management of hospitalized small animals. 1st Edition. Oxford: John Wiley & Sons, Ltd; 2015. p. p234–46.
27. Proenca LM, Mayer J. Prescription Diets for Rabbit. Vet Clin North Am Exot Anim Prac 2014;17:485–502.
28. Latney LV, Toddes BD, Wyre NR, et al. Effects of various diets on the calcium and phosphorus composition of mealworms (Tenebrio molitor larvae) and superworms (Zophobas morio larvae). Am J Vet Res 2017;78(2):178–85.
29. Boyer TH, Scott PW. Nutrition. In: Mader DR, Divers SJ, Stahl SJ, editors. Reptile and Amphibian medicine and Surgery. 3rd edition. St. Louis: WB Saunders; 2019. p. 201–23.
30. Attard L. The development and evaluation of a gut loading diet for feeder crickets formulated to provide a balanced nutrient source for insectivorous amphibians and reptiles. 2013 (Thesis presented to the University of Guelph, Guelph, Ontario, Canada). Available at: https://atrium.lib.uoguelph.ca/xmlui/handle/10214/6653 Accessed on November 23, 2022.
31. Mohan K, Rajan DK, Muralisankar T, et al. Use of black soldier fly (Hermetia illucens L.) larvae meal in aquafeeds for a sustainable aquaculture industry: A review of past and future needs. Aquaculture 2022;553:738095.
32. Boykin KL, Carter RT, Butler-Perez K, et al. Digestibility of black soldier fly larvae (*Hermetia illucens*) fed to leopard geckos (Eublepharis macularius). PLoS One 2020;15(5):e0232496.
33. Dierenfeld ES, King J. Digestibility and mineral availability of phoenix worms, Hermetia illucens, ingested by mountain chicken frogs, Leptodactylus fallax. J Herp Med Surg 2008;18(3):100–5.
34. Wiggans KT, Guzman DS, Reilly CM, et al. Diagnosis, treatment, and outcome of and risk factors for ophthalmic disease in leopard geckos (Eublepharis macularius) at a veterinary teaching hospital: 52 cases (1985–2013). J Am Vet Med Assoc 2018;252(3):316–23.
35. Cojean O, Lair S, Vergneau-Grosset C. Evaluation of β-carotene assimilation in leopard geckos (Eublepharis macularius). J Anim Physiol Anim Nutr 2018; 102(5):1411–8.
36. Hilevski S, Cordero T, Siroski P. Do crocodilians eat plant material? A review of plant nutrients consumed by captive crocodilians. S Am J Herpetol 2022;24(1): 19–25.
37. DiGeronimo PM, Di Girolamo N, Crossland NA, et al. Effects of plant protein diets on the health of farmed american alligators (Alligator mississippiensis). J Zoo Wildl Med 2017;48(1):131–5.
38. Reigh RC, Williams MB. Plant products in compounded diets are effectively utilized by American alligator, Alligator mississippiensis. J World Aquac Soc 2018;49(6):1014–8.
39. Parker VJ, Freeman LM. Comparison of various solutions to dissolve critical care diet clots. J Vet Emerg Crit Care 2013;23(3):344–7.
40. Whittington JK. Esophagostomy feeding tube use and placement in exotic pets. J Exot Pet Med 2013;22(2):178–91.
41. Remillard RL. Parenteral nutrition support in rabbits and ferrets. J Exot Pet Med 2006;15(4):248–54.

42. DeMel D, Gleeson M, Schachterle K, et al. Successful treatment of ivermectin overdose in a bearded dragon (Pogona vitticeps) using gastric lavage and intravenous lipid emulsion. J Vet Emerg Crit Care 2022;32(5):680–4.
43. Perrault JR, Barron HW, Malinowski CR, et al. Use of intravenous lipid emulsion therapy as a novel treatment for brevetoxicosis in sea turtles. Sci Rep 2021; 11(1):1–2.
44. Lubian E, Capitelli R, Nappi S, et al. Use of intralipid emulsion therapy to treat suspected oleander toxicosis in a domestic goose (Anser anser domesticus). J Exot Pet Med 2021;39:78–80.
45. Beaufrère H. Nutrition and Fluid Therapy (Avian). In: Graham JE, Doss GA, Beaufrere H, editors. Exotic animal emergency and critical care medicine. 1st Edition. Hoboken: Wiley-Blackwell; 2021. p. p503–17.
46. Calmarza P, Cordero J. Lipemia interferences in routine clinical biochemical tests. Biochem Med 2011;21(2):160–6.
47. Petritz OA, Antinoff N, Chen S, et al. Evaluation of portable blood glucose meters for measurement of blood glucose concentration in ferrets (Mustela putorius furo). J Am Vet Med Assoc 2013;242(3):350–4.
48. Selleri P, Di Girolamo N, Novari G. Performance of two portable meters and a benchtop analyzer for blood glucose concentration measurement in rabbits. J Am Vet Med Assoc 2014;245(1):87–98.
49. Higbie CT, Eshar D, Bello NM. Evaluation of three point-of-care meters and a portable veterinary chemistry analyzer for measurement of blood glucose concentrations in black-tailed prairie dogs (Cynomys ludovicianus). Am J Vet Res 2015;76(6):532–9.
50. Perrault JR, Arendt MD, Schwenter JA, et al. Comparison of 2 glucose analytical methodologies in immature Kemp's ridley sea turtles: dry chemistry of plasma versus point-of-care glucometer analysis of whole blood. J Vet Diagn Invest 2021;33(3):595–9.
51. Brion L, Zavilowitz B, Suarez C, et al. Metabolic acidosis stimulates carbonic anhydrase activity in rabbit proximal tubule and medullary collecting duct. Am J Physiol Renal Physiol 1994;266(2):F185–95.
52. Mulder P, Shufran A. 2016. Madagascar hissing cockroaches: Information and care. Oklahoma Cooperative Extension Service. Available at: https://extension.okstate.edu/fact-sheets/madagascar-hissing-cockroaches-information-and-care.html.
53. Hill AG. Obesity and Gastrointestinal Impaction in Giant Burrowing Cockroaches (Macropanesthia rhinoceros): A Potential Effect of the Thrifty Phenotype. J Exot Pet Med 2016;25(1):30–3.
54. Canals L, Figueroa D, Torres-Contreras H, et al. Mealworm (Tenebrio molitor) diets relative to the energy requirements of small mygalomorph spiders (Paraphysa sp.). J Exot Pet Med 2012;21(3):203–6.
55. Priestley SM, Stevenson AE, Alexander LG. The influence of feeding frequency on growth and body condition of the common goldfish (Carassius auratus). J Nutr 2006;136(7):1979S, 81S.
56. Lochmann RT, Phillips H. Dietary protein requirement of juvenile golden shiners (Notemigonus crysoleucas) and goldfish (Carassius auratus) in aquaria. Aquaculture 1994;128(3–4):277–85.
57. James R, Sampath K. Effect of feeding frequency on growth and fecundity in an ornamental fish, Betta splendens (Regan). Isr J Aquac Bamidgeh 2004;52(3): 138–47.

58. Mohammadiazarm H, Milad M, Khorshid G, et al. Effects of spirulina powder (Spirulina platensis) as a dietary additive on Oscar fish, Astronotus ocellatus: Assessing growth performance, body composition, digestive enzyme activity, immune-biochemical parameters, blood indices and total pigmentation. Aquac Nutr 2021;27(1):252–60.
59. Dierenfeld ES. Feeding behavior and nutrition of the sugar glider (Petaurus breviceps). Vet Clin North Am Exot Anim Prac 2009;12(2):209–15.
60. Dierenfeld ES. Feeding behavior and nutrition of the african pygmy hedgehog (Atelerix albiventris). Vet Clin North Am Exot Anim Prac 2009;12(2):335–7.
61. Hobbs KJ, DeNotta SL, Gallastegui A, et al. Obstipation in pet pigs: 24 cases. Can Vet J 2021;62(8):843.
62. Helmer PJ, Whiteside DP. Amphibian and physiology. In: O'Malley B, editor. Clinical anatomy and physiology of exotic species. Germany: Elsevier; 2005. p. p3–14.
63. Sales J, Janssens GP. Nutrition of the domestic pigeon (Columba livia domestica). World's Poult Sci J 2003;59(2):221–32.
64. Stockdale B. Passerine birds: nutrition and nutritional diseases. In: BSAVA manual of Raptors, pigeons and passerine birds. BSAVA Publishing; 2008. p. p347–55.
65. Applegate TJ, Fowler J. Backyard poultry nutrition. Backyard poultry medicine and surgery: a guide for veterinary practitioners. John Wiley & Sons, Inc.; 2021. p. 117–30.
66. Kraus VB, Huebner JL, Stabler T, et al. Ascorbic acid increases the severity of spontaneous knee osteoarthritis in a guinea pig model. Arthritis Rheum 2004; 50:1822–31.

Cerebro-Cardiopulmonary Resuscitation and Postarrest Care in Exotic Animal Critical Care

Natalie H. Hall, DVM, Dipl ACZM

KEYWORDS

• Arrest • Cardiopulmonary • CPR • Life support • Resuscitation

KEY POINTS

- Hospital and team preparation for cardiopulmonary resuscitation (CPR) reduces delays and optimizes outcomes.
- The Reassessment Campaign on Veterinary Resuscitation guidelines for basic and advanced life support are appropriate for many nondomestic species until more taxa-specific scientific evidence becomes available.
- Exotic and zoological species may require unique approaches for administering CPR including human safety considerations.
- Postarrest care may be limited by risks of capture myopathy and stressors unique to nondomestic species.
- Rates of positive outcomes for CPR are lower in exotic and zoological species than domestic species; having realistic expectations and staff mental wellness resources supports a team's continued best performance and resiliency.

INTRODUCTION

Cardiopulmonary resuscitation (CPR) is a veterinary practitioner's last opportunity to intervene death in a patient. Historically, evidence-based recommendations for the practice of CPR have been lacking in veterinary medicine. Recently, an exhaustive review of veterinary and human literature was completed by the Reassessment Campaign on Veterinary Resuscitation (RECOVER) initiative, the result of which was generation of the first evidence-based consensus veterinary CPR guidelines.[1] These guidelines are rooted in domestic mammals, yet the techniques have proved useful in exotic and zoological species.[2,3] When using these guidelines, the exotic and zoo practitioner must adapt to unique challenges in patient anatomy and physiology. In addition, human safety precautions often limit delivery of patient care. This article

Disney's Animals, Science and Environment, 1200 North Savannah Circle, EastBay Lake, FL 32830, USA
E-mail address: natalie.h.hall@disney.com

Vet Clin Exot Anim 26 (2023) 737–750
https://doi.org/10.1016/j.cvex.2023.05.010 vetexotic.theclinics.com
1094-9194/23/

serves to review current evidence of CPR principles and provide guidance for adaptation to nondomestic patients. It is important to note that all CPR guidelines are living documents that evolve with time as new scientific evidence in both human and veterinary medicine becomes available. In addition, the presenting circumstances of a patient require assessment and interpretation by the practitioner to select the best course of treatment for optimal outcome. Therefore, these recommendations are not intended to be rigid protocols, but rather a foundation on which to build or adapt a patient care strategy.

For the purposes of this article, the terms avian and bird refer to class Aves; reptile refers to nonavian Sauropsida; lizard refers to non-Serpentes Squamata; snake refers to Serpentes; chelonian refers to Testudines; crocodilian refers to Crocodilia; amphibian refers to Amphibia; mammal refers to Mammalia; and rodent refers to Rodentia.

HOSPITAL AND TEAM PREPARATION

Delays in recognizing cardiopulmonary arrest (CPA) and initiating CPR negatively affect outcomes in neurological status and survival to discharge.[1] Preparing the hospital and field units for rapid emergency assessment is essential for a team's prompt and agile response. Standardizing equipment and medication storage allows teams to respond most efficiently, such as use of in-hospital crash carts and emergency field-grips containing organized and clearly labeled essential supplies.[1] Examinations and diagnostic events on exotic and zoological species are often done under anesthesia. For the briefest of patient procedures in a hospital, a rolling table may be dedicated and prepared with preselected intubation equipment, calculated doses of emergency drugs, vascular access supplies, and monitoring equipment. For small patients where medication waste is negligible, predrawing emergency drugs before a procedure is recommended, as it speeds their administration if needed. Anesthetic reversal drugs should be drawn up before anesthetic induction for the same reason. Keeping reversals close at hand in a standard location, such as a labeled container kept on or next to the anesthetic machine, can ensure any trained staff member can quickly locate and administer them. Clipboards with emergency drug dose sheets, the RECOVER or other CPR algorithm, and CPR data recording sheets may be included for quick reference. Having aids, such as a CPR algorithm poster on the wall, helps teams respond with a readily available, shared plan.[1]

For field procedures with large patients, one can prelabel syringes with emergency drug doses and keep them in a dedicated place, such as in the emergency supply grip. Likewise, reversal drugs can be kept in a small, distinguishable case in a consistent location, for example, the bin containing anesthetic monitoring equipment. A reference sheet with emergency drug doses can be preprinted based on the patient's estimated or actual weight and, similar to a hospital setup, kept on a clipboard with the RECOVER CPR algorithm and CPR recording sheets. Adding a timer to the clipboard helps the recorder to guide the team with timing CPR cycles when a wall-clock may not be present.

Team education can include husbandry personnel, such as kennel technicians and zookeepers that are routinely stationed at the hospital for inpatient care, so that they may provide support in roles such as drawing up emergency drugs, recording CPR data, timing CPR cycles, and, in some cases, performing chest compressions. Team rehearsals and drills speed response time and ensure that everyone is comfortable with both their own skill set as well as working as a team from the same workflow. Practicing techniques such as intraosseous catheter placement on necropsy specimens can build team skill and efficiency.

PATIENT ASSESSMENT

The first step in CPR is patient assessment. In a zoological setting, many patients are required to be under anesthesia for any physical evaluation, so a high percentage of the total CPA events are likely to occur during anesthesia. For prompt CPA recognition during anesthesia, it is important to have effective patient monitoring in place before the CPA event. Establishing standards of care by taxa and procedure (eg, intubation, intravenous [IV] catheter placement, anesthetic monitoring) provides a consistent baseline of patient assessment, ensures mechanisms are in use to recognize and rapidly address a CPA event, and helps staff overcome any hurdles of unfamiliarity with equipment and signal interpretation. In dogs (*Canis lupus familiaris*) and cats (*Felis catus*) undergoing CPR, end-tidal carbon dioxide (ETCO2) and electrocardiogram (ECG) are the primary anesthetic monitoring tools for assessing quality of CPR and patient response to CPR, and, thus, are recommended as a mainstay of anesthetic monitoring in most terrestrial nondomestic species. The practitioner may find other means more effective depending on the patient and working environment, such as cardiac ultrasound in aquatic species. In addition, the expected length of a procedure may dictate practicality of applying anesthetic monitoring equipment. A bird given a brief mask anesthesia solely to facilitate venipuncture may warrant having supplies available but not placed, as the time to apply the monitoring equipment would exceed the venipuncture time itself.

In nonanesthetized patients, access may be limited by safety concerns. Prevention of human injury takes precedence over patient care. When the patient status is unclear, it is preferable to delay approaching the patient to first ensure safety precautions are in place. Before entering any enclosure for an animal that could cause harm, patient mentation should be fully assessed, which may include response to vigorous or humanely noxious stimulus. Staff should don appropriate protective gear, use any indicated protective measures such as baffle boards/shields, and maintain access to enclosure exit points in case a patient suddenly rouses.

Once an unresponsive patient is determined to be safe for approach and handling, a rapid airway, breathing, and circulation assessment can be performed. This assessment is ideally limited to 5 to 10 seconds and then CPR is initiated if indicated.[1] Starting CPR erroneously is preferable to a more prolonged patient assessment.[1] Similar to evaluating mentation, the exotic and zoological practitioner must consider safety during airway assessment. For example, placing hands into the mouth of a possibly responsive animal should be avoided. Note that envenomation can still occur even from animals that are obtunded or deceased. Taxa considerations also include the value of time spent monitoring for respiration. Many air-breathing, aquatic vertebrates (eg, many *Anseriformes*) can exhibit a vagally mediated dive response, resulting in apnea and bradycardia.[4] A prolonged period of respiratory assessment may result in precious lost time. Likewise, because of the low respiratory frequency of many reptiles, time assessing ventilation is often a poor investment. In species that naturally have low respiratory frequency or natural periods of apnea, one may proceed directly to assessing for cardiac contractility and establishing airway access.

There are several means by which the practitioner can assess cardiac contractility. The best method for each patient varies based on anatomy, physiology, and presenting circumstances. Auscultation, whether by exterior or esophageal stethoscope (the latter placed under anesthesia), is the most traditional method and applies to many mammalian and avian species but can be compromised by large size or anatomic structures such as wide ribs, shells, or thick scales. When an ultrasound is at hand, due to preexisting procedure needs or happenstance, it is useful for quick assessment of cardiac contractility in most species, including birds.[5] Broad ribs and large size can preclude the usefulness of ultrasound in some macrofauna (eg, *Ceratotherium simum*). Another alternative for assessing cardiac contractility is via Doppler, although the sound fidelity can be lower quality than when auscultation is a viable option. The Doppler may be placed directly over the region of the heart, which is particularly useful in snakes and amphibians. In some lizards, the heart can be detected with the Doppler placed in the axillary region.[6] In Chelonia, placing a probe (the author prefers a pencil-style) in the cervical fossa medial to the forelimb and angling it toward midline allows for cardiac monitoring.[6] Peripheral pulse may also be assessed by Doppler. In many species, from rhinoceros (family *Rhinocerotidae*) and Nile hippopotamus (*Hippopotamus amphibious*) to small reptiles, the cornea may be lubricated with ultrasound gel and the Doppler placed gently on the cornea to detect retinal flow. In avian species, placing a Doppler over the brachial vessels is effective. With Chelonia and some lizards (eg, *Iguanidae*), the carotid can be monitored using a probe in the cervical region.[6] To the contrary, manual palpation of peripheral pulses is often unreliable and difficult for assessing systemic circulation and may be further inhibited by anesthetic effects.[1]

BASIC LIFE SUPPORT

Once CPA is suspected or confirmed, basic life support (BLS) should be initiated, which includes chest compressions, securing an airway, and providing ventilation. Small domestic species recommendations are to administer high-quality chest compressions at a rate of 100 to 120 per minute, at a depth of one-third to one-half the width of the chest, delivered in uninterrupted cycles of 2 minutes, with ventilation at a rate of 10 breaths/min.[1] Discussion of BLS in zoological species follows in the later section.

Chest compressions should be initiated as soon as possible on recognition of CPA.[1] Historically, airway maintenance was the most prioritized among the processes of CPR. However, human studies on outcomes of CPR with only chest compressions caused a change in the prioritization of CPR steps to circulation-airway maintenance-respiration according to the 2005 American Heart Association guidelines.[7] Based on this evidence, chest compressions are also recommended as the initial step in veterinary CPR. To perform quality chest compressions, the veterinarian must consider patient anatomy, patient positioning, compressor hand placement, and technique.

There are 2 main theories describing how external chest compressions generate blood flow during CPR.[8] In the cardiac pump theory, the cardiac ventricles are directly compressed to generate cardiac output. With patients in dorsal recumbency, this occurs between the sternum and the spine; in lateral recumbency, this occurs between the ribs. The thoracic pump theory suggests that during chest compression, the overall intrathoracic pressure is increased, which compresses the aorta and vena cava, pushing blood out of the thorax; this is followed by elastic recoil of the chest, during which subatmospheric intrathoracic pressure creates a pressure gradient, generating flow of peripheral blood back into the thorax and, therefore, into the lungs. The practitioner can elect either method depending on patient thoracic conformation, and both mechanisms likely have a positive effect on blood flow in many of the studied domestic mammals.[1]

In mammals with very rounded chests or large mammals, direct compression of the heart with external chest compressions is unlikely to be achieved. Therefore, the thoracic pump technique can be performed by compressing over the widest portion of the chest to create an effective increase in intrathoracic pressure followed by allowing elastic recoil.[1] Although compression is performed with the hands in many animals, in very large animals such as giant eland (*Taurotragus derbianus*) or giraffe (*Giraffa spp*), the author has had staff repeatedly sit in a forceful squat (facing away from the patient; immediately caudal to the thoracic limbs) on the mid- to ventral thorax. In one patient, this was observed to generate a rectally palpable aortic pulse. The cardiac pump theory may be used in patients with anatomy that permits direct cardiac compression; this is the recommended compression technique for mammals with a laterally compressed thorax or keel-shaped thorax (eg, *Acinonyx jubatus*) by placing the patient in lateral recumbency (right or left) with the hands directly over the heart.[1] In mammals with a ventrodorsally compressed thorax (eg, *Colobus spp*, *Choloepus spp*), place the patient in dorsal recumbency to administer sternal compressions with the hands or fingers (depending on patient size) placed over the heart. The technique with fingers in small patients is similar to human infant CPR techniques.[1] Lastly, in small mammals (eg, *Suricata suricatta* or *Mustela furo*) with higher thoracic wall compliance, effective cardiac compressions can be achieved using a one-hand technique, with the compressor's fingers wrapped around the sternum at the level of the heart to generate a circumferential cardiac compression.[1]

Conflicting theoretical debate is present in the literature regarding potential impacts of thoracic compressions in birds, given the presence of the large keel, lack of a diaphragm, rigid lung parenchyma, and delicate tissues (note that large Palaeognathae species are generally excluded from these discussions). A recent study in chickens (*Gallus gallus*), however, has shown that sternal (keel) compressions with the chicken in dorsal recumbency paired with interposed caudal coelomic compressions resulted in increases in arterial blood pressure up to 28% of the bird's baseline anesthetized values.[3] Although some chickens experienced cloacal prolapse and/or egg expulsion and, rarely, hepatic fractures due to compressions, there was no gross evidence of pulmonary contusions or follicular rupture. Contrarily, lateral compressions generated significantly less arterial pressure, and another study suggests high rates of grossly visible internal hemorrhage due to lateral compressions in small bird species (*Passer domesticus* and *Sturnus vulgaris*).[3,9] A "wing flap" technique has been proposed in birds to promote blood flow through the vascular flight muscles, but, pilot studies of this have not shown evidence of this generating blood pressure.[3,10] Because of these collective findings, current recommendations for most avian species are to administer sternal compressions.

In the context of nonavian, adiaphragmatic animals such as amphibians and most reptiles, it stands to reason the cardiac pump theory may hold true, where direct, physical compression of the ventricle may generate cardiac output in lieu of spontaneous heart contractility. Given the significant variability in cardiac location between orders, it is important for the clinician to confirm cardiac location before initiating compressions. The heart lies within the thoracic girdle in many lizards, cranial to the liver in snakes, in close proximity to the liver in crocodilians, plus other variations based on behavioral physiology and habitat adaptations.[11] In shelled animals, such as Chelonia, or specimens with significant osteoderms, cardiac compressions may not be feasible.

The quality of cardiac compressions during CPR is important to generate sufficient cardiac output. The staff performing compressions must have proper positioning of their own body in order to perform with best technique; this can include use of a footstool to gain elevation over a patient on an examination table, or the patient may be quickly relocating to the floor. When using a large hydraulic table, the table may need to be lowered and/or the compressor may need to kneel on the table adjacent to the patient. It is also essential (especially in very large and very small patients) to remove all blankets, towels, and padding from beneath the patient receiving compressions, as it is essential to translate all kinetic energy into blood movement rather than compressing materials under the animal. As conscientious veterinary teams often provide very comfortable set-ups for patients before an arrest, remembering to remove these items when CPR is initiated can help assure optimal compressions.

In dogs and cats, the evidence-based recommendation is a compression rate of 100 to 120 per minute.[1] It remains to be explored whether or not a higher rate of chest compressions is appropriate for small mammals (eg, *Oryctolagus sp*) that have higher resting heart rates than studied domestic species.[12] Likewise, avian species may benefit from a higher compression rate, such as 150 bpm.[3] On the other end of the spectrum, some snakes have a relatively low cardiac output due to a low heart rate but with a similar pulmonary and systemic stroke volume compared with mammals and birds, whereas Varanidae are thought to function more similarly to mammals.[13,14] Appropriate cardiac compression rates for taxa with cardiac contractility resting rates significantly different than domestic animals need further exploration. In domestic species, the evidence-based recommendation is to perform deep chest compressions of one-third to one-half the width of the thorax in most patients, which is reasonable to apply to most exotic and zoological species.[1] Of note, studies indicate a common tendency for persons to lean on the patient, preventing full elastic recoil of the thorax between chest compressions and reducing coronary and cerebral perfusion.[1] Regardless of the elected rate, depth, and technique, it is important that thoracic recoil is permitted.

After initiating compressions, securing an airway and providing ventilation are the next steps; this is aimed at reducing both hypoxia and hypercapnia, both of which can lessen the likelihood of return of spontaneous circulation (ROSC). Because pauses in chest compressions can be deleterious to their effectiveness, it is recommended that animals be intubated during active chest compressions.[1] Reviewing intubation techniques for specific nondomestic species is beyond the scope of this article, but there are alternatives to consider that are somewhat unique to these nontraditional patients and useful when intubation is inherently difficult due to patient anatomy. Tight-fitting face masks have been shown to provide effective respiratory support in rabbits (*Oryctolagus cuniculus*) during CPR and is likely applicable to other obligate nasal-breathing species.[2] Using this technique can reduce the delay in starting chest compressions or minimizing interruptions to chest compressions.[2] Laryngeal masks may also be applied if a sufficient seal can be generated; this is an appropriate option in particular avian species for which tracheal strictures secondary to intubation is considered a risk. Verifying endotracheal intubation in a CPR setting can be challenging because ETCO2 measurements are altered. In addition to direct visualization to confirm placement, a Beck Airway Airflow Monitor may be used to confirm placement by airway movement generated during chest compressions. Although mouth-to-snout ventilation has been recommended in domestic species until intubation can be performed, this is not feasible for many nondomestic species due to human safety issues with potentially harmful anatomic structures, zoonotic disease risks, large patient lung volumes exceeding human respiratory capacity, or small patient size rendering this impractical.

Air sac cannulas are an effective alternative to intubation in most avian and some reptile species, and techniques for placement have been well described.[15,16] In a CPA presentation, this can be quickly accomplished using an 18-Ga catheter inserted into the caudal thoracic or abdominal air sac, including very small avian patients.[10] Even with positive pressure ventilation, it is important to avoid pressure on the patient's body so as to allow thoracic skeleton and coelomic expansion for proper ventilatory flow in species with air sacs.[17] In birds, dorsal recumbency can decrease tidal volume, particularly if there are abnormal coelomic structures that may compress the air sacs and reduce their effective volume.[18,19] As a result, upright or ventral recumbency may better promote ventilation and may be appropriate once cardiac/thoracic compressions are no longer needed.[19]

Ventilation rate may also vary between species. A ventilation rate of 10 breaths per minute with a tidal volume of 10 mL/kg and a short inspiratory time of 1 second is recommended in dogs and cats.[1] Exceeding these recommendations in any dimension can increase mean intrathoracic pressure, which reduces venous return and decreases cerebral and coronary perfusion. These effects have been linked with poorer outcomes in people during CPR.[1] However, in small mammals, a respiratory rate of 20 to 30 bpm has been suggested, and appropriate rates in animals with naturally higher ventilation rates need further exploration.[17] For birds, recommendations have been made to ventilate at 10 to 12 breaths per minute. During positive-pressure ventilation, care should be taken to avoid airway pressures greater than 15 to 20 cm H2O to prevent volutrauma to the air sacs.[17] Similarly, reptiles have thinner lung tissues, many with less exterior muscular and skeletal support, so care must be taken not to damage pulmonary tissues by overexpansion during positive-pressure ventilation.[20] Reptile respiratory drive can be reduced by administration of supplemental oxygen.[21] However, in the case of CPR, administering supplemental oxygen is expected to be most beneficial in order to reduce hypoxia. Because positive pressure ventilation is being administered during CPR, the concern for spontaneous respiratory drive is of low priority in the moment of CPR. In addition, the clinician should evaluate the likelihood of cardiopulmonary shunting in reptile patients, which may inhibit the intentions of positive pressure ventilation, discussed further later.[14,22]

If enough staff is present, interposed abdominal compressions can be performed, assuming patient anatomy and positioning permits. In humans with cardiac arrest due to brady-systole or pulseless electrical activity (PEA), intermittent abdominal compressions have been shown to increase “diastolic” arterial pressure.[23] The technique, initially described as a method to increase cardiac output during CPR in domestic dogs, is performed by midabdominal compressions interposed with thoracic compressions, resulting in a depression of the abdomen of at least 50%.[24] In addition to improving arterial pressures, in pigs (*Sus domesticus*), abdominal compressions alone generated significant ventilatory volumes and, when compared with chest compressions, created equivalent, or larger, coronary perfusion pressure.[25] A technique for interposed coelomic compressions (ICC) in birds has also been described with positive results.[3] In birds with anatomy that permits ICC, this technique is a recommended adjunct to keel compressions. Further studies of interposed abdominal compressions are needed, including species with a large rumen or other fermentative stomach, where abdominal compressions may increase the risk of gastric reflux and aspiration.

Human literature shows better survival and neurological outcomes when BLS is performed as uninterrupted cycles of 2 minutes versus shorter cycles with more frequent interruptions to chest compressions.[1] Therefore, veterinary recommendations for dogs and cats are that chest compressions should be performed in 2-minute cycles without interruption in intubated patients. After each 2-minute cycle, a brief patient reassessment can be performed. During this time, rotating the staff performing the chest compressions can help avoid the effects of fatigue that compromise the quality of compressions.[1] Communication between the person performing compressions and the next-in-line staff is helpful for a smooth and fast transition during these breaks. In large patients when using the squat technique, which is very physically demanding, staff may need to trade turns more often due to fatigue. Solid communication including counting compressions aloud in a 3-2-1-swap fashion can minimize any missed "beats" midcycle. Until there is evidence to the contrary, it is appropriate to extrapolate the 2-minute cycle recommendation across nondomestic species as best as possible.

ADVANCED LIFE SUPPORT

After initiating BLS to support systemic circulation, a functional airway, and ventilation, the next steps in CPR include methods for advanced life support (ALS), which include placing patient monitoring equipment. Monitoring enables a team to assess the quality of the CPR, make needed adjustments for optimal CPR administration, tailor CPR to patient presentation, and identify ROSC.

ETCO2 monitoring is applicable to patients of all sizes and helps assess cardiac output being generated during CPR. Familiarity with normal and abnormal waveforms aids in patient respiratory assessment. Direct or side stream methods may be used. For a quick side stream measurement, an 18-gauge needle can be inserted into the lumen of the endotracheal tube, taking care not to obstruct air flow.[26] Nasal capnography is reported to have good correlation with $Paco_2$ in rabbits, suggesting that nasal capnography can be used in obligate nasal breathers when not endotracheally intubated.[27] In small domestic species, the goal of CPR is to produce at least 30% of normal cardiac output, so one can aim for 30% of normal ETCO2 output with quality CPR.[1] If values quickly elevate, this can signal ROSC.

ECG is essential for characterizing cardiac arrhythmias associated with CPA including electromechanical dissociation, now known as PEA, asystole, and ventricular fibrillation.[1] Needle ECG leads are ideal for a wide variety of patients, including small rodents, reptiles, and species with thick, poorly conductive epidermis (eg, *Orycteropus afer, Diceros bicornis*). Needle ECG leads can be purchased as manufactured, or metal alligator clips can be attached to a hypodermic needle placed into the skin. In small patients, this technique is helpful to avoid the use of conductive gels that can cause significant evaporative cooling.[28] Electrocardiographic techniques have been described in avian species, and, similar to small mammals, the leads can be attached via hypodermic needles at the base of each wing and femorotibiotarsal joint.[17] References for ECG lead placement in reptiles have been published, although hypothermia may be a common presenting factor in moribund reptiles that may complicate interpretation.[29]

Some frequently used anesthetic monitoring tools are less helpful during a CPR event. Although blood gases are highly valuable in anesthetic monitoring, during CPR they are expected to be aberrant from normal, and peripheral values may not be reflective of core circulation values. In the author's experience, obtaining peripheral blood gases during CPR has not provided significant benefit more than ETCO2 and ECG. Also, obtaining and testing a sample for blood gases requires labor that is often better expended in other efforts. However, once ROSC occurs, blood gases are very helpful to guide supportive care choices. Peripheral pulse oximetry becomes nonfunctional in a CPA setting because poor peripheral perfusion and lack of pulsatile flow limit functionality of the equipment. Interpretation in a prearrest patient can be complicated by peripheral effects of anesthetics, and finding a functional anatomic location for the probe is difficult in some species. Therefore, pulse oximetry is not recommended for CPR monitoring.

In addition to placing useful patient monitoring equipment, obtaining vascular access is another part of providing advanced life support to permit a rapid route of medication administration. It is ideal to have IV catheter placement as a standard in anesthetized patients to avoid delaying delivery of drugs. However, as CPA can occur at times of anesthetic induction or not in association with anesthesia, this is not always feasible. In addition, some procedures may be so brief that the practitioner must weigh the benefit of IV access versus additional anesthetic time. At minimum, having catheter supplies prepared and readily available next to the patient, such as on a rolling table or in a portable field grip, is recommended as a standard of practice.

Techniques for IV catheters in mammalian, avian, and reptile species have been described, and location varies by species. If readily accessible, an ultrasound for guiding catheter placement is helpful, particularly in species with thick skin or vessels deeply embedded in surrounding tissues. Although immediate metabolism of vasopressors during CPR is not a significant concern, it is important to remember species with a hepatic portal system and/or renal portal system should have vascular access in a location that will not allow excretion or metabolism of administered drugs before systemic delivery.

In animals where IV access is difficult, intraosseous (IO) catheters are a useful alternative. Techniques for IO catheter placement in mammals can be applied for neonates, small mammalian species, or mammals in extreme peripheral circulatory collapse. Intraosseous catheters can be easier to maintain during frequent patient movement, such as during cardiac compressions, because of the protection and stability provided by the medullary cavity.[28] Including IO catheters, such as 25- to 18-gauge needles with wire stylets that are already sterilized, in emergency supplies can speed placement in the critical patient.[28] In rodents, common IO catheter sites include the femur, through the trochanteric fossa, or the tibia, through the tibial crest.[28] In animals large enough, intraosseous catheter drills can be used to facilitate rapid placement; this is particularly useful when animals present in acute hypovolemic shock and rapid IV catheter placement is not feasible.

In birds, IO catheters can be quickly placed in the ulna or tibia, taking care to avoid pneumatized bones. Note that in some avian species (eg, *Pelecanus spp*) the ulna is pneumatized so that medications delivered in this location will not reach systemic circulation as desired. IO catheters can be placed in reptiles also, for example, by using the tibia in crocodilians and lizards.[29] The plastron, at the rostral aspect just lateral to midline, or in the region of the bridge between the plastron and carapace, may be used in Chelonia. Charts have been published for various additional IO and IV locations useful in reptiles.[29] Once vascular access is obtained, vasopressors, anesthetic reversals, and other medications may be administered IV or IO for the most rapid effect.

If IV or IO access cannot be obtained in sufficient time or is not feasible due to extremely small patient size, intratracheal drug administration for epinephrine, vasopressin, or atropine may be performed.[1] Use of a long catheter advanced to or beyond the level of the carina is recommended for administration over use of a shorter catheter or directly administering medication into the endotracheal tube to obtain higher plasma concentrations of drug.[1] If the intratracheal route is used, drugs should be diluted with saline or sterile water to facilitate drug distribution. In addition, increased doses of up to 10x standard doses (in the case of epinephrine) have been suggested.[1] Although intratracheal techniques may be particularly useful for patients of small size, some patients may be too small for the aforementioned techniques, such as the catheter and saline dilution, to be applicable, resulting in infusion through the endotracheal tube being the only practical option for intratracheal administration. Intracardiac administration of medications may be considered if there is no other alternative route available. The benefit of this must be weighed against the pause in chest compressions required for administration.

Literature on pharmacokinetics/dynamics of rescue drugs is intermittent and rare in zoological species. As a general practice, the author follows standard mammalian protocols as described in the RECOVER guidelines.[1] Of note, when a vagolytic effect is desired, glycopyrrolate is recommended for rabbits due to the presence of an atropinase enzyme that can reduce the effect/duration of atropine. However, the significance of this in a CPR context has not been evaluated.[2] The author should also be aware that epinephrine administration in snapping turtles (*Chelydra serpentine*) and alligators (*Alligator mississippiensis*) has been shown to hasten recovery from inhalant anesthetics.[22] Periods of apnea in many reptiles increases pulmonary resistance, which triggers diversion of blood into systemic circulation rather than pulmonary circulation.[14] Administration of epinephrine reverses this effect, likely through abolishing pulmonary to systemic shunting.[22,30] In species for which shunting is a known or suspected mechanism, early administration of epinephrine during CPR is indicated to facilitate ventilation.

An in-depth discussion on defibrillation is beyond the scope of this article. Defibrillation is recommended in certain presentations of CPA and has potential to be beneficial in avian species.[1,3] When considering whether or not to invest in hospital defibrillator, it is important to consider team training and safety. Particularly with large zoological species, a procedure can involve many people who all must be educated on defibrillator safety with clear communication protocols in place before use. It is important to note that many standard defibrillators do not have a range that is low enough for the recommended energy level in small exotic patients.[17] Also worth consideration is the type of CPA presentations that occur in a practice. Some zoological institutions do not have species with significant rates of cardiac disease; therefore, presentations of arrhythmias are rare and most CPAs may present as asystole or PEA. As a result, indications for use of a defibrillator may be extremely rare. When an appropriate defibrillator is not available, administration of a precordial thump is a less-effective but possibly beneficial alternative that may be applied to many nondomestic patients.

Administration of fluids during CPR requires careful consideration. Many nondomestic species presenting on emergency may exhibit extreme dehydration, particularly in settings where husbandry care has been suboptimal. In these cases, fluid administration or transfusion may be appropriate. In euvolemic patients, fluid administration may best be limited to avoid increasing cardiac afterload when the goal is to promote cardiac output. Patients such as those that have already received some fluids as part of their anesthetic plan or those with acute-onset CPR with no fluid loss may benefit most from not having fluids administered during CPR. In patients known to be anemic and when resources are available, transfusion may be preferred to IV fluid administration.

In domestic species, additional drug therapies are described for specific presentations leading to CPA, such as hyperkalemia secondary to urinary obstruction, and similar approaches may apply to nondomestic species. The practitioner must consider the species needs in addition to the presenting conditions to determine additional drug therapies for advanced life support. For example, hypoglycemia in frugivorous species, hypocalcemia in egg-bearing species, and hypomagnesemia in some hoofstock may all be immediately relevant considerations for triage of disease predisposing to CPA. Drugs traditionally used in domestic species may also not be appropriate in particular exotic or zoological species, and the degree of corrective treatment often needs to be done in context with patient metabolic rate. Reptiles and some other poikilotherms have buffering mechanisms in place to withstand high levels of lactic acid accumulation, particularly in diving species.[31] In these patients, exuberant, rapid correction of a lactic acidosis may result in overshooting into an alkalosis, which could be a more challenging physiological state than one for which the animal is naturally adapted to compensate. In this case, a more gradual, titrated treatment of acidosis may be more appropriate. Temperature is an important consideration, particularly for poikilotherms. For example, a cold reptile may have difficulty maintaining cardiac output.[31] Species differences and preferred optimal temperature zones affect emergency treatment such as warming or not warming poikilotherm in shock.

RECOVER guidelines recommend assessing response to CPR no more frequently than at 2-minute intervals, which is based on the need to maintain cardiac compressions for optimizing outcome.[1] The author follows this practice across species, as there is no other evidence at this time in nondomestic taxa. The number of 2-minute "rounds" to pursue CPR is best determined by the veterinarian's evaluation of patient response, treatment needs, and prognosis within the context of husbandry requirements and the patient's history. For example, a bird that will not be able to thrive in an aviary flock and is not amenable to solo housing or frequent handling may be transitioned to a do-not-resuscitate case if an immediate response to CPR is not observed, whereas a pet psittacine may warrant multiple rounds of CPR. Similarly, open-chest CPR is frequently not a viable option for nondomestic patients due to anatomy or the patient being intolerant of the implicit postcare needs.

POSTARREST CARE CONSIDERATIONS

Although some species are excellent candidates for referrals to intensive care centers postarrest, many nondomestic species are not amenable to referral due to stress from handling, habitat change, isolation, or transport. Therefore, zoological institutions should consider the level of care they wish to provide and evaluate on-property facilities to meet these needs, such as padded stalls with hanging fluid options, oxygen-supplemented incubators, and so forth. Prolonged postcardiac arrest care is frequently limited in zoological settings by human safety concerns. A frank discussion with exotic pet owners should also be undertaken to determine their comfort level with prolonged hospitalization and intensive at-home care if their pet requires CPR and survives. Therefore, postarrest monitoring and supportive care must be tailored to each individual patient.

In patients that must promptly be returned to an enclosure with no further handling, it is helpful to confirm all desired treatments have been administered before patient release. These treatments can include hemodynamic optimization strategies, such as blood transfusions. Parenteral administration of long-acting analgesics and long-acting antibiotics is useful in many situations where a patient may not be readily accessible after return to a habitat or enclosure. Neuroleptics can reduce risk of capture myopathy and improve patient tolerance for hospitalization. Capture myopathy effects can be immediate or delayed, which can complicate interpretation of patient response to therapy. In addition, it can make decisions difficult around if and when a repeat of hands-on intervention is indicated. Having a program to proactively train animals for medical behaviors can improve patient tolerance for human interaction and permit more opportunities for providing supportive care interventions or assessments. For example, having large Felidae trained for blood collection from the tail can provide an opportunity for a post-CPA assessment.

OUTCOMES AND TEAM SUPPORT

It is helpful for the nondomestic practitioner to be aware that the reported rates of positive outcomes of CPR in their unique patients differ from domestic species. This knowledge may help manage team expectations and responses to CPR outcomes. In dogs and cats, survival to discharge rates range from 2% to 6%.[32,33] In dogs and cats, patients that arrest in the perianesthetic period have a markedly better prognosis, as high as 47% survival to discharge, than patients that arrest because of other causes.[33] In exotic companion animals the rate to survival to discharge is significantly lower and was recently reported to be 1.3% for animals that entered CPA while at the hospital. It is suggested that the biggest challenges to positive outcomes in nondomestic species might be effective chest compression, airway management, and monitoring as well as establishment of intravenous catheterization routes.[34] As clinical techniques are better honed in zoological species, it is expected that outcomes of CPR will improve.

Providing a debriefing period for staff after a CPR event can be helpful for supporting quality CPR in practice. Techniques such as SWOT (strengths/weaknesses/opportunities/threats) analysis have been shown to improve patient outcomes in human care.[35] In zoos, keepers and veterinary staff often develop intense bonds with animals. With any critical patient event, there can be emotional impacts for the veterinary staff and husbandry teams. Support for team's mental wellness is vital to team's long-term resiliency and continued best performance. Small domestic animal clinics are more and more engaging the services of social workers that would also undoubtedly benefit exotic owners as well. Resources to promote mental well-being (eg, GRAZE for zoo and aquarium employees) and providing access to grief counselors for processing patient loss can promote team recovery in times when CPR is not successful. Reassurance for the team can be gained by practicing evidence-based CPR so it is known by the team that the opportunity for best possible outcome is provided by and for all.

CLINICS CARE POINTS

- Preparation for anesthesia includes being ready for a possible CPA event, including drawing up anesthetic reversal drugs, calculating emergency drug doses, and having intubation equipment prepared even for mask-only or injectable-only procedures.
- The RECOVER CPR algorithm may be applied to most zoological species.
- When the species permits, $ETCO_2$ monitoring and ECG are most useful to guide CPR administration.
- Before approaching any zoological patient, human safety precautions should be in place. Patient mentation should be fully evaluated before entering enclosures of potentially dangerous species.
- Many zoo species may have natural periods of apnea or low respiratory rates, making a ventilation assessment difficult or impractical. The initial patient assessment should be brief at 5 to 10 seconds before proceeding to CPR if indicated.
- For most species, apply RECOVER guidelines to compress the chest at a rate of 100 to 120 per minute and a depth of 1/3 to ½ the chest width, in 2-minute cycles, with a ventilation rate of 10 breaths per minute.
- Place IV or IO catheters for administration of emergency drugs. Intratracheal administration is a less-preferred but potentially effective route of administration.
- In patients with pulmonary to systemic shunting, such as crocodilians and turtles, early epinephrine administration is indicated to facilitate effective ventilation.
- Human safety and patient accessibility for intensive treatment in a post-CPR setting will guide care and timelines for stopping resuscitative efforts in zoological species.
- Team debriefs and mental wellness support after CPR events are vital for team resiliency and sustaining best performance.

DISCLOSURE

The author has no affiliations to disclose.

REFERENCES

1. Fletcher D., Boller M., Brainard B., et al., RECOVER evidence and knowledge gap analysis on veterinary CPR. Part 7: Clinical guidelines, *J Vet Emerg Crit Care*, 22 (S1), 2012, 102–131.
2. Buckley G, DeCubellis J, Sharp C, et al. Cardiopulmonary resuscitation in hospitalized rabbits: 15 cases. J Exot Pet Med 2011;20:46–50.
3. Eisenbarth J., Cummings C., Rozanski E., et al., Evaluation of cardiac compression techniques for cardiopulmonary resuscitation in laying hens (Gallus gallus). In: IVECCS Forum Proceedings, September 7-11, 2022, San Antonio, Texas.
4. Butler P, Jones D. Onest of and recovery from diving bradycardia in ducks. J Vet Physiology 1968;196:255–72.
5. Straub J, Forbes N, Pees M, et al. Pulsed-wave Doppler-derived velocity of diastolic ventricular inflow and systolic aortic outflow in raptors. Vet Rec 2004;154: 145–7.
6. Music M, Strunk A. Reptile critical care and common emergencies. Vet Clin Exot Anim 2016;19:591–612.
7. Iwami T., Kawamura T., Hiraide A., et al., Effectiveness of bystander-initiated cardiac-only resuscitation for patients with out-of-hospital cardiac arrest, *Circulation*, 116, 2007, 2900–2907.
8. Tucker KJ, Savitt MA, Idris A, et al. Cardiopulmonary resuscitation. Historical perspectives, physiology, and future directions. Arch Intern Med 1994;154(19): 2141–50.
9. Paul-Murphy JR, Engilis A Jr, Pascoe PJ, et al. Comparison of intraosseous pentobarbital administration and thoracic compression for euthanasia of anesthetized sparrows (*Passer domesticus*) and starlings (*Sturnus vulgaris*). Am J Vet Res 2017;78(8):887–99.
10. Crawford A., Ableson A., Gladden J., et al., Retrospective evaluation of cardiopulmonary arrest and resuscitation in hospitalized birds: 41 cases (2006-2019), *J Vet Emerg Crit Care*, 32, 2022, 491–499.
11. Jacobson E. Overview of reptile biology, anatomy, and histology. In: Jacobson E, editor. Infectious diseases and pathology of reptiles. Boca Raton: CRC; 2007. p. 1–130.
12. Marano G, Grigioni M, Tiburzi F, et al. Effects of isoflurane on cardiovascular system and sympathovagal balance in New Zealand white rabbits. J Cardiovasc Pharmacol 1996;28:513–8.
13. Jensen B, Moorman A, Wang T. Structure and function of the hearts of lizards and snakes. Biol Rev 2014;89:302–36.
14. Burggren W, Farrell A, Lillywhite H. Vertebrate cardiovascular systems. In: Dantzler W, editor. Comprehensive physiology. Hoboken: John Wiley & Sons, Inc; 1998. p. 215–308.
15. Myers D, Wellehan J, Isaza R. Saccular lung cannulation in a ball python (*Python regius*) to treat a tracheal obstruction. J Zoo Wildl Med 2009;40:214–6.
16. Gunkel C, Lafortune M. Current Techniques in Avian Anesthesia. Sem Av Exot Pet Med 2005;14:263–76.
17. Costello M. Principles of cardiopulmonary cerebral resuscitation in special species. Sem Av Exot Pet Med 2004;13:132–41.

18. King A, Payne D. The maximum capacities of the lungs and air sacs of *Gallus domesticus*. J Anat 1962;96:495–503.
19. Gonzalez M, Carrasco D. Emergencies and critical care of commonly kept fowl. Vet Clin Exot Anim 2016;19:543–65.
20. Sladky K, Mans C. Clinical anesthesia in reptiles. J Exot Pet Med 2012;12:17–31.
21. Schumacher J. Reptile respiratory medicine. Vet Clin Exot Anim 2003;6:213–31.
22. Goe A., Shmalberg J., Gatson B., et al., Epinephrine or GV-26 electrical stimulation reduces inhalant anesthetic recovery time in common snapping turtles (*Chelydra serpentine*), *J Zoo Wildl Med*, 47, 2016, 501–507.
23. Groeneveld A. Haemodynamic effect of intermittent abdominal compression during cardiopulmonary resuscitation in the critically ill. Clin Intensive Care 2003;14: 25–30.
24. Ralston S, Babbs C. Cardiopulmonary resuscitation with interposed abdominal compression in dogs, . Weldon School of Biomedical Engineering Faculty Publications, Paper 38. West Lafayette, Indiana: Purdue University; 1982.
25. Pargett M, Geddes L, Otlewski M, et al. Rhythmic abdominal compression CPR ventilates without supplemental breaths and provides effective blood circulation. Resuscitation 2008;79:460–7.
26. Allweiler S. How to improve anesthesia and analgesia in small mammals. Vet Clin Exot Anim 2016;19:361–77.
27. Evans J, Hogg M, Rosen M, et al. Correlation of alveolar PCO_2 estimated by infrared analysis and arterial PCO_2 in the human neonate and the rabbit. Br J Anaesth 1977;49:761–4.
28. Hawkins M, Graham J. Emergency and critical care of rodents. Vet Clin Exot Anim 2007;10:501–31.
29. Martinez-Jimenez D, Hernandez-Divers S. Emergency care of reptiles. Vet Clin Exot Anim 2007;10:557–85.
30. Gatson B, Goe A, Granone T, et al. Intramuscular epinephrine results in reduced anesthetic recovery time in American alligators (*Alligator mississippiensis*) undergoing isoflurane anesthesia. J Zoo Wildl Med 2017;48:55–61.
31. Long S. Approach to reptile emergency medicine. Vet Clin Exot Anim 2016;19: 567–90.
32. Kass P, Haskins S. Survival following cardiopulmonary resuscitation in dogs and cats. J Vet Emerg Crit Care 1992;2:57–65.
33. Hofmeister E, Brainard B, Egger C, et al. Prognostic indicators for dogs and cats with cardiopulmonary arrest treated by cardiopulmonary cerebral resuscitation at a university teaching hospital. J Am Vet Med Assoc 2009;235:50–7.
34. Onuma M, Kondo H, Ono S, et al. Retrospective investigation of cardiopulmonary resuscitation outcome in 146 exotic animals. J Vet Med Sci 2017;79:1611–4.
35. Wu C, Wu L, Jin P. Effect of SWOT analysis combined with the medical and nursing integration emergency nursing process on emergency treatment efficiency and prognosis of patients with acute myocardial infarction. Emerg Med Int 2022;2022:6.

Coagulation Disorders, Testing, and Treatment in Exotic Animal Critical Care

Kathryn L. Perrin, BVetMed, PhD, DACZM, DECZM (Zoo Health Management)

KEYWORDS

• Coagulation • Coagulopathy • DIC • Fibrinolysis • Hemostasis • Thrombosis • Transfusion

KEY POINTS

- Disorders of the 3 components of hemostasis; the vasculature, coagulation proteins, and platelets, can affect any vertebrate species.
- Hemostatic disorders are underrecognized in exotic animal medicine due to a lack of access to validated diagnostic assays.
- Advances in understanding of hemostasis in veterinary patients allow better recognition and management of coagulopathies.

INTRODUCTION

Hemostasis is the complex system through which perfusion of blood is maintained in the event of vascular injury. Interactions between the vasculature, platelets/thrombocytes, and plasma proteins result in primary hemostasis, secondary hemostasis and fibrinolysis.[1] Coagulopathy is a broad term covering a spectrum of disorders with increased risk of bleeding and/or increased risk of thrombosis. Coagulopathies result from an imbalance between clot formation and breakdown, a process which is tightly controlled in the healthy individual. The primary trigger for *coagulation*, the formation of a fibrin-platelet clot or thrombus, is the exposure of circulating platelets and proteins to sub-endothelial tissue factor. Coagulation serves to seal a localized vascular lesion to prevent further blood loss. The clot is then broken down via *fibrinolysis*, as soon as possible to prevent unnecessary impedance to blood flow. A disturbance in the hemostatic system can cause hypercoagulable, hypocoagulable and/or hyper- or hypofibrinolytic states, which may result in detrimental clotting or bleeding.[1] While differences in hemostatic pathways do exist between taxonomic groups, the fundamental principles of coagulation are conserved across vertebrate taxa.[2] There is a perception that

San Diego Zoo Wildlife Alliance, Veterinary Services, 15500 San Pasqual Valley Road, Escondido, CA 92027, USA
E-mail address: Klperrin01@gmail.com

Vet Clin Exot Anim 26 (2023) 751–769
https://doi.org/10.1016/j.cvex.2023.05.006

coagulopathies are rare in exotic species; however, most clinicians have managed anticoagulant rodenticide exposures, bacterial sepsis, or a patient with hepatic disease that bled for longer than expected after blood sampling (**Box 1**). Coagulopathies are likely under-recognized in exotic animal medicine due to a variety of factors, including the lack of access to validated diagnostic tests. Understanding the basic principles of hemostasis and hemostatic disorders will guide the clinician in selecting appropriate diagnostics in order to identify and manage coagulopathies.

PHYSIOLOGIC HEMOSTASIS AND COAGULOPATHY

Hemostasis, both coagulation and fibrinolysis, is conserved to varying degrees across vertebrate taxa.[2] There are continual advances in understanding of hemostasis in humans and animals, and only basic principles will be outlined here. Recent reviews of avian[3] and small mammal[4] hemostasis are available, while only preliminary investigations have been performed in reptiles.[5–7] In a healthy individual, physiologically active tissue factor is only expressed on cells outside of blood vessels.[8,9] The initiation phase of coagulation occurs when damage to a blood vessel exposes circulating platelets and proteins to *tissue factor*, a protein cofactor expressed on the surface

Box 1
Examples of potential causes of hemostatic disorders in non-domestic animals

Degenerative
- Hepatopathy
- Chronic kidney disease

Anomalous
- Hyperestrogenism
- Congenital clotting factor deficiencies

Metabolic
- Heat stroke/hyperthermia
- Hypothermia
- Shock

Neoplastic

Nutritional
- Hypervitaminosis E

Infectious and inflammatory
- Sepsis – bacterial, viral, fungal
- Viral - Rabbit hemorrhagic disease, influenza viruses, herpesviruses
- Parasitic - Rickettsial disease, hepatic coccidiosis

Traumatic
- Trauma
- Thermal burns

Toxic
- Anticoagulant rodenticides
- Drugs – Benzimidazoles, aspirin, chloramphenicol, polysulfated glycosaminoglycans
- Envenomation
- Aflatoxin

Vascular
- Cardiac disease
- Vasculitis
- Vitamin C deficiency
- Ischemia

of many extravascular cells.[10] Procoagulant plasma proteins, often referred to as clotting factors, circulate as inactive proenzymes (zymogens) which require activation.[2] The exception to this is factor VII for which a small percentage is circulating in the active form, VIIa. The cascade model of coagulation (**Fig. 1**) outlines the series of plasma protein reactions that occur during the coagulation of plasma samples, but does not account for the influence of cells, particularly tissue factor-bearing cells, endothelial cells, and platelets. The extrinsic pathway occurs on tissue-factor bearing extracellular cells, while the intrinsic and common pathways are localized on activated platelets.[11] The cell-based model of coagulation (**Box 2**) describes how these reactions are mediated by exposure to, and on the surface of, these cells.

Many mechanisms localize coagulation only to the site of vascular injury to avoid excessive clot formation, or more generalized disseminated intravascular coagulation (DIC).[4,9,11] For example, clotting factors that diffuse away in plasma are inactivated by inhibitors, or do not have access to activated cell membranes upon which they can promote coagulation.[9,11] Negative feedback loops also limit coagulation, such as when thrombin is produced and binds to receptors on endothelial cells, which then inactivate cofactors essential for further thrombin generation.[4]

A recent review of fibrinolysis describes the complicated initiation and control of fibrin clot breakdown.[13] Tissue plasminogen activator or urokinase cleave plasminogen to form plasmin, which is primarily responsible for fibrinolysis. Tissue plasminogen activator is released by endothelial cells during secondary hemostasis[4] and has a short half-life due to inhibitors in the plasma. Circulating plasmin is also rapidly inhibited, but it is protected when bound to fibrin, which allows fibrinolysis to proceed. Fibrin and fibrinogen also exert a positive feedback effect on fibrinolysis as they convert plasminogen to plasmin. As the thrombus is broken down, fibrin degradation products, including d-dimers, are released into the circulation.[4]

DIAGNOSTIC APPROACH

Diagnosis of coagulopathy starts with a thorough history and physical exam.[4] Owner reports of frank hemorrhage, for example, epistaxis, are indicators of a potential coagulopathy, but often signs will be more subtle and non-specific. Exposure to anticoagulant rodenticides or treatment with benzimidazoles, aspirin, or chloramphenicol has

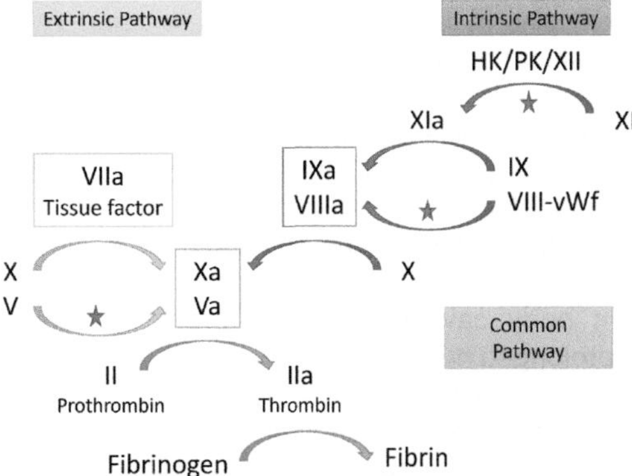

Fig. 1. The extrinsic and intrinsic pathways of the cascade model. HK - high-molecular-weight kininogen, PK – prekallikrein, vWf – von Willebrand factor. Boxes indicate a complex is formed; VIIa/tissue factor, IXa/VIIIa tenase complex and Xa/Va prothrombinase complex. Thrombin catalyzes reactions indicated with a star.

Box 2
The cell-based model of coagulation,[10] summarized from reviews by Smith[9] and Hoffman.[11]

Initiation

- Damage to the blood vessel endothelium exposes circulating blood, particularly platelets and large proteins (eg, von Willebrand factor-factor VIII complex), to tissue factor on the surface of extravascular cells.
- Active factor VIIa from the blood binds with tissue factor, forming a complex that activates more factor VII, as well as factors IX to IXa and X to Xa.
- Factor Xa slowly activates factor V to Va, and then binds to these Va molecules, forming the prothrombinase (Xa/Va) complex. First responder platelets also release a form of factor V that is resistant to inactivation.
- Prothrombinase cleaves factor II, prothrombin, to produce limited amounts of factor IIa, also known as thrombin.

Amplification

- Platelets are activated to their procoagulant state by binding with extravascular collagen, binding with thrombin, and platelet release of procoagulant granules.
- Factors V, VIII, and XI are activated on the platelet surface by thrombin and other procoagulant signals. Factor VIII is activated by cleavage from von Willebrand factor. Factors V and XI activation are accelerated in the presence of granules released from activated platelets.

Propagation

- Activated platelet granules attract more platelets, which form aggregates at the site of vascular injury. Avian thrombocytes do not aggregate, but rather form a sheet of cells.[12]
- Factor IXa from the initiation phase is relatively resistant to inactivation, so can travel to activated platelets and bind to the surface, along with factors Va, VIIIa and XIa.
- Factors IXa and VIIIa form a tenase complex on the platelet, rapidly activating more X to Xa.
- Factors Xa and Va (from the amplification stage) form the prothrombinase complex, activating more prothrombin to thrombin. By this stage a large amount of thrombin is rapidly produced, which cleaves fibrinogen to fibrin. Fibrin cross links to form strands, stabilizing the platelet clot. Thrombin enhances clot stabilization by the inhibition of fibrinolysis factors, activation of factor XIII and incorporation into the clot to trigger further coagulation if the clot is disturbed. Thrombin also further activates factors V, VIII and XI.

been associated with thrombocytopenia and/or coagulopathy.[4] Aflatoxin, found in poor quality feed, is a hepatotoxin that can cause hypocoagulation in a wide range of species. Some examples of the many infectious and non-infectious diseases that have the potential to affect hemostasis are listed in **Box 1**.

Clinical signs of thrombosis can include reduced or absent tissue perfusion, necrotic extremities, loss of pulses, and regional pain or loss of nociception. Hypocoagulation may present as prolonged bleeding after minor trauma such as phlebotomy, or non-traumatic blood loss. Disorders of primary hemostasis (platelet/thrombocyte plug formation) often cause petechial or mucosal hemorrhage, whereas secondary hemostatic disorders (failure of fibrin clot stabilization) cause hematomas and large bleeds in body cavities including the thorax, abdomen/coelom and joints.[4,14] Severe or prolonged hemorrhage may result in anemia, hypovolemia, pallor, hypothermia, and/or lethargy. DIC affects both primary and secondary hemostasis, as well as fibrinolysis, and can therefore present with a broad range of clinical signs. Non-overt, or compensated DIC causes hypercoagulation, which, if not corrected, can progress to overt DIC, severe hypocoagulation and bleeding. Less severe or early stage coagulopathies can be more difficult to detect, and may only be identifiable via diagnostic testing. When a coagulopathy is suspected, blood work is highly recommended.

Currently, there is no single test that comprehensively evaluates the main components of coagulation – the endothelium, coagulation proteins and platelets. Traditional coagulation panels rely on plasma-based tests to evaluate clotting times, alongside a platelet or thrombocyte count, and fibrinogen concentration. Viscoelastic testing is able to evaluate the performance of whole blood coagulation and, in some assays, fibrinolysis, and has been shown to better reflect hemostatic status in the patient. Recent reviews of hemostatic[4] and viscoelastic[15] testing in exotic animals are available, and summarized in **Tables 1** and **2**. A good starting point is a complete blood count to evaluate platelet numbers, as well as for evidence of infection, inflammation, and anemia. Sequential assessment of platelets may be helpful to identify clinically significant downwards trends.[4] Serum or plasma chemistry is useful to evaluate organ function, particularly of the liver and kidneys. There is a close relationship between the innate immune system, inflammation, the acute phase response and hemostasis.[17] Fibrinogen concentration may increase as part of the inflammatory acute phase response, but can also decrease due to consumption in a hypercoagulable state.

Blood collection technique is important when assessing coagulation. Phlebotomy should be performed with minimal tissue trauma to avoid excessive tissue factor contamination of the sample. Excessive aspiration pressure can activate coagulation and should be avoided. Most tests require anticoagulated blood, with the choice of anticoagulant dependent on the assay and species. For many species, ethylenediaminetetraacetic acid (EDTA) is the anticoagulant of choice to evaluate cell morphology and prevent platelet/thrombocyte aggregates. However in some avian and reptile species, EDTA will cause cell lysis, and heparin is preferred. Potassium citrate tubes must be adequately filled to avoid spurious results due to the incorrect ratio of blood to anticoagulant. While viscoelastic testing can be performed on plasma samples, whole blood samples are preferred in order to evaluate platelet numbers and function.[18]

The basic principle of clot-based coagulation testing is to reactivate coagulation and measure parameters of clot formation in a blood sample. Potassium citrate and other anticoagulants chelate calcium, thereby inhibiting clot formation in patient blood samples. Addition of calcium and assay-specific clotting activators enables analysis of specific reactions within the hemostatic system.[19] Results from different assays and reagents are not comparable. Thromboplastin is a source of tissue factor and phospholipids, and is used to activate the extrinsic clotting pathway in the prothrombin time (PT) and some TEG assays. Tissue factor can be a recombinant product, or sourced from brain, lung, and placental tissue.[20] It has long been recognized that species-specific thromboplastin results in efficient clotting, which may not be replicated when thromboplastin from another species is utilized.[5,21,22] For example, recombinant human tissue factor and rabbit thromboplastin did not activate sea turtle coagulation, whereas sea turtle thromboplastin did,[22] and reptile thromboplastin resulted in shorter PT in iguanas compared to avian thromboplastin.[5] Use of species-specific activators, particularly for birds and reptiles, may result in more useful assays. Thromboplastin obtained from brain tissue can be stored frozen and offers a promising species-specific activator for exotic animals.[5,22]

The intrinsic pathway, measured by the activated partial thromboplastin time (APTT) and other assays, is activated by the addition of phospholipids without tissue factor, and a surface activator such as kaolin, Celite, or silica. Commercially available reagents source phospholipid from brain or plant tissues, and the amount of lipid content can be variable between reagents.[19] Birds and reptiles do not have an intrinsic pathway equivalent to mammals, therefore assays validated to evaluate the mammalian intrinsic pathway tend to produce variable and potentially unhelpful results in nonmammalian species.

Table 1
Common hemostatic assays[4]

Assay	Evaluates	Sample Type	Comments
Platelet/thrombocyte count	Number of platelets/thrombocytes	Native or anticoagulated whole blood	Automated counts should be checked with a manual blood smear evaluation.
Flow cytometry	Platelet/thrombocyte function	Anticoagulated whole blood	Limited availability.[16]
Buccal mucosal bleeding time (BMBT)	Platelet/thrombocyte function Von Willebrand disease	Mucosa in-vivo	Thrombocytopenia will prolong BMBT
Activated clotting time (ACT)	Intrinsic (FXI, IX, VIII) Common (FX, V, II, fibrinogen)	Native whole blood	Thrombocytopenia will prolong ACT
Prothrombin time (PT)	Extrinsic (FVII) Common (FX, V, II, fibrinogen)	Citrated plasma	
Activated partial thromboplastin time (APTT)	Intrinsic (FXI, IX, VIII) Common (FX, V, II, fibrinogen)	Citrated plasma	
Fibrin degradation products	Fibrinolysis	Citrated plasma	Serum samples will also contain fibrinogen degradation products so results are not specific for fibrinolysis.
D-dimer	Fibrinolysis	Citrated plasma	Species test validation is required.

Table 2
Selected visocoelastic assays[14]

Parameter	Evaluates	Sample	Comments
TEG Reaction time (R) TEM Clotting time (CT)	Initial fibrin formation (clotting factors)	Native or citrated whole blood or citrated plasma	
TEG K time and alpha angle TEM clot formation time (CFT) and alpha angle Sonoclot clot rate (CR)	Rate of clot formation, dependent on fibrinogen concentration, factor XIII, platelets/thrombocytes	Citrated whole blood or citrated plasma (TEG, TEM) Native whole blood (Sonoclot)	Platelets/thrombocytes not assessed in plasma samples.
TEG maximum amplitude (MA) TEM maximum clot firmness (MCF)	Platelet/thrombocyte number and function, fibrinogen	Native or citrated whole blood or citrated plasma	Platelets not assessed in plasma samples.
Lysis at 30 min TEG LY30 TEM LI30	Rate of fibrinolysis dependent on plasmin	Native or citrated whole blood or citrated plasma	
Sonoclot platelet function score	Platelet/thrombocyte function	Native whole blood	
Platelet mapping (TEG)	Platelet/thrombocyte function	Citrated and heparinized whole blood	

Abbreviations: TEG, thromboelastography; TEM, thromboelastometry.

An additional factor to consider when assessing coagulation is temperature. Many assays are performed at 37°C to replicate mammalian body temperature. Avian body temperature is typically higher than this, and ectothermic species experience wide variations in body temperature. TEG performed at 30°C on cold-stunned sea turtles resulted in hypocoagulable thromboelastograms, however as body temperature was reported to be as low as 1.9°C, these results are unlikely to truly reflect the patient's hemostatic status. Optimization of existing assays for exotic species will help in accurately detecting coagulopathies in the future.

DISORDERED HEMOSTASIS

Coagulation Protein Disorders

Various proteins are essential for pro- and anticoagulation. Von Willebrand factor is a protein produced by endothelial cells and megakaryocytes in mammals and is crucial for initiating platelet aggregation during primary hemostasis.[23] Platelet/thrombocyte plug stabilization is the end point of secondary hemostasis, where a cascade of plasma coagulation protein activations results in the production of a stable network of cross-linked fibrin. The liver synthesizes all the procoagulant plasma clotting proteins (except von Willebrand factor) and many proteins associated with fibrinolysis.[1,24] Birds have lost the ability to produce factor XII and there are conflicting studies on the presence of factor XI in birds and reptiles.[7,25] Clotting factor deficiencies can prolong plasma clotting times; however, the effect on bleeding tendency in the patient is variable. Factor VII deficiency is rarely associated with bleeding, factor XI deficiencies may or may not result in bleeding and deficiencies of factors VIII or IX will usually cause bleeding.[11] Congenital clotting factor deficiencies are rarely reported in animals other than dogs, and the exotic animal clinician is far more likely to encounter acquired clotting factor deficiencies.

Because of the liver's role in synthesizing hemostatic proteins, coagulopathy due to reduced liver function can occur secondary to any hepatopathy.[1,24] Hemostasis will often stay balanced due to decreases in both pro- and anticoagulant proteins, but is less able to respond effectively to tissue damage caused by phlebotomy, intravenous catheter placement or other trauma. Examples of hepatopathies affecting coagulation include hepatic coccidiosis in rabbits,[26] fatty liver hemorrhagic syndrome in backyard chickens[27] and hepatic lipidosis, hepatic neoplasia, and end-stage liver disease in reptiles.[28] Identifying the underlying etiology of a hepatopathy often relies on obtaining a liver biopsy for histopathology and other analyses, but must be weighed up against the risk of hemorrhage. Assessment of coagulation status prior to liver biopsy is routinely recommended, however prolonged PT and APTT do not correlate well with the clinical risk of bleeding in the patient.[29,30] Viscoelastic testing is showing promise in human medicine as a more accurate indicator of bleeding risk.[24]

Vitamin K is a co-factor that carboxylates glutamate residues on some clotting factors, without which they cannot bind to form active procoagulant complexes.[3] Vitamin K-dependent clotting factors include factors II, VII, IX and X. Factor VII has the shortest half-life and will become deficient first and can be diagnosed by a prolonged PT. Excess vitamin E competes with vitamin K and can result in a relative Vitamin K deficiency and a subsequent hypocoagulopathy. Over-supplementation of vitamin E, and possibly other fat soluble vitamins, was responsible for prolonged clotting times, widespread hemorrhages and death in pink-backed pelicans.[31] Correction of dietary vitamin E levels and parenteral supplementation of vitamin K was successful in treating surviving pelicans.[31]

A more common cause of vitamin K deficiency is anticoagulant rodenticide consumption, a potential threat to a wide range of mammal, avian and reptile species. Anticoagulant rodenticides inactivate vitamin K epoxide reductase, which is required for the synthesis of biologically active vitamin K.[32] Identification of the type rodenticide, where possible, is important to determine the duration of action. Second-generation anticoagulant rodenticides brodifacoum and difenacoum are more potent and suppress coagulation for longer than first-generation rodenticides such as warfarin.[33] Cholecalciferol and bromethalin rodenticides do not cause anticoagulation, and therefore require different therapeutic approaches following accidental ingestion.[34]

Exposure to anticoagulant rodenticides can be acute or chronic, direct through the consumption of bait, or secondary through the consumption of target rodents and non-target species. Absorption through the skin and respiratory tract is possible.[35] Second-generation rodenticides are slowly metabolized and can bioaccumulate over time.[35] Free-ranging birds of prey frequently present to rehabilitation facilities with evidence of secondary rodenticide exposure.[36] Toxicity in any species can be assumed in cases of confirmed anticoagulant rodenticide exposure and compatible clinical signs, including weakness, pallor, anemia, bruising or hemorrhage. In acute exposure, decontamination with gastric lavage or emesis may be indicated. Factor VII will decrease first, resulting in a prolonged PT within 72 hours. The risk of bleeding increases as factor IX becomes deficient.[34] The severity of PT prolongation has been shown to correlate with bleeding tendency in Japanese quail.[37] Treatment should be initiated immediately, rather than waiting to monitor clotting times. Vitamin K supplementation is indicated for 2 to 6 weeks or more, and PT should be reassessed 48 hours after the cessation of therapy. Plasma or whole blood transfusions for temporary replacement of clotting factors may be necessary if vitamin K therapy is delayed and active bleeding is present.

Fatal hemorrhagic diathesis has been reported in birds treated with parenteral polysulfated glycosaminoglycans (PSGAG) to manage osteoarthritis.[38] Hypocoagulability is caused by the heparinoid-like effects of PSGAG, although the exact mechanism of action is unknown. Heparin inhibits thrombin and factor Xa resulting in anticoagulation and prolonged clotting times.[38] Affected birds presented with severe pectoral muscle hemorrhage shortly after an intramuscular administration of 0.5 to 100 mg/kg PSGAG. Doses were administered at varying time intervals between q.48 hours to q.4 weeks. The total number of doses ranged from 2 to 10. A subsequent study in chickens suggests that 1 mg/kg administered subcutaneously may be safe, while higher doses induced hypocoagulability in flamingo plasma.[39] As there are significant differences between the effects of PSGAG on coagulation in various mammalian species, further studies are warranted in exotic species to determine if there are other species of concern when prescribing PSGAG.

Platelet Disorders

Both platelet/thrombocyte number and function are important for plug formation during primary hemostasis. Initial evaluation should include a platelet count to check for thrombocytopenia, taking into account any platelet clumping. Very low platelet counts can be associated with spontaneous bleeding. Establishing the cause of thrombocytopenia is the next step – is this a congenital or acquired condition? Congenital thrombocytopenia is rarely recognized in veterinary patients, and the author is not aware of any reports in non-domestic species. In contrast, acquired thrombocytopenia due to reduced platelet production and/or increased consumption is common. Mammalian platelets originate from megakaryocytes while avian and reptile thrombocytes originate from thromboblast precursor cells.[40] Both megakaryocytes and thromboblasts are primarily located in bone marrow.[41] Toxic effects on bone marrow caused by benzimidazole administration have been reported in rabbits and other small mammals,[42] birds[43] and reptiles.[44] Persistent estrus in female ferrets causes bone marrow hypoplasia and thrombocytopenia.[45] Neoplasia and chemotherapeutic agents have been associated with thrombocytopenia in birds and small mammals.[46,47] Many bacterial, viral (eg, polyoma virus in parrots[48]), parasitic (eg, *Eimeria* infections in rabbits[26]) and fungal (eg, histoplasmosis in an African pygmy hedgehog[49]) infections can cause platelet depletion. Thrombocytopenia is a diagnostic criterion for DIC.[50] Thrombocytopenia and thrombopathia can occur concurrently.

Platelet function assays include flow cytometry,[21] Sonoclot platelet function score, thromboelastography platelet mapping, and the eponymous platelet function assay. Buccal mucosal bleeding time evaluates the time for a platelet/thrombocyte clot to form in vivo.[14] It's easily accessible, but somewhat crude, and may be difficult to perform and interpret in birds and reptiles. Congenital thrombopathia is rarely recognized in animals aside from Chediak-Higashi syndrome, a genetic condition that results in abnormal granules in platelets and other cells, affects platelet function and can result in bleeding diathesis. Aleutian mink and blue foxes have been described with an analogous condition.[51,52] Platelet function can be affected by a wide range of diseases including hepatic and renal dysfunction, neoplasia, infectious diseases, toxins, venoms and therapy with non-steroidal anti-inflammatories or synthetic colloids.[14]

Venomous snake bites are a common cause of thrombocytopenia, thrombopathia, bleeding, and activation of fibrinolysis without DIC.[53] Most venomous snake bites in North America are caused by Crotalinae species (pit vipers) in the Viperidae family. In the absence of observing the bite, puncture wounds with associated pain, edema, tissue necrosis and hemorrhage are suggestive of envenomation. Treatment with antivenom, intravenous isotonic fluids, and opioid analgesia should be immediately initiated. Successful treatment with equine-derived Crotalidae polyvalent immune F(ab')2 antivenins has been reported in sandhill cranes,[54] a red-tailed hawk[55] and a ferret.[56] Non-steroidal anti-inflammatories are generally avoided because of their potential effects on platelet function. The use of plasma and other blood products is controversial and should only be considered if antivenom therapy does not adequately control bleeding. Fresh frozen plasma administration resulted in persistent afibrinogenemia in a small study investigating brown snake (*Pseudonaja affinis*) envenomation in dogs, and 2/6 dogs in the plasma group died compared to 0/5 dogs in the control group.[57] However, delayed treatment with fresh frozen plasma, after antivenom therapy, has been associated with improved clotting times and shorter recovery times in envenomated humans.[58]

Vascular Diseases

Vasculitis due to systemic inflammation, sepsis, and tick-borne diseases can cause activation of hemostasis and eventual consumption of platelets and clotting factors.[14] Abnormal collagen synthesis secondary to vitamin C deficiency causes ultrastructural changes to blood vessel walls, leading to hemorrhage.[59] Susceptible species include those that cannot synthesize vitamin C: teleost fish, old and new world primates, some bats, guinea pigs and most passerine birds.[60] Treatment for guinea pigs includes 50 to 100 mg vitamin C parenterally to stabilize the patient, and then oral supplementation and correction of the diet.[61]

Disseminated Intravascular Coagulation and Fibrinolysis

A wide variety of diseases can cause DIC, a syndrome where both the coagulation and fibrinolytic systems are activated.[50,62] Microthrombi are a consistent feature of hypercoagulation however the degree of hyperfibrinolysis varies depending on the underlying cause of DIC.[63] When clot breakdown cannot balance clot formation, a primarily thrombotic syndrome will be observed, which can cause ischemic organ damage. Increased bleeding tendency occurs when fibrinolysis is upregulated more than coagulation. In some cases coagulation and fibrinolysis are balanced, and will cause minimal clinical signs until platelets and clotting factors are consumed, eventually resulting in severe hypocoagulation.

Many diseases affecting exotic companion animals can potentially cause DIC. Animal models of DIC include mice, rats, and guinea pigs.[62] Sepsis and neoplasia are the most common causes in humans, and trauma, shock, acute pancreatitis, severe infections, burns, vasculitis, hepatitis and many other conditions have also been associated with DIC.[50,63] Diagnosis can be challenging and relies on a panel of tests in patients with a pre-existing disease that can cause DIC. Human scoring systems have been adapted for use in dogs and rabbits.[64,65] Trends over time may be more informative than stand-alone values, although severe thrombocytopenia with prolonged clotting times and elevated fibrin-related markers (eg, d-dimer) are likely indicative of overt DIC.[50] Lack of access to diagnostic tests, lack of validated assays, difficulty interpreting results and small sample volumes can make the diagnosis of DIC difficult for exotic species. The primary goal of management of DIC is to address the underlying cause as early as possible. Specific therapy will vary depending on the causative pathology but may include antibiosis, anti-inflammatory therapy, and analgesia. Supportive therapy includes plasma or platelets for bleeding-type DIC and anticoagulant therapy for thrombotic-type DIC.[62]

Infectious diseases associated with coagulopathy and DIC in birds include bacterial (*Escherichia coli*, *Salmonella* spp., *Erysipelothrix rhusiopathiae*, *Streptococcus zooepidemicus*) and viral (infectious bursal disease in chickens, eastern encephalitis virus, psittacine polyomavirus, reovirus, Newcastle disease, avian herpesviruses and avian reoviruses) diseases.[3] Highly pathogenic avian influenza (HPAI), a zoonotic and World Organization for Animal Health (OIE) reportable disease, has been shown to cause severe coagulopathy within hours of experimental infection in chickens.[66] Viral replication in endothelial cells and monocytes/macrophages is associated with the upregulation of tissue factor gene expression, resulting in widespread thrombosis, thrombocytopenia and clotting factor deficiency due to consumption coagulopathy.[66] HPAI can also cause consumption coagulopathy and death in experimentally infected ferrets, while human seasonal influenza infection causes ferret endothelial cell activation, transient prolongations of clotting times and increases in d-dimer concentrations.[67]

Rabbit hemorrhagic disease virus targets European rabbit (*Oryctolagus cuniculus*) hepatocytes, phagocytic and endothelial cells, leading to hepatocellular necrosis, DIC, and death.[68,69] Cases may present as peracute death, acute lethargy, pyrexia and respiratory or neurologic signs, or more chronic lethargy, jaundice, and death in 1 to 2 weeks.[68] Thrombocytopenia, prolonged PT and APTT, and hypofibrinogenemia, indicative of consumption coagulopathy, may be seen shortly prior to death.[70] Treatment is usually limited to supportive care. Commercially available vaccines are recommended, although break-through disease has been observed.[71]

Sporadic reports of DIC in reptiles include an eastern spiny softshell turtle with acute mycobacteriosis,[72] oak toxicity in an African spurred tortoise,[73] cold-stunned sea turtles[6] and *Nannizziopsiaceae* fungal infection in a Galapagos tortoise.[74]

Hyper- and hypofibrinolysis can cause hemorrhage and thrombosis, respectively. Evaluation of fibrinolysis is indicated when primary and secondary hemostatic disorders have been ruled out in the face of a persistent hemostatic disorder.[75] Reported causes of hyperfibrinolysis in dogs and cats include trauma, *Angiostrongylus vasorum*

Table 3
Blood products used for the management of coagulopathies[91]

Blood Product	Contains	Indication	Storage
Whole blood	Coagulation factors, platelets, RBC, WBC, albumin	Severe hemorrhage Anemia with coagulopathy	See Brooks et al[89]
Platelet-rich plasma	Coagulation factors, platelets, albumin	Severe thrombocytopenia resulting in hemorrhage	Room temperature for 5 d under constant agitation
Platelet concentrate	Platelets		As above
Lyophilized platelets	Platelets		1–6°C for 24 mo
Fresh frozen plasma	Coagulation factors, albumin	Coagulopathy with hemorrhage, or prior to an invasive procedure	−18°C for 12 mo
Cryoprecipitate	Factors VIII, XIII, vWf, fibrinogen, fibronectin	Deficiency of specific factors	−18°C for 12 mo
Cryosupernatant	Factors II, V, VII, IX, X, XI	Deficiency of specific factors	−18°C for 12 mo

Abbreviation: RBC, red blood cells; vWf, von Willebrand factor; WBC, white blood cells.

infection, snake envenomation, hepatic disease, cavitary effusions and DIC.[75] The fibrinolytic system is not well understood in birds and reptiles,[76,77] and antifibrinolytic therapy has only been reported in laboratory settings in small mammals and birds.

Thrombosis

Cardiovascular disease is a risk factor for thrombosis due to endothelial cell injury and turbulent or static blood flow associated with valve or chamber pathology.[78] Mammalian platelets do not contain a nucleus and quickly form three-dimensional platelet aggregates in response to endothelial injury. Nucleated avian thrombocytes are unable to aggregate in the same way, rather spreading to form a sheet of cells.[12] Avian clots take longer to form, but also do not tend to shear off and cause thrombotic disease.

Cardiovascular disease and atrial thrombosis are reported in aged Syrian hamsters and African hedgehogs.[79,80] Radiography and echocardiography are useful to assess heart size and function, and empiric treatment with angiotensin-converting enzyme inhibitors, diuretics, and anticoagulants have been suggested.[81] Non-bacterial thrombotic endocarditis has been reported in the ferret[82] but thromboemboli are generally considered rare in this species.[83]

Bacteremia can cause endothelial cell activation, providing a procoagulant surface for the formation of a fibrin clot with bacteria on cardiac valves.[84] Endocarditis has been associated with orthopedic injuries in birds[85–87] and with pododermatitis in birds and mammals.[86,88]

Treatment of Acquired Coagulopathies

For acquired coagulopathies the mainstay of treatment is to aggressively address the underlying cause, while providing supportive care. Blood product transfusions are indicated for platelet, plasma protein and erythrocyte deficiencies (**Table 3**). Blood banking procedures are not established in exotic animal medicine, although collection and maintenance of plasma for common species should be achievable for many practices. Whole blood transfusion using freshly harvested blood is a relatively common treatment for severe anemia in exotic animal practice,[89] and the same principles can be used for the management of coagulopathies. Donors are usually selected by convenience and availability, and should ideally be a healthy adult of the same genus and species as the recipient. Cross-matching is recommended for all species, except first transfusions in ferrets as this species does not appear to have blood types.[89,90] Subsequent ferret blood transfusions should be cross-matched. The health status of donor animals should be evaluated with a physical exam, complete blood count, biochemistry panel, and infectious disease testing.[89] The volume collected from each donor should not exceed 1% of body weight, and in some species, the safe volume is considerably less. Multiple donors may be required to provide a large enough volume for the recipient. Blood can be administered intravenously or intraosseously through a filter, taking care to avoid pneumatized avian bones. Transfusion reactions may be detected through increases in heart rate, respiratory rate or temperature, or skin erythema and swelling. Administration of blood products should be slowed or stopped.[89] If no reaction is detected, the rate can be increased to 10 to 20 mL/kg/h. Sedation may be appropriate for donors and recipients.

SUMMARY

Recognition that disorders of hemostasis are possible in any species, and a systematic approach to patient evaluation and management will go a long way towards improving case outcomes, despite the lack of evidence-based medicine specific to exotic species. Clinicians are encouraged to consider the presence of coagulopathies, particularly in critically sick patients, and use basic principles to address underlying causes and provide supportive care.

CLINICS CARE POINTS

- The first step in evaluating coagulation status is to obtain a complete history and perform a thorough clinical exam.
- Evaluation of a blood smear is important when interpreting platelet counts, as clumping often occurs in heparinized blood samples.
- Whole blood assays are more reflective of the in-vivo hemostatic status when compared to plasma-based assays.
- Trends in diagnostic testing results over time can be useful to evaluate disease progression and response to treatment.
- Treatment of hemostatic disorders in exotic companion animals is extrapolated from domestic species.

DISCLOSURE

The author has previously received support from Peter Fischer, a distributor of thromboelastography machines, in the form of use of equipment and discounted consumables for research and diagnostic purposes.

REFERENCES

1. Webster CRL. Hemostatic disorders associated with hepatobiliary disease. Vet Clin North Am Small Anim Pract 2017;47(3):601–15.
2. Gentry PA. Comparative aspects of blood coagulation. Veterinary J 2004;168(3): 238–51.
3. Russell KE, Heatley JJ. Avian hemostasis. In: Brooks MB, Harr KE, Seelig DM, et al, editors. Schalm's veterinary Hematology. Hoboken, NJ: John Wiley & Sons, Ltd; 2022. p. 865–74.
4. Kaye S, Stokol T. Hemostatic testing in companion exotic mammals. Vet Clin North Am Ex Anim Pract 2022;25(3):613–30.
5. Sladakovic I, Brainard BM, Divers SJ, et al. Coagulation testing in green iguanas (Iguana iguana) with development of prothrombin time assays using reptile and avian thromboplastin. J Vet Emerg Critl Care 2022;32(5):685–9.
6. Barratclough A, Tuxbury K, Hanel R, et al. Baseline plasma thromboelastography in Kemp's ridley (Lepidochelys kempii), green (Chelonia mydas) and loggerhead (Caretta caretta) sea turtles and its use to diagnose coagulopathies in cold-stunned Kemp's ridley and green sea turtles. J Zoo Wildl Med 2019;50(1):62–8.
7. Ribeiro ÂM, Zepeda-Mendoza ML, Bertelsen MF, et al. A refined model of the genomic basis for phenotypic variation in vertebrate hemostasis. BMC Evol Biol 2015;15(1):1–8.
8. Mann KG, Krudysz-Amblo J, Butenas S. Tissue factor controversies. Thromb Res 2012;129(SUPPL. 2):S5–7.
9. Smith SA. The cell-based model of coagulation. J Vet Emerg Crit Care 2009; 19(1):3–10.

10. Hoffman M, Monroe DM. A cell-based model of hemostasis. Thromb Haemost 2001;85(6):958–65.
11. Hoffman M. Cell-mediated hemostasis. In: Moore HB, Moore EE, Neal MD, editors. Trauma induced coagulopathy. 2nd edition. Handel, Switzerland: Springer Nature Switzerland AG; 2021. p. 31–41.
12. Schmaier AA, Stalker TJ, Runge JJ, et al. Occlusive thrombi arise in mammals but not birds in response to arterial injury: evolutionary insight into human cardiovascular disease. Blood 2011;118(13):3661–9.
13. Chapin JC, Hajjar KA. Fibrinolysis and the control of blood coagulation. Blood Rev 2015;29(1):17–24.
14. Jandrey KE. Assessment of platelet function. J Vet Emerg Crit Care 2012;22(1):81–98.
15. Cummings CO, Eisenbarth J, deLaforcade A. Viscoelastic coagulation testing in exotic animals. Vet Clin North Am Ex Anim Prac 2022;25(3):597–612.
16. Weiss DJ. Application of flow cytometric techniques to veterinary clinical hematology. Vet Clin Pathol 2002;31(2):72–82.
17. Cray C. Biomarkers of inflammation in exotic pets. J Exot Pet Med 2013;22(3):245–50.
18. Perrin KL, Krogh AK, Kjelgaard-Hansen M, et al. Thromboelastography in the healthy Asian elephant (Elephas maximus): Reference intervals and effects of storage. J Zoo Wildl Med 2018;49(1).
19. Kitchen S, Cartwright I, Woods TAL, et al. Lipid composition of seven APTT reagents in relation to heparin sensitivity. Br J Haematol 1999;106(3):801–8.
20. Bates SM, Weitz JI. Coagulation assays. Circulation 2005;112(4):e53–60.
21. Janson TL, Stormorken H, Prydz H. Species specificity of tissue thromboplastin. Pathophysiol Haemost Thromb 1984;14(5):440–4.
22. Barratclough A, Hanel R, Stacy NI, et al. Establishing a protocol for thromboelastography in sea turtles. Vet Rec Open 2018;5(1):e000240.
23. Ruggeri ZM. The role of von Willebrand factor in thrombus formation. Thromb Res 2007;120(SUPPL. 1):S5–9.
24. Kujovich JL. Coagulopathy in liver disease: A balancing act. Hematology 2015;2015(1):243–9.
25. Ponczek MB, Shamanaev A, LaPlace A, et al. The evolution of factor XI and the kallikrein-kinin system. Blood Adv 2020;4(24):6135–47.
26. Jing J, Liu C, Zhu SX, et al. Pathological and ultrastructural observations and liver function analysis of Eimeria stiedai-infected rabbits. Vet Parasitol 2016;223:165–72.
27. Trott KA, Giannitti F, Rimoldi G, et al. Fatty iver hemorrhagic syndrome in the backyard chicken: A retrospective histopathologic case series. Vet Pathol 2014;51(4):787–95.
28. Parkinson L, Kierski K, Mans C. Coagulopathy secondary to chronic hepatopathy in three lizards. J Herpetol Med Surg 2021;31(4):296–301.
29. Reece J, Pavlick M, Penninck DG, et al. Hemorrhage and complications associated with percutaneous ultrasound guided liver biopsy in dogs. J Vet Intern Med 2020;34(6):2398–404.
30. Pavlick M, Webster CRL, Penninck DG. Bleeding risk and complications associated with percutaneous ultrasound-guided liver biopsy in cats. J Feline Med Surg 2019;21(6):529–36.
31. Nichols DK, Wolff MJ, Phillips LG, et al. Coagulopathy in pink-backed pelicans (Pelecanus rufescens) associated with hypervitaminosis E. J Zoo Wildl Med 1989;20(1):57–61.

32. Rattner BA, Mastrota FN. Anticoagulant rodenticide toxicity to non-target wildlife under controlled exposure conditions. In: van den Brink N, Elliott J, Shore R, et al, editors. Emerging Topics in Ecotoxicology, vol. 5. Cham (Switzerland): Springer; 2018. p. 45–86.
33. Park BK, Leck JB. A comparison of vitamin K antagonism by warfarin, difenacoum and brodifacoum in the rabbit. Biochem Pharmacol 1982;31(22):3635–9.
34. Lichtenberger M, Richardson JA. Emergency care and managing toxicoses in the exotic animal patient. Vet Clin North Am Ex An Pract 2008;11(2):211–28.
35. Redig PT, Arent LR. Raptor toxicology. Vet Clin North Am Ex An Pract 2008;11(2): 261–82.
36. Murray M. Anticoagulant rodenticide exposure and toxicosis in four species of birds of prey in Massachusetts, USA, 2012–2016, in relation to use of rodenticides by pest management professionals. Ecotoxicology 2017;26(8):1041–50.
37. Webster KH, Harr KE, Bennett DC, et al. Assessment of toxicity and coagulopathy of brodifacoum in Japanese quail and testing in wild owls. Ecotoxicology 2015;24(5):1087–101.
38. Anderson K, Garner MM, Reed HH, et al. Hemorrhagic diathesis in avian species following intramuscular administration of polysulfated glycosaminoglycan. J Zoo Wildl Med 2013;44(1):93–9.
39. Wonn AM, Brooks MB, Hu H, et al. Hypocoagulability effect of adequan in domestic chickens (Gallus gallus) and Chilean flamingos (Phoenicopterus chilensis). J Zoo Wildl Med 2022;53(1):126–32.
40. Scanes CG. Blood. In: Scanes CG, Dridi S, editors. Sturkie's avian Physiology. 7th ed. Hoboken, NJ: Academic Press; 2022. p. 293–326.
41. Wasserkrug-Naor A. Platelet kinetics and laboratory evaluation of thrombocytopenia. In: Brooks MB, Harr KE, Seelig DM, et al, editors. Schalm's veterinary Hematology. 7th edition. Hoboken, NJ: John Wiley & Sons, Ltd; 2020. p. 675–85.
42. Graham JE, Garner MM, Reavill DR. Benzimidazole toxicosis in rabbits: 13 cases (2003 to 2011). J Exot Pet Med 2014;23(2):188–95.
43. Weber MA, Terrell SP, Neiffer DL, et al. Bone marrow hypoplasia and intestinal crypt cell necrosis associated with fenbendazole administration in five painted storks. J Am Vet Med Assoc 2002;221(3):417–9.
44. Neiffer DL, Lydick D, Burks K, et al. Hematologic and plasma biochemical changes associated with fenbendazole in Hermann's tortoises (Testudo hermanni). J Zoo Wildl Med 2005;36(4):661–72.
45. Sherrill A, Gorham J. Bone marrow hypoplasia associated with estrus in ferrets. Lab Anim Sci 1985;35(3):280–6.
46. Harrison TM, Kitchell BE. Principles and applications of medical oncology in exotic animals. Vet Clin North Am Ex An Pract 2017;20(1):209–34.
47. Ammersbach M, DeLay J, Caswell JL, et al. Laboratory findings, histopathology, and immunophenotype of lymphoma in domestic ferrets. Vet Pathol 2008;45(5): 663–73.
48. Phalen DN, Radabaugh CS, Dahlhausen RD, et al. Viremia, virus shedding, and antibody response during natural avian polyomavirus infection in parrots. J Am Vet Med Assoc 2000;217(1):32–6.
49. Snider TA, Joyner PH, Clinkenbeard KD. Disseminated histoplasmosis in an African pygmy hedgehog. J Am Vet Med Assoc 2008;232(1):74–6.
50. Taylor FB Jr, Toh CH, Hoots WK, et al. Towards definition, clinical and laboratory criteria, and a scoring system for disseminated intravascular coagulation. Thromb Haemost 2001;86(5):1327–30.

51. Sjaastad Ov, Blom AK, Stormorken H, et al. Adenine nucleotides, serotonin, and aggregation properties of platelets of blue foxes (Alopex lagopus) with the Chediak-Higashi syndrome. Am J Med Genet 1990;35(3):373–8.
52. Windhorst DB, Padgett G. The Chediak-Higashi syndrome and the homologous trait in animals. J Invest Derm 1973;60(6):529–37.
53. Armentano RA, Schaer M. Overview and controversies in the medical management of pit viper envenomation in the dog. J Vet Emerg Crit Care 2011;21(5):461–70.
54. Field CL, Maclean RA, Grillo JF. Treatment of snakebite envenomation in sandhill cranes (Grus canadensis). Vet Rec Case Rep 2016;4(1):e000323.
55. Masri A, Berg KJ, Paul-Murphy J, et al. Crotalid polyvalent F(ab)2 antivenom treatment in a red-tailed hawk (Buteo jamaicensis). J Avian Med Surg 2022;36(1):63–9.
56. Loredo AI, Bauman JE, Wells RJ. The first report of crotalid envenomation in a domesticated ferret (Mustela furo) and successful treatment with a novel F(AB') 2 antivenom. J Zoo Wildl Med 2018;49(2):497–500.
57. Jelinek GA, Smith A, Lynch D, et al. The effect of adjunctive fresh frozen plasma administration on coagulation parameters and survival in a canine model of antivenom-treated Brown Snake envenoming. Anaesth Intensive Care 2005;33(1):36–40.
58. Holla SK, Rao HA, Shenoy D, et al. The role of fresh frozen plasma in reducing the volume of anti-snake venom in snakebite envenomation. Tropical Doct 2018;48(2):89–93.
59. Kim JCS. Ultrastructural studies of vascular and muscular changes in ascorbic acid deficient guinea-pigs. Lab Anim 2016;11(2):113–7.
60. Drouin G, Godin JR, Page B. The genetics of vitamin C loss in vertebrates. Curr Genomics 2011;12(5):371–8.
61. Pignon C, Mayer J. Guinea Pigs. In: Quesenberry KE, Orcutt CJ, Mans C, et al, editors. Ferrets, rabbits, and rodents. 4th edition. Philadelphia, PA: W.B. Saunders; 2021. p. 270–97.
62. Berthelsen LO, Kristensen AT, Tranholm M. Animal models of DIC and their relevance to human DIC: A systematic review. Thromb Res 2011;128(2):103–16.
63. Asakura H. Classifying types of disseminated intravascular coagulation: clinical and animal models. J Intensive Care 2014;2(1):20.
64. Goggs R, Mastrocco A, Brooks MB. Retrospective evaluation of 4 methods for outcome prediction in overt disseminated intravascular coagulation in dogs (2009-2014): 804 cases. J Vet Emerg Crit Care 2018;28(6):541–50.
65. Olrik Berthelsen L, Thuri Kristensen A, Wiinberg B, et al. Implementation of the ISTH classification of non-overt DIC in a thromboplastin induced rabbit model. Thromb Res 2009;124(4):490–7.
66. Muramoto Y, Ozaki H, Takada A, et al. Highly pathogenic H5N1 influenza virus causes coagulopathy in chickens. Microbiol Immunol 2006;50(1):73–81.
67. Goeijenbier M, van Gorp ECM, van den Brand JMA, et al. Activation of coagulation and tissue fibrin deposition in experimental influenza in ferrets. BMC Microbiol 2014;14(1):1–13.
68. Harcourt-Brown N, Silkstone M, Whitbread TJ, et al. RHDV2 epidemic in UK pet rabbits. Part 1: clinical features, gross post mortem and histopathological findings. J Small An Pract 2020;61(7):419–27.
69. Ueda K, Park JH, Ochiai K, et al. Disseminated intravascular coagulation (DIC) in rabbit haemorrhagic disease. Jpn J Vet Res 1992;40(4):133–41.

70. Bonvehí C, Ardiaca M, Montesinos A, et al. Clinicopathologic findings of naturally occurring Rabbit Hemorrhagic Disease Virus 2 infection in pet rabbits. Vet Clin Pathol 2019;48(1):89–95.
71. Hänske GG, König P, Schuhmann B, et al. Death in four RHDV2-vaccinated pet rabbits due to rabbit haemorrhagic disease virus 2 (RHDV2). J Small Anim Pract 2021;62(8):700–3.
72. Murray M, Waliszewski NT, Garner MM, et al. Sepsis and disseminated intravascular coagulation in an eastern spiny softshell turtle (Apalone spinifera spinifera) with acute mycobacteriosis. J Zoo Wildl Med 2009;40(3):572–5.
73. Rotstein DS, Lewbart GA, Kristen Hobbie D, et al. Suspected oak, Quercus, toxicity in an African spurred tortoise, Geochelone sulcata. J Herpetol Med Surg 2003;13(3):20–1.
74. Christman JE, Alexander AB, Donnelly KA, et al. Clinical manifestation and molecular characterization of a novel member of the Nannizziopsiaceae in a pulmonary granuloma from a Galapagos tortoise (Chelonoidis nigra). Front Vet Sci 2020;7:24.
75. Birkbeck R, Humm K, Cortellini S. A review of hyperfibrinolysis in cats and dogs. J Small Anim Pract 2019;60(11):641–55.
76. Chudzinski-Tavassi AM, Polizello ACM, Gonçalves LRC, et al. High inhibitory activity on proteases in a reptile plasma (Bothrops jararaca snake) impairs its intrinsic fibrinolytic-like mechanism. Fibrinolysis 1995;9(2):79–85.
77. Tentoni J, Polini NN, Casanave EB. Comparative vertebrate fibrinolysis. Comp Clin Path 2010;19(3):225–34.
78. Robinson WF, Robinson NA. Cardiovascular System. In: Maxie MG, editor. Jubb, Kennedy & Palmer's pathology of domestic animals, vol. 3, 6th edition. St. Louis, MO: Elsevier Inc.; 2016. p. 1–101.
79. Raymond JT, Garner MM. Cardiomyopathy in captive African hedgehogs (Atelerix albiventris). J Vet Diag Invest 2000;12(5):468–72.
80. Sichuk G, Bettigole RE, Der BK, et al. Influence of sex hormones on thrombosis of left atrium in Syrian (golden) hamsters. Am J Phys 1965;208:465–70.
81. Miwa Y, Mayer J. Hamsters and gerbils. In: Quesenberry KE, Orcutt CJ, Mans C, et al, editors. Ferrets, rabbits, and rodents. 4th edition. Philadelphia, PA: W.B. Saunders; 2021. p. 368–84.
82. Kottwitz JJ, Luis-Fuentes V, Micheal B. Nonbacterial thrombotic endocarditis in a ferret (Mustela putorius furo). J Zoo Wildl Med 2006;37(2):197–201.
83. van Zeeland YRA, Schoemaker NJ. Ferret cardiology. Vet Clin North Am Ex Anim Pract 2022;25(2):541–62.
84. Liesenborghs L, Meyers S, Vanassche T, et al. Coagulation: At the heart of infective endocarditis. J Thromb Haemost 2020;18(5):995–1008.
85. Lemon MJ, Pack L, Forzán MJ. Valvular endocarditis and septic thrombosis associated with a radial fracture in a red-tailed hawk (Buteo jamaicensis). Canadian Vet J 2012;53(1):79–82.
86. Suárez-Santana CM, Fernández A, Quesada-Canales Ó, et al. Bacteremia and aortic valvular endocarditis in a Eurasian stone-curlew (Burhinus oedicnemus distinctus) due to Streptococcus dysgalactiae. J Wildl Dis 2022;58(3):697–700.
87. Vielmo A, Bianchi RM, Argenta FF, et al. Thromboembolic encephalitis secondary to bacterial valvular endocarditis in a red-billed curassow (Crax blumenbachii). Braz J Vet Path 2018;11(1):28–31.
88. Bumblefoot Blair J. A comparison of clinical presentation and treatment of pododermatitis in rabbits, rodents, and birds. Vet Clin North Am Ex Anim Pract 2013;16(3):715–35.

89. Brooks MB, Harr KE, Seelig DM, et al. Blood transfusion in exotic species. In: Schalm's veterinary Hematology. 7th edition. Hoboken, NJ: John Wiley & Sons, Ltd; 2020. p. 933–9.
90. Hohenhaus AE. Importance of blood groups and blood group antibodies in companion animals. Transfus Med Rev 2004;18(2):117–26.
91. Walker JM. Component therapy. In: Yagi K, Holowaychuk MK, editors. Manual of veterinary transfusion medicine and blood banking. Hoboken, NJ: John Wiley & Sons, Ltd; 2016. p. 13–26.

9780323939959